CW00793687

Lippincott P

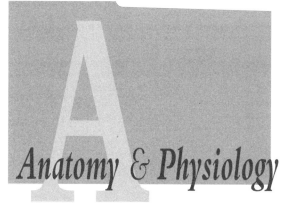

Anatomy & Physiology

Second Edition

Lippincott Professional Guides

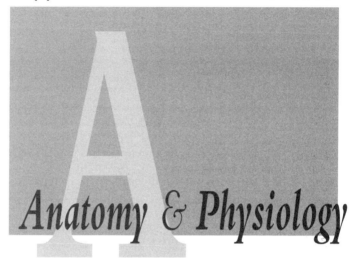

Anatomy & Physiology

Second Edition

LIPPINCOTT WILLIAMS & WILKINS
A **Wolters Kluwer** Company
Philadelphia • Baltimore • New York • London
Buenos Aires • Hong Kong • Sydney • Tokyo

Staff

Publisher
Judith A. Schilling McCann, RN, MSN

Editorial Director
David Moreau

Clinical Director
Joan M. Robinson, RN, MSN

Senior Art Director
Arlene Putterman

Editors
Jaime L. Stockslager (senior associate editor), Raphe Cheli, Kevin Haworth

Clinical Editors
Collette Bishop Hendler, RN, CCRN (clinical project manager); Amy Poling Bishop, RN, BSN

Copy Editors
Peggy Williams (copy supervisor), Kimberly Bilotta, Heather Ditch, Pamela Wingrod

Designers
Mary Ludwicki (art director)

Illustrators
Mike Adams, John Carlance, John Cymerman, Jacalyn Facciolo, Dan Fione, Jean Gardner, Francis Grobelny, Bob Jackson, BJ Krim, Cynthia Mason, Bob Neumann, Judy Newhouse

Associate Editor (Electronic)
Liz Schaeffer

Electronic Production Services
Diane Paluba (manager), Joyce Rossi Biletz, Richard Eng

Manufacturing
Patricia K. Dorshaw (senior manager), Beth Janae Orr

Editorial Assistants
Danielle J. Barsky, Beverly Lane, Linda Ruhf

Indexer
Karen C. Comerford

Printed in the United States of America.

LPGAP2- D N O S A J J M A
04 03 02 10 9 8 7 6 5 4 3 2 1

Library of Congress Cataloging-in-Publication Data

Anatomy & physiology.—2nd ed.
p. ; cm. — (Lippincott professional guides)
Includes bibliographical references and index.
1. Human physiology—Handbooks, manuals, etc.
2. Human Anatomy—Handbooks, manuals, etc.
3. Allied health personnel—Handbooks, manuals, etc. I. Title: Anatomy and physiology. II. Series.
[DNLM: 1. Anatomy—Handbooks. 2. Physiology—Handbooks. QS 39 A535 2002]
QP35 .A537
612—dc21
ISBN 1-58255-180-4 (alk. paper) 2001050828

Contents

Contributors

James Agostinucci, ScD
Associate Professor
University of Rhode Island
Kingston

Cheryl L. Brady, RN, MSN
Adjunct Faculty
Kent State University
East Liverpool, Ohio

Darlene Nebel Cantu, RNC, MSN
Director
Baptist Health System
School of Professional Nursing
San Antonio, Tex.

Nancy H. Haynes, RN, MSN, CCRN
Assistant Professor of Nursing
Saint Luke's College
Kansas City, Mo.

Lourdes "Cindy" Santoni-Reddy, MSN, MEd, NP-C, CPP, FAAPM
Faculty, Nurse Practitioner, Pain Management Practitioner
Reddy Associates, PC
Newtown, Pa.

Paul Keith Small, PhD, MS, BSc
Professor of Biology
Eureka (Ill.) College

Foreword

Every health care professional requires a basic understanding of anatomy and physiology. The vast details associated with these subjects can be overwhelming at times, and you probably have moments when you need to double-check a critical fact about the structure and function of the human body. As you know, you can't afford to waste time futilely searching for answers in large, cumbersome textbooks. Instead, you need a handy reference that quickly and concisely summarizes these concepts — one that's accurate, succinct and, best of all, user-friendly.

Lippincott Professional Guides: Anatomy & Physiology, Second Edition, offers all of these features and more in a portable, pocket-sized guide. The multilevel presentation of the subject matter — using both a systems approach and a functional approach to the study of anatomy and physiology — will appeal to you whether you're a student or a health care provider.

The material is logically organized, beginning with chapter 1, which provides an overview of the anatomy of the human body, including cell structure, cell division, and cellular physiology. This information, like the DNA of a cell, serves as the building block for the more detailed examinations of the body systems that you'll find in later chapters. Chapter 2 continues to build with its discussion of basic chemical processes that are vital to life and necessary for an understanding of the normal physiologic functions covered in this book. Key terms are italicized throughout the text and defined in the glossary, making the book even easier to use.

Chapters 3 through 16, give a thorough overview of the integumentary, musculoskeletal, nervous, endocrine, cardiovascular, hematologic, immune, respiratory, GI, urinary, and reproductive systems, including expanded coverage of complex topics, such as nutrition and metabolism; fluid, electrolyte, and acid-base balance; and fertilization, pregnancy, labor, and lactation.

The final chapter in the book reviews the normal aging process and its effects on anatomy and physiology, a topic of growing importance given the rapid rise in the elderly population. It includes a valuable chart of age-related changes in diagnostic test values.

Lippincott Professional Guides: Anatomy & Physiology is loaded with anatomic illustrations, schematic representations, tables, and flow charts that complement and reinforce the written material throughout the text. In addition, a 32-page color section with nearly 75 illustrations depicts details of anatomy and important physiologic processes, providing even more detailed coverage.

Features new to the second edition include:

- *A structural view* — sidebars that illustrate and detail structures of the human anatomy
- *Focus on function* — sidebars that depict and elaborate on important physiologic processes
- expanded coverage of exercise physiology.

An important returning feature is the *Point to remember,* which emphasizes important anatomic and physiologic concepts.

Whether you're a student or a health care practitioner, *Lippincott Professional Guides: Anatomy & Physiology*, Second Edition, is a valuable and convenient reference. As a student, you'll find clearly presented, concise, essential information that will help you through your anatomy and physiology courses. As a practitioner, you'll find a handy reference that you'll use again and again for quick reviews of numerous subjects encountered daily in your clinical practice.

Joyce King, RN, PhD, CNM, FNP
Assistant Professor
Nell Hodgson Woodruff School of Nursing
Emory University
Atlanta

1 The human body

The practice of any health care profession requires a basic understanding of anatomy and physiology. *Anatomy* is the study of the structure of the body and the relationship of its parts. *Physiology* is the study of how body parts function; it includes the chemical and physical processes of the body.

Branches of anatomy include gross anatomy, microanatomy, developmental anatomy, applied anatomy, and pathologic anatomy.

Gross anatomy (also called macroscopic anatomy) is the study of anatomic structures visible to the unaided eye.

Microanatomy is the study of anatomic structures using a microscope. It's subdivided into cytology and histology. *Cytology* is the study of the origin, structure, function, and pathology of individual cells. *Histology* is the study of tissues (groups of cells). It involves mounting thin tissue sections on slides; frozen sections or prepared tissues can be used.

Developmental anatomy is the study of structural changes from conception through old age. It includes embryology and gerontology.

Applied anatomy refers to the use of anatomic findings to diagnose and treat medical disorders.

Pathologic anatomy is the study of diseased, abnormal, or injured tissue.

Anatomic terms

Anatomic terms useful in health care practice include those that describe directions within the body and those that describe the body's planes, cavities, and regions.

Directional terms

Directional terms help to describe the exact location of a structure in relation to another. *Superior* means toward the head; *inferior*, toward the lower part of the body. *Anterior* means toward the front of the body; *posterior*, toward the back of the body.

Medial means toward the body's midline; *lateral*, away from the midline. *Proximal* indicates closest to the point of origin of a part, or to the trunk; *distal* indicates farthest from the point of origin of a part, or from the trunk. *Superficial* means toward or at the body surface; *deep*, away from the body surface.

Body planes and sections

Imaginary lines called planes are used to section the body and its structures. The three major body reference planes are the sagittal, frontal, and transverse planes. (See *Body reference planes*, page 2.)

A *sagittal* plane runs lengthwise (longitudinally) and divides the body into right and left regions. When exactly midline, it's called a *median sagittal plane* or a *midsagittal plane.* When not exactly midline, it's called a *parasagittal plane.*

A *frontal* (coronal) plane also runs lengthwise but at a right angle to a sagittal plane. It divides the body into anterior and posterior regions. A *transverse* plane runs horizontally at a right angle to the vertical axis. It divides the body into superior and inferior regions. An *oblique* section is a slanted plane situated between a horizontal plane and a vertical plane. Such sections are

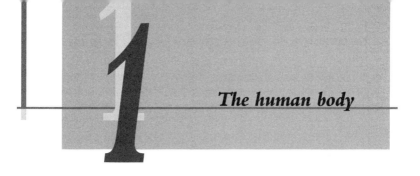

Body reference planes

Body reference planes are used to indicate the locations of body structures. Shown here are the median sagittal, frontal, and transverse planes, which lie at right angles to one another.

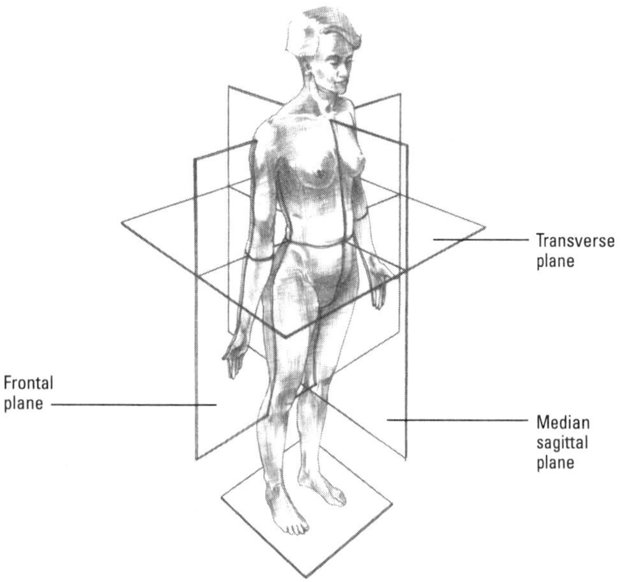

typically confusing and aren't commonly used.

Body cavities

Body cavities are spaces within the body that contain the internal organs. The dorsal and ventral cavities are the two major closed cavities. (See *Locating body cavities.*)

Dorsal cavity

Located in the posterior region of the body, the dorsal cavity is subdivided into the cranial and vertebral cavities. The *cranial cavity* (skull) encases the brain. The *vertebral cavity* (also called the *spinal cavity* or *vertebral canal*) extends down the vertebral column and encloses the spinal cord. Because the spinal cord is connected to the brain, the cranial and spinal cavities are continuous with one another.

Ventral cavity

Found in the anterior region of the trunk, the ventral cavity is subdivided into the *thoracic cavity* and the *abdominopelvic cavity.* A thin membrane, the *serosa*, covers the walls of the ventral cavity and the outer surface of its organs. The portion of the membrane lining the walls is called the *parietal serosa;* the portion covering the organs is termed the *visceral serosa.*

Thoracic cavity

Located superior to the abdominopelvic cavity, the thoracic cavity is surrounded

Locating body cavities

The dorsal cavity, in the posterior region of the body, is divided into the cranial and vertebral cavities. The ventral cavity, in the anterior region, is divided into the thoracic and abdominopelvic cavities.

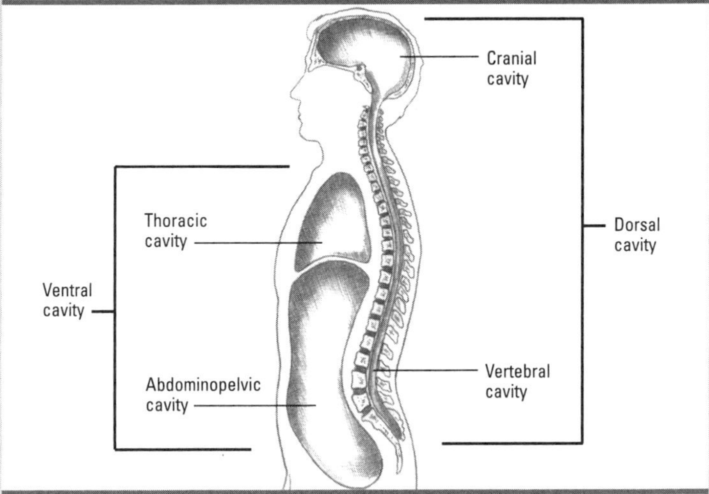

by the ribs and chest muscles. It's subdivided into the *pleural cavities*, which each contain a lung, and the *mediastinum*. The mediastinum contains the pericardial cavity, which encloses the heart. It surrounds the large vessels of the heart, trachea, esophagus, thymus, and lymph nodes as well as other blood vessels and nerves.

The serosa in the pleural cavities is called the *pleura;* in the mediastinum, it's called the *pericardium*.

Abdominopelvic cavity

The abdominopelvic cavity is subdivided into two regions: the *abdominal cavity* and the *pelvic cavity*. The abdominal cavity contains the stomach, the intestines, the spleen, the liver, and other organs. The pelvic cavity, inferior to the abdominal cavity, contains the bladder, some of the reproductive organs, and the rectum.

No muscles or membranes physically separate the abdominal and pelvic cavities. The serosa in these cavities is called the *peritoneum*.

Other cavities

The body also contains an oral cavity (the mouth), a nasal cavity (located in the nose), orbital cavities (which house the eyes), middle ear cavities (which contain the small bones of the middle ear), and synovial cavities (enclosed within the capsules surrounding certain joints).

Abdominopelvic regions

Because the abdominopelvic cavity is large and contains many organs, it's helpful to divide it into smaller regions for study. One method used by health care personnel divides the abdominopelvic cavity into four quadrants. (See *Abdominal quadrants,* page 4.)

Abdominal quadrants

The quadrant method divides the abdominopelvic cavity into four quadrants.

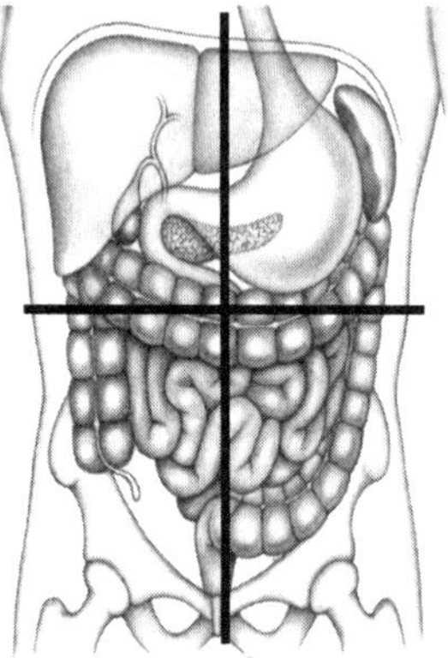
RIGHT UPPER QUADRANT
▸ Right lobe of the liver
▸ Gallbladder
▸ Pylorus
▸ Duodenum
▸ Head of the pancreas
▸ Hepatic flexure of the colon
▸ Portions of the ascending and transverse colons
RIGHT LOWER QUADRANT
▸ Cecum and appendix
▸ Portion of the ascending colon
LEFT UPPER QUADRANT
▸ Left lobe of the liver
▸ Stomach
▸ Body of the pancreas
▸ Splenic fixture of the colon
▸ Portions of the transverse and descending colon
LEFT LOWER QUADRANT
▸ Sigmoid colon
▸ Portion of the descending colon

A more complex method divides the cavity into nine body regions. Like other anatomic terms, the terms applied to these body regions help describe the locations of various body structures. The abdominal regions include the umbilical, epigastric, hypogastric, right and left iliac, right and left lumbar, and right and left hypochondriac regions. (See *Anterior view of the abdominal regions.*)

The *umbilical region* — the area around the umbilicus — includes sections of the small and large intestines, inferior vena cava, and abdominal aorta.

The *epigastric region,* superior to the umbilical region, contains the pancreas and portions of the stomach, liver, inferior vena cava, abdominal aorta, and duodenum.

The *hypogastric region* (pubic area) lies inferior to the umbilical region. Prominent structures include a portion of the sigmoid colon, urinary bladder and ureters, and portions of the small intestine.

The *right* and *left iliac regions* (inguinal regions) are situated on either side of the hypogastric region. They include portions of the small and large intestines.

The *right* and *left lumbar regions* (loin regions) are located on either side of the umbilical region. Their structures include portions of the small and large intestines and portions of the right and left kidneys.

The *right* and *left hypochondriac regions,* located on either side of the epigastric region, contain the diaphragm, portions of the kidneys, the right side of the liver, the spleen, and part of the pancreas.

Cells

The *cell* is the basic structural and functional unit of all living organisms. Human cells vary widely, ranging from the simple squamous epithelial cell to the highly specialized neuron. Generally, the simpler the cell, the greater its power to regenerate. The more specialized the cell, the weaker its regenerative power. Cells with greater regenerative power have a shorter life span than those with less regenerative power.

Anterior view of the abdominal regions

The illustration here shows the abdominal regions from the front.

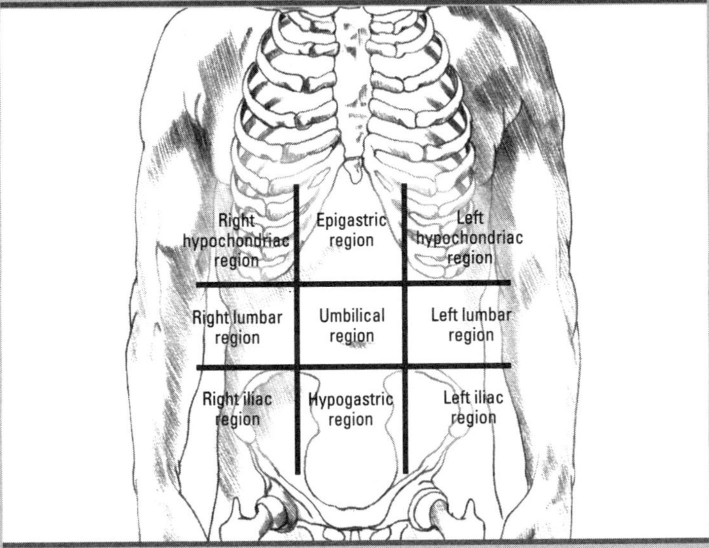

Cell structure

The three basic components of a typical cell are the cytoplasm, plasma membrane, and nucleus. Some cells also contain cilia and flagella.

Cytoplasm

A viscous, translucent, watery material, *cytoplasm* is the primary component of cells. It contains a large percentage of water, inorganic ions (potassium, calcium, magnesium, and sodium), and naturally occurring organic compounds (such as proteins, lipids, and carbohydrates).

Cytoplasm surrounds and supports the cellular structures. The area where most cellular activities take place, the cytoplasm contains cytosol, organelles, and inclusions.

Cytosol

Cytosol is a viscous, semitransparent fluid that's 70% to 90% water. It contains proteins, salts, and sugars.

Organelles

Organelles are the cell's metabolic units. Each organelle performs a specific function to maintain the life of the cell. Organelles include mitochondria, ribosomes, endoplasmic reticulum, Golgi apparatus, lysosomes, peroxisomes, cytoskeleton, and centrosomes:

- A *mitochondrion,* which is known as the "powerhouse" of the cell, is a threadlike structure within the cytoplasm that provides most of the body's adenosine triphosphate (ATP). ATP is an enzyme that fuels many cellular activities. (See *Fuel for exercise,* page 6.) The number of mitochondria in a particular cell reflects that cell's energy requirements. Active cells, such as muscle and liver cells, have hundreds of mitochondria. Relatively inactive cells, such as lymphocytes, have only a few.
- *Ribosomes* are the sites of protein synthesis.
- The *endoplasmic reticulum* is an extensive network of membrane-enclosed

Fuel for exercise

During exercise, muscle cells require the breakdown of adenosine triphosphate (ATP) to provide energy for muscle contraction. However, as a person exercises, ATP is quickly depleted. Creatine phosphate, a high-energy molecule stored in muscles, regenerates ATP while other body processes adjust to the sudden demand for ATP. Creatine phosphate and ATP both become depleted when the body fatigues.

tubules. Rough endoplasmic reticulum, covered with ribosomes, produces certain proteins; smooth endoplasmic reticulum contains enzymes that synthesize lipids.

- Each *Golgi apparatus* modifies, concentrates, and packages proteins produced by rough endoplasmic reticulum. Each protein is then delivered to a specific area in the cell. It also packages enzymes into membranous sacs called lysosomes.
- *Lysosomes* are digestive bodies that break down foreign or damaged material in cells. A membrane surrounding each lysosome separates its digestive enzymes from the rest of the cytoplasm. The enzymes digest matter brought into the cell by the action of *phagocytes*—special cells that surround and engulf matter and transport it through the cell membrane. The membrane of the lysosome fuses with the membrane of the cytoplasmic spaces surrounding the phagocytized material; this allows the lysosomal enzymes to digest the engulfed material.
- *Peroxisomes* are membranous sacs that contain *oxidases*, enzymes capable of reducing oxygen to hydrogen peroxide and hydrogen peroxide to water.
- The *cytoskeleton* is an elaborate series of rods that runs through the cytosol. It supports cellular structures and generates cell movements.
- *Centrosomes* contain *centrioles,* short cylinders adjacent to the nucleus that take part in cell division.

Inclusions

Inclusions are nonfunctioning units made up of chemical substances. They may or may not be present, depending on the cell type. For example, *melanin* in epithelial cells is an inclusion.

Cilia

Cilia are short, hairlike extensions that occur in large numbers on the outer surface of certain cells. Cilia produce a wavelike motion that moves substances in one direction across the cell's surface. For example, cells that contain cilia line the respiratory tract and propel mucus-containing dust particles and bacteria away from the lungs.

Flagella

Long projections formed by centrioles, called *flagella,* propel the cell itself. One example of a cell that contains a fagellum is the sperm.

Plasma membrane

The semipermeable *plasma membrane* (cell membrane) serves as the cell's external boundary, separating it from other cells and from the external environment. It consists of a double layer of phospholipids with protein molecules. The protein molecules provide structural support, act as binding sites, and form channels that allow water and dissolved substances to flow through.

Nucleus

The cell's control center, the *nucleus* plays a role in cell growth, metabolism, and reproduction. Within it lies the *nucleolus*, a dark-staining structure that synthesizes *ribonucleic acid* (RNA), a complex polynucleotide that controls protein synthesis. A nucleus may contain one or more nucleoli. The nucleus also contains *chromosomes,* which control cellular activities and direct protein synthesis through ribosomes in the cytoplasm.

Deoxyribonucleic acid

Deoxyribonucleic acid (DNA) is a large molecule that carries genetic information and provides the blueprint for protein synthesis. Its basic structural unit, the *nucleotide,* consists of a phosphate group linked to a five-carbon sugar—deoxyribose—joined to a nitrogen-containing compound called a *base.* Four different DNA bases exist:

- *Adenine* and *guanine* are double-ring compounds classified as purines.
- *Thymine* and *cytosine* are single-ring compounds classified as pyrimidines.

Nucleotides are joined into long chains by chemical bonds between the phosphate group of the nucleotide and a carbon atom in the deoxyribose molecule of the adjacent nucleotide. Existing in pairs, DNA chains are held together by weak chemical attractions between the nitrogen bases on adjacent chains. Because of the chemical shape of the bases, adenine bonds only with thymine and guanine bonds only with cytosine. Bases that can link with each other are called *complementary.*

Linked DNA chains form a spiral structure, or *double helix,* that resembles a spiral staircase; the deoxyribose and phosphate groups form the railings, while the nitrogen base pairs form the steps. The sequence of nucleotide bases in DNA chains forms a series of coded messages called the *genetic code.* Each group of three bases, called a *codon,* directs the synthesis of a specific amino, which is carried to the ribosomes to synthesize protein.

Ribonucleic acid

Like DNA, RNA consists of nucleotide chains, except some of its components differ. RNA transfers genetic information from nuclear DNA to ribosomes in the cytoplasm, where protein synthesis occurs. This process involves several types of RNA.

- *Ribosomal RNA* is used to make ribosomes in the endoplasmic reticulum of the cytoplasm, where the cell produces proteins.
- *Messenger RNA* directs the arrangement of amino acids to make proteins at the ribosomes. Its single strand of nucleotides is complementary to a segment of the DNA chain that contains instructions for protein synthesis. Its chains pass from the nucleus into the cytoplasm, attaching to ribosomes there.
- *Transfer RNA* consists of short nucleotide chains, each of which is specific for an individual amino acid.

POINT TO REMEMBER

RNA serves as the genetic material for many viruses.

Chromosomes

Composed of DNA and protein, chromosomes appear as a network of chromatin granules in the nondividing cell. Except in the *gametes* (germ cells), chromosomes exist in pairs. One chromosome from each pair comes from the male germ cell (*spermatozoon*); the other, from the female germ cell (*ovum*).

Normal human cells contain 23 pairs of chromosomes. In these cells, 22 pairs, called *homologous chromosomes,* are sets containing genetic information that controls the same characteristics or functions. The 23rd pair contains sex (X and Y) chromosomes. The composition of these chromosomes determines gender: XX produces a genetic female; XY, a genetic male.

In the female, the genetic activity of both X chromosomes is essential only during the first few weeks after conception. Later development requires just one functional X chromosome. The other X chromosome is inactivated and appears as a dense chromatin mass called a *Barr body* (sex chromatin body) that's attached to the nuclear membrane in the cells of a normal female. In the cells of a normal male, who has only one functional X chromosome, the Barr body is absent.

Genes

Arranged in a line on the chromosomes, *genes* are segments of chromosomal DNA chains that determine the properties of a cell. The *gene locus* is the location of a specific gene on a chromosome. *Alleles* are alternate forms of a gene that can occupy a particular gene locus; only one allele can occupy a specific locus.

Because chromosomes are paired, genes also occur in pairs on homologous chromosomes, with one allele at its locus on both homologous chromosomes. If the alleles for a particular gene are the same on both chromosomes, the person is *homozygous* for that gene. If the alleles differ, the person is *heterozygous* for that gene.

Genes account for inherited traits, their effects varying with the gene. *Gene expression* refers to a gene's effect on cell structure or function.

POINT TO REMEMBER

A dominant gene, such as the one for dark hair, is expressed even if only one parent transmits it to the offspring. In contrast, a recessive gene, such as the one for blond hair, is expressed only when both parents transmit it to the offspring. Codominant genes allow expression of both alleles, as in the genes that direct specific types of hemoglobin synthesis in red blood cells.

Sex-linked genes are carried on sex chromosomes. Almost all appear on the X chromosome and are recessive. In the male, sex-linked genes behave like dominant genes because no second X chromosome exists.

Cell division

Each cell must replicate itself for life to continue. Cells divide by mitosis or meiosis.

Before a cell divides, its chromosomes are duplicated. During this process, the double helix separates into two DNA chains; each serves as a template for constructing a new chain. Individual DNA nucleotides are linked into new strands with bases complementary to those in the originals. In this way, two identical double helices are formed, each containing one of the original strands and a newly formed complementary strand. These double helices are duplicates of the original DNA chain. (See *DNA duplication: Two double helices from one.*)

Mitosis

Mitosis is the equal division of material in the nucleus (*karyokinesis*) followed by division of the cell body (*cytokinesis*). This process yields two exact duplicates of the original cell.

All cells of the human body except gametes undergo mitosis. In mitosis, cell division occurs in five phases: an inactive phase called interphase and four active phases (prophase, metaphase, anaphase, and telophase).

Mitosis results in two daughter cells, each containing 23 pairs of chromosomes (46 chromosomes). This is called the *diploid number*. (See *Five steps of mitosis,* page 10.)

Meiosis

Only gametes (ova and spermatozoa) undergo meiosis. In this type of cell division, genetic material between homologous chromosomes is intermixed, and the number of chromosomes in the four daughter cells diminishes by half. Meiosis has two divisions separated by a resting phase.

First division

The first division, which has six phases, begins with one parent cell and ends with two daughter cells, each containing the haploid number of chromosomes.

During *interphase,* the first phase of meiosis, chromosomes replicate, each forming a double strand attached at the center by a centromere. Chromosomes appear as an indistinguishable matrix within the nucleus; centrioles (in animal cells only) appear outside the nucleus.

The nucleolus and nuclear membrane disappear during *prophase I,* the second phase. Chromosomes become distinct, and chromatids remain attached by a centromere. Homologous chromosomes move close together and intertwine; exchange of genetic information (genetic recombination) may occur. Centrioles separate, and spindle fibers appear.

During *metaphase I,* pairs of synaptic chromosomes line up randomly

DNA duplication: Two double helices from one

The nucleotide—the basic structural unit of deoxyribonucleic acid (DNA)—contains a phosphate group, deoxyribose, and a nitrogen base made of adenine (A), guanine (G), thymine (T), or cytosine (C). A double helix of a DNA molecule forms from the twisting of many nucleotide strands (shown here).

During duplication, linked DNA chains separate and new complementary chains form and link to the originals (parents). The result is two identical double helices—parent and daughter.

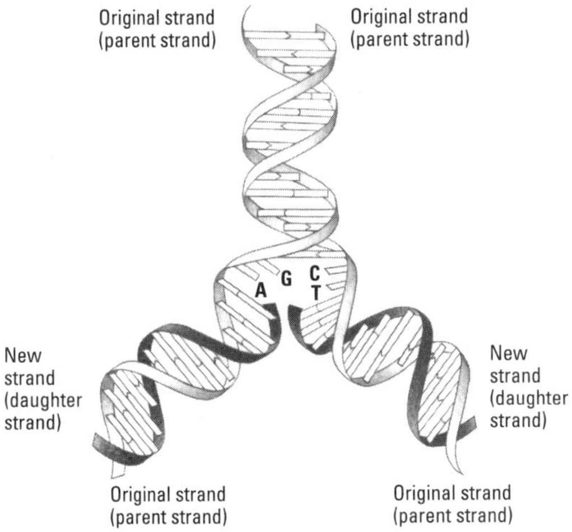

along the metaphase plate, and spindle fibers attach to each chromosome pair.

Synaptic pairs separate during the next phase, *anaphase I.* Spindle fibers pull the homologous, double-stranded chromosomes to opposite ends of the cell. Because the centromeres haven't divided, the chromatids remain attached.

A nuclear membrane forms around each end of the cell during the fifth phase, *telophase I.* Spindle fibers and chromosomes disappear. The cytoplasm compresses and divides the cell in half; each new cell contains the haploid number of chromosomes.

During *interkinesis,* the last phase of the first division, the nucleus and nuclear membrane are well defined, the nucleolus is prominent, and each chromosome consists of two chromatids that don't replicate.

Second division

Second division is a four-phase division that resembles mitosis. It starts with two new daughter cells, each containing the haploid number of chromosomes, and ends with four new haploid cells. In each cell, the two chromatids of each chromosome separate to form new daughter cells. However, because each cell entering the second division has only 23 chromosomes, each daughter cell formed has only 23 chromosomes.

During *prophase II,* the first phase, the nuclear membrane disappears and

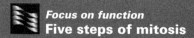

Focus on function

Five steps of mitosis

In mitosis—used by all cells except gametes (sex cells)—the nuclear contents of a cell reproduce and divide, resulting in the formation of two new daughter cells. The five steps, or phases, of this process are illustrated below.

Interphase

The nucleus and nuclear membrane are well defined and the nucleolus is prominent. Chromosomes replicate, each forming a double strand that remains attached at the center by a centromere; they appear as an indistinguishable matrix within the nucleus. Centrioles (in animal cells only) appear outside the nucleus.

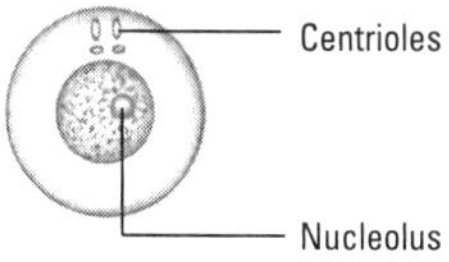

Prophase

Now the nucleolus disappears and chromosomes become distinct. Halves of each duplicated chromosome (chromatids) remain attached by a centromere. Centrioles move to opposite sides of the cell and radiate spindle fibers.

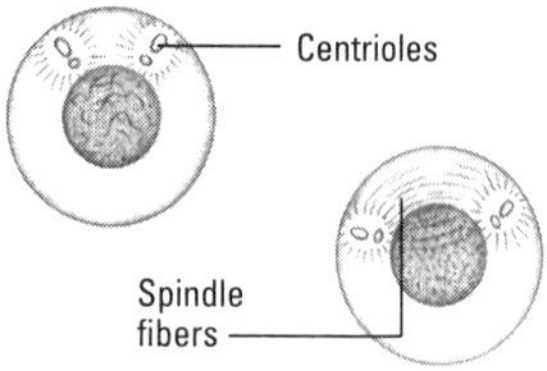

Metaphase

Chromosomes line up randomly in the center of the cell between spindles, along the metaphase plate. The centromere of each chromosome replicates.

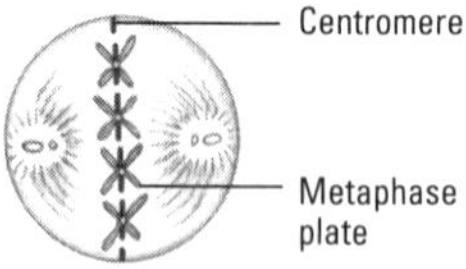

Anaphase

Centromeres move apart, pulling the separate chromatids (now called chromosomes) to opposite ends of the cell. The number of chromosomes at each end of the cell equals the original number.

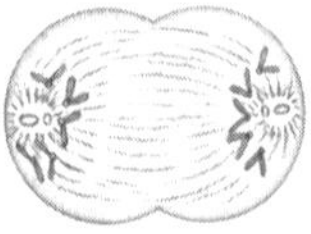

Telophase

A nuclear membrane forms around each end of the cell and spindle fibers disappear. The cytoplasm compresses and divides the cell in half. Each new cell contains the diploid number of chromosomes.

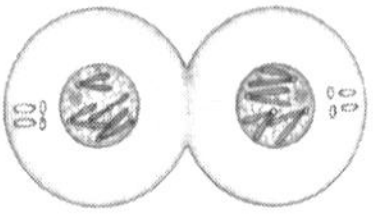

spindle fibers form. Double-stranded chromosomes, which don't synapse, appear as thin threads.

Chromosomes line up along the metaphase plate and centromeres replicate during the next phase, *metaphase II.*

Then, during *anaphase II,* chromatids separate; each is now a single-stranded chromosome. Also, chromosomes move away from each other and move to opposite ends of the cell.

Telophase II, the last phase, is characterized by formation of a nuclear membrane around the end of each cell and disappearance of chromosomes and spindle fibers. The cytoplasm compresses and divides the cells in half, leaving four daughter cells, each of which contain the haploid number of chromosomes.

Thus, at the end of the second meiotic division, each parent cell has produced four daughter cells genetically different from the parent cell.

Cellular energy generation

All cellular function depends on energy generation and transportation of substances within and among cells.

How ATP generates energy

ATP serves as the chemical fuel for cellular processes. ATP consists of a nitrogen-containing compound (adenine) joined to a five-carbon sugar (ribose), forming adenosine; adenosine is joined to three phosphate groups. Chemical bonds between the first and second and the second and third phosphate groups contain abundant energy. When the terminal high-energy phosphate bond ruptures, ATP is converted to *adenosine diphosphate* (ADP).

Liberation of the third phosphate releases energy stored in the chemical bond. Mitochondrial enzymes reconvert ADP and the liberated phosphate to ATP. To obtain the energy needed for this reattachment, mitochondria oxidize food nutrients, making the recycled ATP available again for energy production.

How substances move across the cell membrane

Each cell interacts with body fluids through the interchange of substances. Several transport methods — diffusion, osmosis, active transport, and endocytosis — move substances between cells and body fluids. Filtration, another transport method, transfers fluids and dissolved substances across capillaries into *interstitial fluid* (fluid in the spaces between cells and tissues).

Diffusion

In *diffusion,* dissolved particles, or *solutes,* move from an area of higher concentration to one of lower concentration. Diffusion is a *passive transport method* — one that requires no cellular energy.

Several factors influence the rate of diffusion:

- concentration gradient (the difference in particle concentration on either side of the plasma membrane) — the greater the concentration gradient, the faster diffusion takes place
- particle size — small particles diffuse faster than large ones
- lipid solubility — lipid-soluble particles diffuse more rapidly through the lipid layers of the cell membrane.

The electrical charge of the diffusing particles also affects the diffusion rate. Electrically charged particles (*ions*) of unlike charge are attracted to each other, whereas ions with the same electrical charge repel each other. For this reason, ions on one side of the membrane diffuse more rapidly when ions on the other side have the opposite electrical charge.

Facilitated diffusion, a special type of diffusion, occurs when a carrier molecule in the cell membrane picks up the diffusing substance on one side of the membrane and deposits it on the other side. This process is faster than simple diffusion.

Osmosis, the diffusion of a solvent, occurs when molecules move from a solution of higher molecular concentration to one of lower concentration. Osmosis involves the movement of a water (solvent) molecule across the cell membrane from a dilute solution (one with a high concentration of water molecules) to a concentrated one (one with a lower concentration).

Osmosis is influenced by the *osmotic pressure* of a solution. Osmotic pressure reflects the water-attracting property of a solution. It's determined by the number of dissolved particles in a given volume of solution — not by their size or electrical charge. A calcium chloride molecule, for instance, ionizes in solution into three particles: one calcium ion and two chloride ions. Its osmotic pressure exceeds that of a larger glucose molecule, which doesn't dissociate into ions when dissolved in solution.

Water movement in and out of cells by osmosis depends on the difference in osmotic pressure between intracellular and extracellular fluids. Normally, intracellular and extracellular osmotic pressures are equal, so the water content of cells doesn't change. However, osmotic pressure changes in body fluids cause water to shift between cells and extracellular fluids, impairing or disrupting cell functions. When the osmotic pressure of extracellular fluid falls below that of intracellular fluid, water enters the cells, making them swell and possibly rupture. When the situation is reversed (osmotic pressure of extracellular fluid exceeds that of intracellular fluid), water moves into extracellular fluid, causing the cells to shrink.

Active transport

Unlike passive transport methods, *active transport* requires energy. Usually, this mechanism moves a substance across the cell membrane against the *concentration gradient* — from an area of lower concentration to one of higher concentration.

However, active transport can also move a substance *with* the concentration gradient. In this process, a carrier molecule in the cell membrane combines with the substance, transports it through the membrane, and deposits it on the other side.

Unlike facilitated diffusion, which also uses a carrier molecule, active transport requires energy from ATP breakdown to transport substances across cell membranes.

Endocytosis is an active transport method in which a substance is engulfed by the cell, rather than passed through the cell membrane. The cell surrounds the substance with part of the cell membrane, which separates to form a *vacuole* (cavity) that moves to the cell's interior.

Endocytosis involves either phagocytosis or pinocytosis. *Phagocytosis* refers to engulfment and ingestion of particles too large to pass through the cell membrane. *Pinocytosis* resembles phagocytosis but occurs only to engulf dissolved substances or small particles suspended in fluid.

Filtration

Fluid and dissolved substances also may move across a cell membrane by *filtration*. In this method, pressure applied to a solution on one side of the cell membrane forces fluid and dissolved particles through the membrane. The filtration rate (the rate at which substances pass through the membrane) depends on the amount of pressure.

Filtration promotes the transfer of fluids and dissolved materials from the blood across the capillaries into the interstitial fluid; the pressure of capillary blood provides the filtration force.

POINT TO REMEMBER

Urine formation depends on fluid filtration from blood flowing through the capillaries in the kidneys.

Tissues

Tissues are groups of cells with the same general structure and function. The human body contains four basic types of tissue — epithelial, connective, muscle, and nervous tissue.

Epithelial tissue

Epithelial tissue (*epithelium*) is a continuous cellular sheet that covers the body's surface, lines body cavities, and forms certain glands. It contains at least two types of epithelial cells.

Epithelial tissue with a single layer of squamous cells attached to a basement membrane is called *endothelium.* Such tissue lines the cavities of the cardiovascular, GI, and respiratory systems. Epithelial tissues protect underlying tissues from injury and bacterial invasion and contain nerve endings that respond to various stimuli, such as pressure and heat. The tissue that lines the GI tract absorbs substances, and the epithelial tissue found in the kidneys performs specialized functions, such as absorption, filtration, secretion, and excretion.

Types of epithelial tissue

Epithelial tissue is classified by the number of cell layers it has and the shape of cells on its surface. Based on the number of cell layers, epithelial tissue may be simple, stratified, or pseudostratified. *Simple* epithelial tissue has only one layer, *stratified* epithelial tissue has two or more layers, and *pseudostratified* epithelial tissue has one layer but appears to have more.

Based on the shape of its surface cells, epithelial tissue may be squamous, columnar, or cuboidal. *Squamous* epithelial tissue has flat surface cells; *columnar* epithelial tissue has tall, cylindrical, prism-shaped surface cells; and *cuboidal* epithelial tissue has cube-shaped surface cells. (See *Distinguishing types of epithelial tissue,* page 14.)

Some epithelial tissues have certain other characteristics:

- In the lining of the intestines, some columnar epithelial cells have vertical striations, forming a *striated border.* In the tubules of the kidneys, borders of columnar epithelial cells have tiny, brushlike structures (*microvilli*) called a *brush border.*
- *Stereociliated epithelial cells,* which line the epididymis, have long, piriform (pear-shaped) tufts.
- *Ciliated epithelial cells* possess *cilia,* fine hairlike protuberances on the free border. Larger than microvilli, cilia move fluid and particles through the cavity of an organ.
- In some epithelial tissues, such as the mucous tissue that lines the nasal passages, branches of sensory nerves pierce the underlying layer (*basement membrane*) of the tissue.
- *Wandering cells* are macrophages (phagocytes) that enter the epithelium from connective tissue.
- Some types of epithelium are *desquamated* (shed) and regenerate continuously by transformation of cells from deeper layers.

Glandular epithelium

Organs that produce secretions consist of a special type of epithelium called *glandular epithelium.* Many glands are enclosed in a dense capsule of connective tissue; these capsules are divided into *lobes*, then into smaller units called *lobules*.

Exocrine and endocrine glands

Depending on how it secretes its products, a gland is classified as *exocrine* or *endocrine. Secretion* — the process of producing a specific substance — may involve separation of an element of the blood or production of a totally new chemical substance (such as the urine secreted by the kidneys). *Excretion,* in contrast, is the elimination of a product from the body. The urinary bladder, for example, excretes urine.

Endocrine glands release their secretions into the blood or lymph. For instance, the medulla of the adrenal gland secretes epinephrine and norepinephrine into the bloodstream. (For more information on endocrine glands, see chapter 6, Endocrine system.)

Exocrine glands discharge their secretions onto external or internal surfaces. An example is sweat, which sweat glands secrete onto the surface of the skin.

Mixed glands contain both endocrine and exocrine cells. The pancreas, a mixed gland, contains alpha and beta

Distinguishing types of epithelial tissue

Epithelial tissue (epithelium) is classified by the number of cell layers and the shape of surface cells. Thus, epithelium may be *simple* (one-layered), *stratified* (multilayered), or *pseudostratified* (one-layered but appearing to be multilayered) and *squamous* (containing flat surface cells), *columnar* (containing tall, cylindrical surface cells), or *cuboidal* (containing cube-shaped surface cells).

The top left illustration shows how the basement membrane of simple squamous epithelium joins the epithelium to underlying connective tissues. The other illustrations show five additional types of epithelial tissue.

SIMPLE SQUAMOUS EPITHELIUM

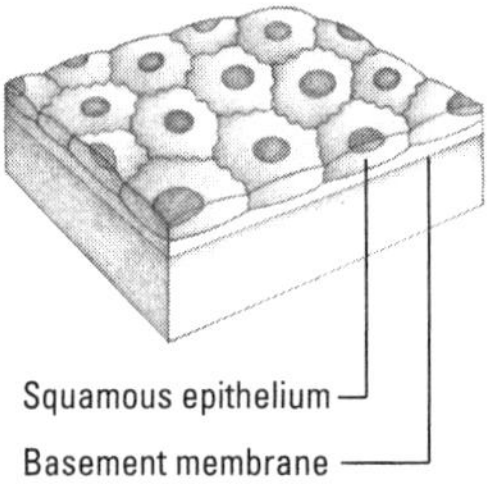

STRATIFIED COLUMNAR EPITHELIUM

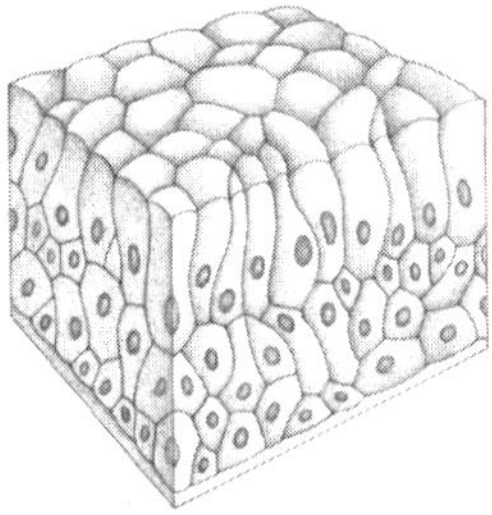

SIMPLE CUBOIDAL EPITHELIUM

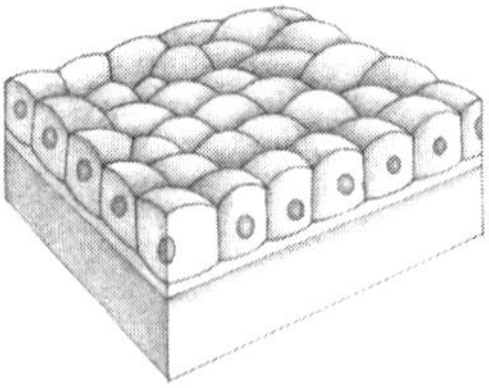

STRATIFIED SQUAMOUS EPITHELIUM

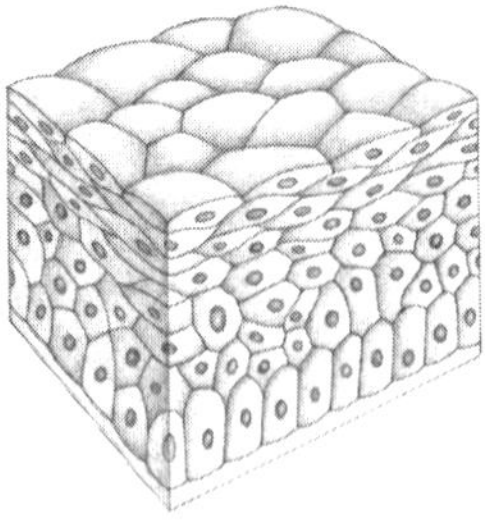

SIMPLE COLUMNAR EPITHELIUM

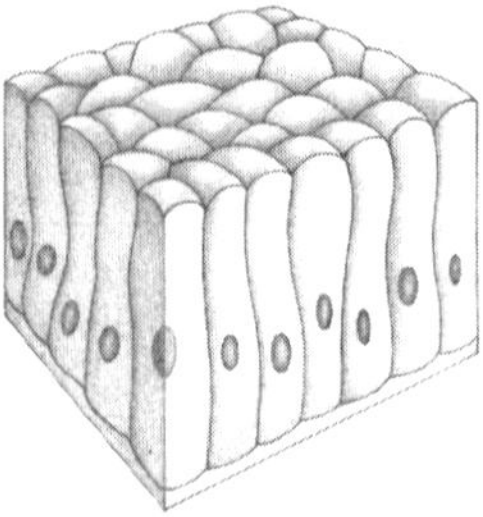

PSEUDOSTRATIFIED COLUMNAR EPITHELIUM

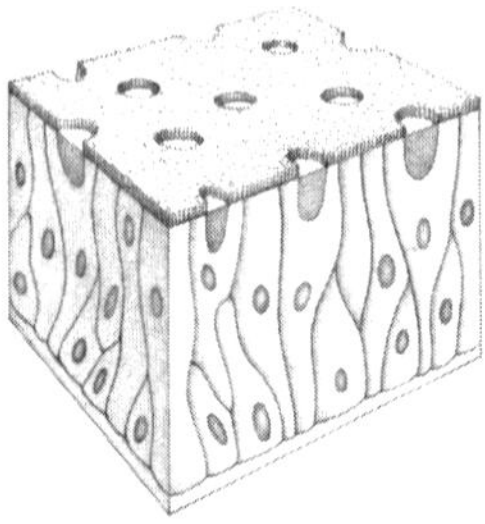

cells (in the islets of Langerhans); these endocrine cells produce glucagon and insulin, respectively. The pancreas also contains acinar cells, exocrine cells that secrete digestive juices.

Connective tissue

Connective tissue — a category that includes bone, cartilage, blood, and adipose (fatty) tissue — binds together and supports body structures. Three types of fibers are found in connective tissue: collagen, reticular, and elastic fibers.

Collagenous fibers are soft, flexible, white fibers consisting of *collagen,* a protein. Present in all types of connective tissue, these fibers are highly resistant to pulling forces. *Reticular* fibers are immature collagenous fibers. They form delicate networks that surround small blood vessels and support the soft tissues of organs. *Elastic* fibers are yellowish fibers with an elastic quality that can be found in the lungs, blood vessel walls, and skin.

Connective tissue cells may be fixed or wandering. *Fixed cells* are typical cells that remain in place, whereas *wandering cells* may move from one site to another.

Types of connective tissue

Connective tissue is classified as loose or dense. *Loose (areolar) connective tissue* has large spaces separating the fibers and cells and contains much intercellular fluid.

Dense connective tissue, which provides structural support, has greater fiber concentration. Dense tissue is further subdivided into dense regular and dense irregular connective tissue:

- *Dense regular* connective tissue consists of tightly packed fibers arranged in a consistent pattern. It includes tendons, ligaments, and *aponeuroses* (flat fibrous sheets that attach muscles to bones or other tissues).
- *Dense irregular* connective tissue has tightly packed fibers arranged in an inconsistent pattern. It's found in the dermis, submucosa of the GI tract, fibrous capsules, and fascia.

Adipose tissue

Commonly called fat, *adipose tissue* is a specialized type of loose connective tissue in which a single lipid (fat) droplet occupies most of each cell. It cushions internal organs, acts as a reserve supply of energy, and helps protect the body from temperature extremes. Adipose tissue is widely distributed subcutaneously.

POINT TO REMEMBER

The distribution of adipose tissue varies with sex and age. In men, subcutaneous fat appears mainly in the nape of the neck, the regions overlying the seventh cervical vertebra, deltoid and triceps muscles, lumbosacral region, and buttocks. In women, subcutaneous fat occurs chiefly in the breasts, buttocks, and thighs. In both sexes, fat accumulates extensively in the abdominal region.

Blood

A special type of connective tissue, *blood* is an opaque, viscous fluid that circulates through the heart and blood vessels. Blood is classified as a connective tissue because it consists of blood cells, surrounded by a nonliving fluid, *plasma.* The fibers in blood are soluble protein molecules that become visible during clotting.

Special properties

Connective tissue in some parts of the body has special properties. For instance, mucous connective tissue of the umbilical cord (Wharton's jelly) is a temporary tissue that supports the umbilical cord until after birth. Elastic connective tissue of the vocal cords permits speech, whereas reticular connective tissue of the spleen forms a soft skeleton for support of other cells. (Some cells of this tissue are phagocytic, protecting the body against foreign materials.) Finally, pigmented connective tissue of the sclera gives the eyeball its white color.

Muscle tissue

Muscle tissue consists of muscle cells with a generous blood supply. Measur-

Smooth-muscle tissue sites

Smooth-muscle tissue is located throughout the body, including the following sites:
- walls of internal organs such as those of the GI tract from the middle of the esophagus to the internal anal sphincter
- walls of the respiratory passages from the trachea to the alveolar ducts
- urinary and genital ducts
- walls of arteries and veins
- walls of larger lymphatic trunks
- arrectores pilorum
- iris and ciliary body of the eye.

ing up to several centimeters long, muscle cells have an elongated shape that enhances their *contractility* (ability to contract).

Types of muscle tissue

The three basic types of muscle tissue are skeletal, cardiac, and smooth.

Skeletal muscle tissue

Skeletal muscle tissue is striped, or *striated,* in appearance. Its fibers, which contain masses of cytoplasm with many nuclei, receive stimulation from cerebrospinal nerves. All skeletal muscle tissue is capable of voluntary contraction. (For more information on skeletal muscles, see chapter 3, Integumentary system.)

Skeletal muscles contain specialized *myofibrils,* bundles of fine fibers made up of even finer fibers called thin and thick filaments. Thin filaments contain the contractile protein *actin,* whereas thick filaments contain the contractile protein *myosin.*

Cardiac muscle tissue

The muscle tissue of the heart, cardiac muscle tissue is sometimes classified as striated, rather than placed in a separate category. However, it differs from other striated tissue in two ways:
- Its fibers are separate cellular units, which (unlike other striated muscle fibers) don't contain many nuclei.
- It contracts involuntarily.

Smooth-muscle tissue

Lacking the striped pattern of striated tissue, smooth-muscle tissue consists of long, spindle-shaped cells. Its activity, stimulated by the autonomic nervous system, isn't under voluntary control.

Smooth-muscle tissue lines the walls of many internal organs and other structures. (See *Smooth-muscle tissue sites.*)

In the skin, smooth-muscle fibers form the *arrectores pilorum,* tiny muscles whose contraction causes the hair to stand erect. In the mammary glands, smooth muscle causes the nipples to become erect; in the scrotum, it wrinkles the skin to help raise the testes.

Smooth muscle in the ciliary body of the eye plays a part in *accommodation* (focusing the eye for clear vision at various distances). In the iris, smooth-muscle contraction results in pupil dilation.

Nervous tissue

The main function of nervous tissue is communication. Its primary properties are *irritability* (the capacity to react to various physical and chemical agents) and *conductivity* (the ability to transmit the resulting reaction from one point to another).

Types of nervous tissue cells

Nervous tissue cells may be neurons or neuroglia. Highly specialized cells, *neurons* generate and conduct nerve impulses. A typical neuron consists of a cell body with cytoplasmic extensions — numerous dendrites on one pole and a single axon on the opposite pole. These extensions allow the neuron to conduct impulses over long distances.

Neuroglia form the support structure of nervous tissue, insulating and protecting neurons. They're found only in the central nervous system. (For more information on neurons and neuroglia, see chapter 5, Nervous system.)

2 Chemical organization

The human body is composed of chemicals, and all its activities are chemical in nature. Thus, knowledge of chemistry is basic to an understanding of the human body and its functions.

The chemical level is the simplest and most important level of structural organization. Body cells — and eventually the body itself — would die without the proper chemicals in the proper amounts.

Principles of chemistry

Every cell contains thousands of different chemicals. Far from constituting an inert mixture, these chemicals constantly interact with each another.

Differences in chemical composition differentiate types of body tissue. What's more, the blueprints of heredity are encoded in chemical form. (See *Chemical makeup of the human body,* page 18.)

Matter and energy

Matter is anything that has mass and occupies space. It may be a solid, liquid, or gas.

Energy is the capacity to do work — to put mass into motion. It may be potential (stored) energy or kinetic energy (the energy of motion). Types of energy include chemical, electrical, and radiant.

POINT TO REMEMBER
Neither matter nor energy can be created or destroyed. However, matter can be converted to energy.

Molecules and compounds

A *molecule* is the smallest unit of matter than can exist alone and still display the characteristic chemical properties of a particular element or compound. It's composed of two or more atoms held together by chemical forces.

A *compound* is a substance made up of two or more different elements joined by chemical bonds to form molecules.

Chemical elements

An *element* is matter that can't be broken down into simpler substances by normal chemical reactions. All forms of matter are composed of chemical elements. Each of the 109 chemical elements in the periodic table has a chemical symbol such as Ca (the chemical symbol for calcium). (See *Periodic table of elements,* pages 20 and 21.)

Carbon, hydrogen, nitrogen, and oxygen account for 96% of the body's total weight. Calcium and phosphorus account for another 2.5%.

Atomic structure

An *atom* is the smallest unit of matter that can take part in a chemical reaction. Atoms of a single type constitute an element.

Each atom has a dense central core called a *nucleus,* plus one or more surrounding energy layers called *electron shells*. Atoms consist of three basic subatomic particles: protons, neutrons, and electrons.

Protons

Protons (p^+) are closely packed particles in the atom's nucleus that have a

Chemical makeup of the human body

This chart lists the 22 chemical elements of the human body, shown in descending order from most to least plentiful.

Element	Percentage in human body
Oxygen	65%
Carbon	18.5%
Hydrogen	9.5%
Nitrogen	3.3%
Phosphorus	1%
Calcium	0.5%
Potassium	0.4%
Sulfur	0.3%
Chlorine	0.2%
Sodium	0.2%
Magnesium	0.1%
Iron	0.004%
Iodine	0.00004%
Silicon	Trace
Fluorine	Trace
Copper	Trace
Manganese	Trace
Zinc	Trace
Selenium	Trace
Cobalt	Trace
Molybdenum	Trace
Boron	Trace

positive charge. The number of protons is unique for each element and determines the element's *atomic number.* For example, all carbon atoms — and *only* carbon atoms — have 6 protons; therefore, the atomic number of carbon is 6. Hydrogen's atomic number is 1 because its nucleus contains 1 proton.

The positive charge of a nucleus equals the number of its protons. For instance, because a carbon atom contains 6 protons, the positive charge of its nucleus is 6 ($6p^+$). A proton weighs nearly the same as a neutron (n); a proton and a neutron each weigh 1,836 times as much as an electron (e^-).

An atom's *atomic weight* (atomic mass) equals the total mass of its protons, neutrons, and electrons (p + n + e). An atom's *mass number* is the sum of its protons and neutrons (p + n). Electrons have little mass; for this reason, an atom's mass number may nearly equal its atomic mass.

Neutrons

Neutrons are uncharged, or neutral, particles in the atom's nucleus. Not all the atoms of an element necessarily have the same number of neutrons. Those with a different number of neutrons (and a different atomic weight) than most of the atoms of an element are called *isotopes*.

Electrons

Electrons are negatively charged particles that orbit the nucleus in different electron shells. They play a key role in chemical bonds and reactions.

The number of electrons in an atom equals the number of protons in its nucleus. The electrons' negative charges cancel out the protons' positive charges, making atoms electrically neutral.

Each electron shell can hold a maximum number of electrons. The innermost shell can accommodate two electrons at most, whereas the outermost shells can hold many more.

An atom with single (unpaired) electrons orbiting in its outermost electron shell can be chemically active — that is, it's able to take part in chemical reactions. An atom whose outer shell contains no single electrons but only pairs of electrons is chemically inactive, or stable.

An atom's *valence* equals the number of unpaired electrons in its outer shell. For example, sodium (Na^+) has a plus-one valence because its outer shell contains one unpaired electron.

POINT TO REMEMBER
When one atom combines with or breaks apart from another, a chemical reaction occurs.

Chemical bonds

A *chemical bond* is a force of attraction that binds the atoms of a molecule together. Formation of a chemical bond usually requires energy, whereas breakup of a chemical bond usually releases energy.

Types of bonds

Several types of chemical bonds exist. An *ionic (electrovalent) bond* occurs when valence electrons transfer from one atom to another. A *covalent bond* forms when atoms share pairs of valence electrons. (See *Picturing ionic and covalent bonds,* page 22.) A *hydrogen bond* occurs when two atoms associate with a hydrogen atom; oxygen and nitrogen, for instance, commonly form hydrogen bonds.

Chemical reactions

A *chemical reaction* involves unpaired electrons in the outer shells of atoms. In this reaction, one of two events occurs:

- unpaired electrons from the outer shell of one atom transfer to the outer shell of another
- one atom shares its unpaired electrons with another atom.

Energy, particle concentration, speed, and orientation determine whether a chemical reaction will occur. The four basic types of chemical reactions are synthesis, decomposition, exchange, and reversible reactions. (See *Comparing chemical reactions,* page 23.)

Synthesis reaction

A *synthesis reaction* combines two or more substances (reactants) to form a new, more complex substance (product); this results in a chemical bond. Many such reactions occur in the body. Collectively, synthesis reactions are called *anabolism.*

Decomposition reaction

In a *decomposition reaction,* a substance decomposes, or breaks down, into two or more simpler substances, leading to the breakdown of a chemical bond. Thus, a decomposition reaction is the opposite of a synthesis reaction. *Catabolism* is the collective term for the body's many decomposition reactions.

POINT TO REMEMBER
An example of a decomposition reaction is the breakdown (digestion) of large fat molecules into two simpler substances — glycerol and fatty acids.

Exchange reaction

A combination of a decomposition and a synthesis reaction, an *exchange reaction* occurs when two complex substances decompose into simpler substances, and the simple substances then join (through synthesis) with different simple substances to form new complex substances.

An example of an exchange reaction occurs in the blood between lactic acid and sodium bicarbonate. Both substances decompose in exchange for synthesis of sodium lactate and carbonic acid.

Reversible reaction

In a *reversible reaction,* the product reverts to its original reactants, and vice versa. Reversible reactions may necessitate special conditions, such as heat or light.

Inorganic compounds

Although most biomolecules (molecules produced by living cells) form organic compounds, some form *inorganic compounds*. Usually small and lacking carbon, inorganic compounds include water and inorganic acids, bases, and salts.

Water

The body's most abundant substance, water performs a host of vital functions — many of them related to its

(Text continues on page 22.)

Periodic table of elements

In the periodic table, all the known chemical elements are arranged in order of increasing proton number. This arrangement reveals the similarities of elements with similar electronic configuration (indicated by the same number of electrons in the outermost shell). The elements fall into vertical columns, or groups. The atoms of elements in the same group all have the same outer shell structure but an increasing number of inner

Metals
Metalloids
Nonmetals
Noble gases

TRANSITION METALS

	1 1A	2 2A	3 3B	4 4B	5 5B	6 6B	7 7B	8 8B	9 8B
1	1 H Hydrogen 1.008								
2	3 Li Lithium 6.941	4 Be Beryllium 9.012							
3	11 Na Sodium 22.99	12 Mg Magnesium 24.312							
4	19 K Potassium 39.098	20 Ca Calcium 40.08	21 Sc Scandium 44.956	22 Ti Titanium 47.88	23 V Vanadium 50.942	24 Cr Chromium 51.996	25 Mn Manganese 54.938	26 Fe Iron 55.847	27 Co Cobalt 58.933
5	37 Rb Rubidium 85.468	38 Sr Strontium 87.62	39 Y Yttrium 88.906	40 Zr Zirconium 91.22	41 Nb Niobium 92.906	42 Mo Molybdenum 95.94	43 Tc Technetium (98)	44 Ru Ruthenium 101.07	45 Rh Rhodium 102.906
6	55 Cs Cesium 132.905	56 Ba Barium 137.33	57 La Lanthanum 138.906	72 Hf Hafnium 178.49	73 Ta Tantalum 180.948	74 W Tungsten 183.85	75 Re Rhenium 186.207	76 Os Osmium 190.2	77 Ir Iridium 192.22
7	87 Fr Francium (223)	88 Ra Radium 226.025	89 Ac Actinium 227.028	104 Rf Rutherfordium (261)	105 Db Dubnium (261)	106 Sg Seaborgium (263)	107 Bh Bohrium (262)	108 Hs Hassium (265)	109 Mt Meitnerium (266)

INNER TRANSITION METALS

Lanthanide series

58 Ce Cerium 140.12	59 Pr Praseodymum 140.908	60 Nd Neodymium 144.24	61 Pm Promethium (145)	62 Sm Samarium 150.36
90 Th Thorium 232.038	91 Pa Protactinium 231.036	92 U Uranium 238.029	93 Np Neptunium 237.0482	94 Pu Plutonium (244)
1	2	3	4	5

Actinide series

KEY:

1 — Atomic number
H — Symbol
Hydrogen — Name
1.008 — Atomic weight

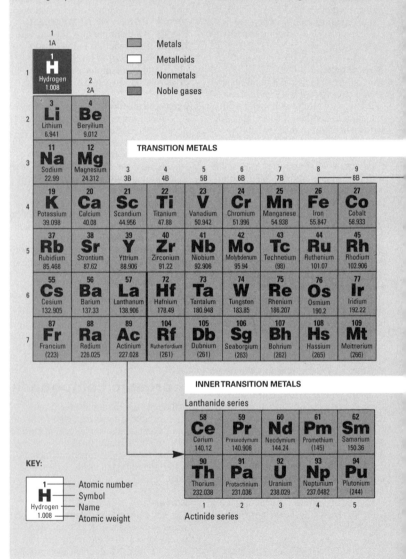

shells. Horizontal rows in the table are called periods. Within a period, atoms of all the elements have the same number of shells but a steadily increasing number of electrons in the outer shell. *Note:* An atomic mass shown in parentheses is the mass number of the isotope of longest half-life for that element.

10	11 1B	12 2B	13 3A	14 4A	15 5A	16 6A	17 7A	18 8A
								2 **He** Helium 4.003
			5 **B** Boron 10.811	6 **C** Carbon 12.011	7 **N** Nitrogen 14.007	8 **O** Oxygen 15.999	9 **F** Fluorine 18.998	10 **Ne** Neon 20.179
			13 **Al** Aluminum 26.982	14 **Si** Silicon 28.086	15 **P** Phosphorus 30.974	16 **S** Sulfur 32.064	17 **Cl** Chlorine 35.453	18 **Ar** Argon 39.948
28 **Ni** Nickel 58.69	29 **Cu** Copper 63.546	30 **Zn** Zinc 65.38	31 **Ga** Gallium 69.72	32 **Ge** Germanium 72.59	33 **As** Arsenic 74.922	34 **Se** Selenium 78.96	35 **Br** Bromine 79.904	36 **Kr** Krypton 83.80
46 **Pd** Palladium 106.42	47 **Ag** Silver 107.868	48 **Cd** Cadmium 112.41	49 **In** Indium 114.82	50 **Sn** Tin 118.69	51 **Sb** Antimony 121.75	52 **Te** Tellurium 127.60	53 **I** Iodine 126.905	54 **Xe** Xenon 131.30
78 **Pt** Platinum 195.08	79 **Au** Gold 196.967	80 **Hg** Mercury 200.59	81 **Tl** Thallium 204.383	82 **Pb** Lead 207.2	83 **Bi** Bismuth 208.980	84 **Po** Polonium (209)	85 **At** Astatine (210)	86 **Rn** Radon (222)

63 **Eu** Europium 151.96	64 **Gd** Gadolinium 157.25	65 **Tb** Terbium 158.925	66 **Dy** Dysprosium 162.50	67 **Ho** Holmium 164.930	68 **Er** Erbium 167.26	69 **Tm** Thulium 168.934	70 **Yb** Ytterbium 173.04	71 **Lu** Lutetium 174.967
95 **Am** Americium (243)	96 **Cm** Curium (247)	97 **Bk** Berkelium (247)	98 **Cf** Californium (251)	99 **Es** Einsteinium (252)	100 **Fm** Fermium (257)	101 **Md** Mendelevium (258)	102 **No** Nobelium (259)	103 **Lr** Lawrencium (260)
6	7	8	9	10	11	12	13	14

Picturing ionic and covalent bonds

In an ionic bond, an electron is transferred from one atom to another. In the example illustrated below, an electron transfers from a sodium (Na) atom to a chlorine (Cl) atom. The result is a molecule of sodium chloride (NaCl).

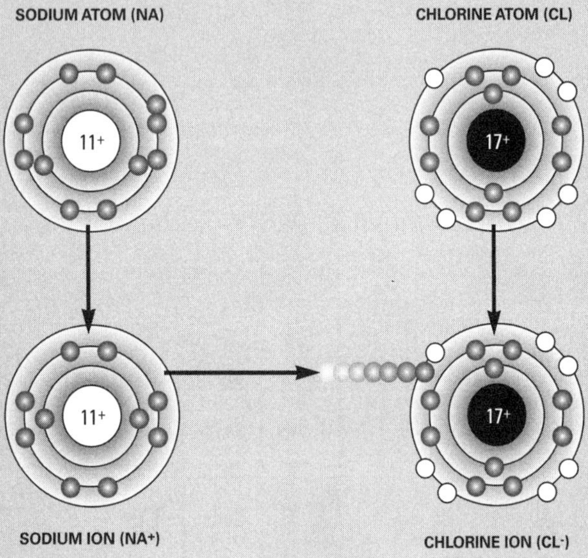

In a covalent bond, atoms share a pair of electrons. The diagram below shows what happens when two hydrogen (H) atoms form a covalent bond.

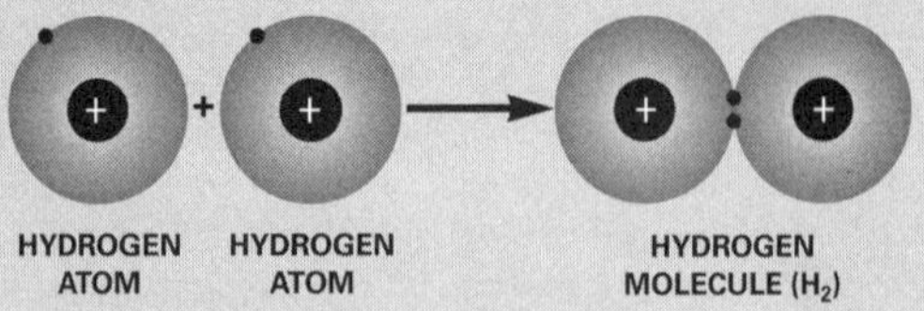

ability to dissolve substances. These functions include:

- easily forming polar covalent bonds
- acting as a lubricant in mucus and other body fluids
- entering into chemical reactions such as nutrient breakdown during digestion
- enabling the body to maintain a relatively constant temperature (by absorbing and releasing heat slowly).

Inorganic acids, bases, and salts

Acids, bases, and salts are *electrolytes* — compounds whose molecules consist of positively charged ions (cations) and negatively charged ions (anions) and that ionize (separate into ions) in solution. In water, electrolytes dissociate into cations and anions.

Acids are compounds that ionize into hydrogen ions (H^+) and anions. For example, hydrochloric acid (HCl) dissociates into H^+ and the anion Cl^-.

Bases, in contrast, ionize into hydroxide ions (OH^-) and cations. For example, potassium hydroxide (KOH) dissociates into OH^- and the cation K^+.

Salts are compounds that form when acids react with bases. In water, salts ionize into cations and anions, but not H^+ or OH^- ions; for example, potassium chloride (KCl) dissociates into the cation K^+ and the anion Cl^-.

Body fluids must attain *acid-base balance* to maintain homeostasis. A solution's acidity is determined by the number of hydrogen ions it contains; the more hydrogen ions present, the more acidic the solution. Conversely, the more OH^- a solution contains, the more basic (alkaline) it is.

The term *pH* refers to the hydrogen ion concentration of a solution. The acidity or alkalinity of body fluids is measured on the *pH scale*. A neutral solution — one with a pH of 7 — contains equal amounts of H^+ and OH^-. An acidic solution — one with a pH below 7 — contains more H^+ than OH^-. A basic (alkaline) solution has a pH above 7 and contains more OH^- than H^+.

Along with respiratory and kidney mechanisms, buffers maintain pH in the body. (For more information on acid-base balance and buffer systems, see chapter 14, Fluid, electrolyte, and acid-base balance.)

Organic compounds

Most biomolecules form *organic compounds*. These compounds, which contain carbon and hydrogen, use covalent bonds. Organic compounds include:

- carbohydrates — sugars, starches, glycogen, cellulose
- lipids — water-insoluble organic biomolecules
- proteins — polypeptides made up of amino acids
- nucleic acids — compounds consisting of a phosphate group, a pentose sugar, and a nitrogenous base.

Comparing chemical reactions

The formulas below reflect the four basic types of chemical reactions.

Synthesis reaction
$A + B \rightarrow AB$

Decomposition reaction
$AB \rightarrow A + B$

Exchange reaction
$AB + CD \rightarrow AD + BC$

Reversible reaction
$A + B \leftrightarrow AB$

Carbohydrates

The main functions of carbohydrates are to release and store energy. The three types of carbohydrates are monosaccharides, disaccharides, and polysaccharides.

Monosaccharides, such as ribose and deoxyribose, are sugars with three to seven carbon atoms. *Disaccharides*, such as lactose and maltose, contain two monosaccharides. *Polysaccharides*, such as glycogen, are large carbohydrates with many monosaccharides.

Through dehydration synthesis, monosaccharides combine to form disaccharides or polysaccharides. Hydrolysis uses water to break down disaccharides and polysaccharides (large molecules) into monosaccharides (smaller molecules).

Lipids

The major lipids are triglycerides, phospholipids, steroids, lipoproteins, and eicosanoids.

Triglycerides

The most abundant lipid both in food and in the body, *triglycerides* are neutral fats that insulate and protect. They also serve as the body's most concentrated energy source. Triglycerides contain three molecules of a fatty acid chemically joined to one molecule of glycerol.

Phospholipids
The major structural components of cell membranes, *phospholipids* consist of one molecule of glycerol, two molecules of a fatty acid, and a phosphate group. A common phospholipid is phosphatidylcholine (lecithin).

Steroids
Steroids are simple lipids with no fatty acids in their molecules. They fall into four main categories, each of which performs different functions.

- *Bile salts* emulsify fats during digestion and aid the absorption of fat-soluble vitamins (vitamins A, D, E, and K).
- *Male and female sex hormones* are responsible for sexual characteristics and reproduction.
- *Cholesterol,* a part of animal cell membranes, is needed to form all other steroids.
- *Vitamin D* helps to regulate the body's calcium concentration.

Lipoproteins and eicosanoids
Lipoproteins help transport lipids to various parts of the body. *Eicosanoids* include *prostaglandins* and *leukotrienes.* Prostaglandins have varied functions, such as modifying hormone responses, promoting the inflammatory response, and opening the airways. Leukotrienes play a part in allergic and inflammatory responses. (See *Other energy sources.*)

Proteins
The most abundant organic compound in the body, proteins are composed of building blocks called *amino acids.* Amino acids are linked together by *peptide bonds* — chemical bonds that join the carboxyl group of one amino acid to the amino group of another.

A small peptide of six amino acids

Proteins differ from the simple polypeptide chain shown below by having hundreds of thousands of amino acids linked through peptide bonds; note that for peptides and proteins, the two end functional groups are usually different; one end group is usually an amine group (the N-terminal) and the other is usually a carboxyl group (the C-terminal).

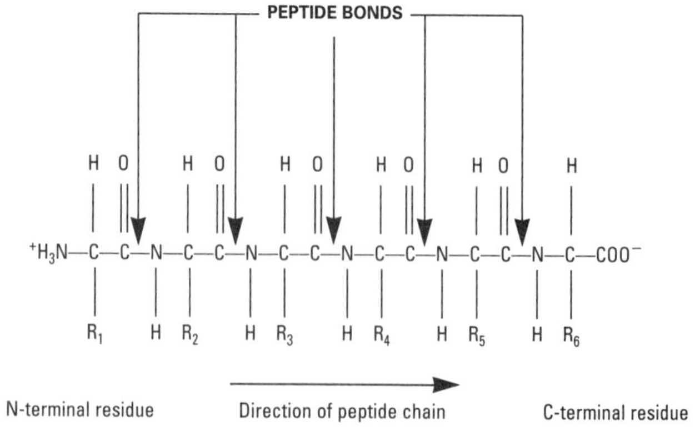

Many amino acids linked together form a *polypeptide.* One or more polypeptides in turn form a protein. The sequence of amino acids in a protein's polypeptide chain dictates its shape, which in turn determines the protein's functions. (See *A small peptide of six amino acids.*)

The functions of proteins include providing structure and protection, promoting muscle contraction, transporting various substances, regulating processes, and serving as enzymes. *Enzymes,* the largest group of proteins, act as catalysts for crucial chemical reactions.

Other energy sources

During exercise, the body requires water, carbohydrates, and lipids. Water, the most plentiful substance in the body, regulates body temperature by slowly absorbing and releasing heat. Carbohydrates, in turn, supply the body with an immediate source of energy. As exercise continues, lipids become the secondary source of energy. Stored fat represents the body's most plentiful source of energy. Relative to other nutrients, the quantity of fat available for energy is almost unlimited.

Nucleic acids

The nucleic acids *deoxyribonucleic acid* (DNA) and *ribonucleic acid* (RNA) are composed of nitrogenous bases, sugars, and phosphate groups. The primary hereditary molecule, DNA contains two long chains of deoxyribonucleotides, which coil into a double-helix shape. Deoxyribose and phosphate units alternate in the "backbone" of the chains. Holding the two chains together are base pairs of adenine-thymine and guanine-cytosine. Each human DNA molecule contains a specific sequence of more than 100 million base pairs. (See *Base pairs: Links between DNA strands.*)

Base pairs: Links between DNA strands

Hydrogen bonds between the two members of each base pair (shown below) hold together the two polynucleotide chains of a deoxyribonucleic acid (DNA) molecule. A DNA molecule contains only two types of base pairs: adenine-thymine and guanine-cytosine.

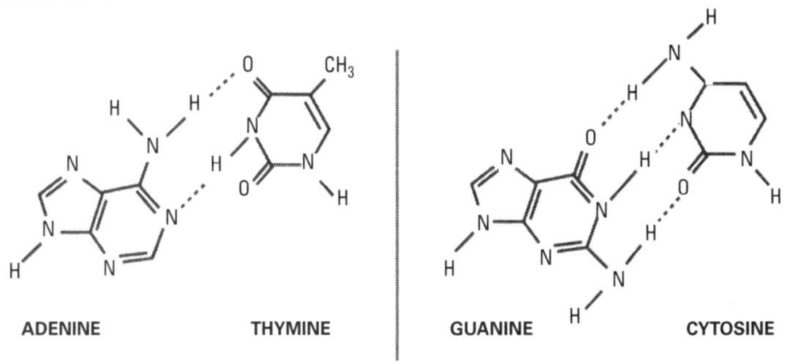

Key:
H = hydrogen N = nitrogen O = oxygen C = carbon

POINT TO REMEMBER
The base pair sequence is identical in all the DNA of one individual — and different from that of all other individuals.

Unlike DNA, RNA has a single-chain structure. It contains ribose instead of deoxyribose and replaces the base thymine with uracil. RNA transmits genetic information from the cell nucleus to the cytoplasm; in the cytoplasm, it guides protein synthesis from amino acids.

3 Integumentary system

The largest body system, the integumentary system includes the skin and accessory structures (the hair, nails, and sebaceous and sweat glands). The integumentary system covers an area measuring $10\ ^3/_4$ to $21\ ^1/_2$ square feet (1 to 2 m^2) and accounts for about 15% of body weight.

Functions

The integumentary system performs many vital functions, including protection of inner body structures, sensory perception, and regulation of body temperature and blood pressure.

Protection

The skin's top layer protects the body against traumatic injury, noxious chemicals, and bacterial and microorganismal invasion. *Langerhans' cells,* specialized cells in this skin layer, enhance the body's immune response by helping lymphocytes to process antigens entering the skin.

Melanocytes, another type of skin cell, protect the skin by producing the brown pigment *melanin,* which helps filter ultraviolet light (irradiation); exposure to ultraviolet light can stimulate melanin production.

The skin also protects the body by limiting water and electrolyte excretion. It prevents body fluids from escaping while eliminating body wastes through more than 2 million pores.

Sensory perception

Sensory nerve fibers originate in the nerve roots along the spine and supply specific areas of the skin known as *dermatomes.* These nerve fibers carry impulses from the skin to the central nervous system. Autonomic nerve fibers carry impulses to smooth muscle in the walls of the skin's blood vessels, to the muscles around the hair roots, and to the sweat glands.

POINT TO REMEMBER

Through autonomic nerve fibers, the skin transmits various sensations, including temperature, touch, pressure, pain, and itching.

Temperature and blood pressure regulation

Abundant nerves, blood vessels, and eccrine glands within the skin's deeper layer aid *thermoregulation,* or control of body temperature. When the skin is exposed to cold or the internal body temperature falls, blood vessels constrict in response to stimuli from the autonomic nervous system. This leads to a decrease in blood flow through the skin and conservation of body heat. When the skin is too hot or the internal body temperature rises, small arteries in the second skin layer dilate; increased blood flow through these vessels then reduces body heat. If this doesn't adequately lower temperature, the eccrine glands act to increase sweat production and subsequent evaporation cools the skin.

Dermal blood vessels aid regulation of the systemic blood pressure by *vasoconstriction* (constriction of blood vessels). (See *How skin protects during exercise,* page 28.)

How skin protects during exercise

Skin plays an important role during exercise through temperature regulation. Resting body temperatures typically range between 97.7° to 99.5° F (36.5° to 37.5° C). During exercise, body temperature can quickly rise to 104° F (40° C). The skin works to lower body temperature through three mechanisms: blood vessel dilation, which causes radiant heat loss; the excretion and evaporation of sweat; and the conduction and convection of heat directly through the skin.

Vitamin synthesis

When stimulated by ultraviolet light, the skin synthesizes vitamin D_3 (cholecalciferol).

Excretion

The skin is also an excretory organ; the sweat glands excrete sweat, which contains water, electrolytes, urea, and lactic acid.

Maintenance of body surface integrity

The skin maintains the integrity of the body surface by migration and shedding. It can repair surface wounds by intensifying normal cell-replacement mechanisms.

POINT TO REMEMBER

Skin regeneration can't occur if the dermal layer is destroyed.

The sebaceous glands produce *sebum*, a mixture of keratin, fat, and cellulose debris. Combined with sweat, sebum forms a moist, oily, acidic film that's mildly antibacterial and antifungal and that protects the skin surface.

Skin layers

Two distinct layers of skin, the *epidermis* and *dermis,* lie above a third layer of subcutaneous fat (sometimes called the *hypodermis*). (See *Close-up view of the skin.*)

Epidermis

The outermost layer, the epidermis varies in thickness from less than 0.1 mm on the eyelids to more than 1 mm on the palms and soles. It's composed of avascular, stratified, squamous (scaly or platelike) epithelial tissue, which contains several layers — the stratum corneum, stratum lucidum, stratum granulosum, stratum spinosum, and stratum basale.

Stratum corneum

The stratum corneum, the outermost part of the epidermis, consists of tightly arranged layers of cellular membranes and *keratin,* a protein. After mitosis (cell division) occurs in the germinal layer, epithelial cells undergo a series of changes as they travel to the stratum corneum.

Langerhans' cells are interspersed among the keratinized cells below the stratum corneum. Epidermal cells are usually shed from the surface as epidermal dust. Differentiation of cells from the basal layer to the stratum corneum takes up to 28 days.

Stratum basale

Also called the *basal layer,* the stratum basale produces new cells to replace the superficial keratinized cells that are continuously shed or worn away. It also contains melanocytes, which produce and disperse melanin to the surrounding epithelial cells.

Dermis

The skin's second layer, the dermis (also called the *corium*) is an elastic system that contains and supports blood vessels, lymphatic vessels, nerves, and epidermal appendages.

Most of the dermis is made up of extracellular material called *matrix*. Matrix contains connective tissue fibers — collagen, elastin, and reticular fibers. *Collagen,* a protein, gives strength to the dermis; *elastin* makes the skin pliable; and *reticular fibers*

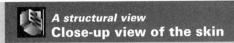

A structural view
Close-up view of the skin

Major components of the skin include the epidermis, dermis, and epidermal appendages.

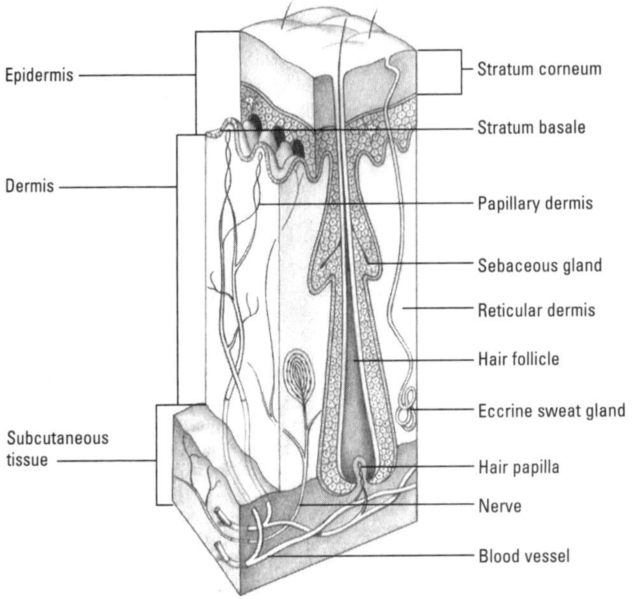

bind the collagen and elastin fibers together.

Matrix and connective tissue fibers are produced by *dermal fibroblasts*, spindle-shaped connective tissue cells that become part of the matrix as it forms. In the papillary dermis, fibers are loosely arranged; in the deeper reticular dermis, they're more tightly packed.

The dermis itself has two layers — the superficial *papillary dermis* and the *reticular dermis*.

Papillary dermis

The papillary dermis has fingerlike projections (*papillae*) that nourish epidermal cells. The epidermis lies over these papillae and bulges downward to fill the spaces. A collagenous membrane called the *basement membrane* separates the epidermis and dermis, holding them together.

Reticular dermis

The reticular dermis covers a layer of subcutaneous tissue (the adipose layer, or *panniculus adiposus*), a specialized layer primarily composed of fat cells. Besides insulating the body to conserve heat, the reticular dermis provides energy and serves as a mechanical shock absorber.

Epidermal appendages

Numerous epidermal appendages occur throughout the skin. They include the hair, nails, sebaceous glands, and two types of sweat glands — eccrine glands (located over most of the body except the lips) and apocrine glands (found under the arms and in the groin near hair follicles).

Hair

The hairs are long, slender shafts composed of keratin. At the expanded lower end of each hair is a bulb or root. On its undersurface, the root is indented by a *hair papilla,* a cluster of connective tissue and blood vessels.

Each hair lies within an epithelial-lined sheath called a *hair follicle.* A bundle of smooth-muscle fibers (*arrector pili*) extends through the dermis to attach to the base of the follicle. When these muscles contract, the hair stands on end. Hair follicles also have a rich blood and nerve supply.

Nails

Situated over the distal surface of the end of each finger and toe, nails are specialized types of keratin. The nail plate, surrounded on three sides by the nail folds (cuticles), lies on the nail bed. The nail plate is formed by the nail matrix, which extends proximally for about 1/4″ (5 mm) beneath the nail fold.

The distal portion of the matrix shows through the nail as a pale crescent-moon-shaped area, called the *lunula*. The translucent *nail plate* distal to the lunula exposes the nail bed. The vascular bed imparts the characteristic pink appearance under the nails.

Sebaceous glands

Sebaceous glands occur on all parts of the skin except the palms and soles. They're most prominent on the scalp, face, upper torso, and genitalia.

Sebaceous glands produce sebum, a lipid substance, and secrete it into the hair follicle through the sebaceous duct. Sebum then exits through the hair follicle opening to reach the skin surface.

POINT TO REMEMBER
Sebum may help to waterproof the hair and skin, may promote the absorption of fat-soluble substances into the dermis, and may be involved in vitamin D_3 production. It may also have an antibacterial function.

Sweat glands

Sweat glands are located throughout the entire skin surface (except the nipples and parts of the external genitalia). There are two types of sweat glands: eccrine and apocrine.

Widely distributed throughout the body, the eccrine glands produce an odorless, watery fluid with a sodium concentration equal to that of plasma. A duct from the coiled secretory portion passes through the dermis and epidermis, opening onto the skin surface.

Eccrine glands in the palms and soles secrete fluid mainly in response to emotional stress such as occurs while taking a test. The remaining 3 million eccrine glands respond primarily to thermal stress, effectively regulating temperature.

Located chiefly in the axillary and anogenital areas, the apocrine glands have a coiled secretory portion that lies deeper in the dermis than that of the eccrine glands. A duct connects an apocrine gland to the upper portion of the hair follicle.

Apocrine glands begin to function at puberty. However, they have no known biological function. As bacteria decompose the fluids produced by these glands, body odor occurs.

Ceruminous glands are modified apocrine glans found in the lining of the external ear canal. They secrete a yellow, waxy substance called *cerumen* or earwax. Cerumen protects the ear from insects and other foreign materials.

4 Musculoskeletal system

The musculoskeletal system consists of the muscles, tendons, ligaments, bones, cartilage, joints, and bursae. These structures work together to produce skeletal movement.

Muscles

The three major types of muscle in the human body are classified by the tissue they contain. *Visceral (involuntary)* muscle contains smooth-muscle tissue, *skeletal (voluntary)* muscle consists of striated tissue, and *cardiac (heart)* muscle is made up of a specialized type of striated tissue.

This chapter discusses only skeletal muscle — the type attached to bone. The human body has about 600 skeletal muscles. Skeletal muscle is voluntary, meaning that its contractions are controlled at will. (See *Viewing the major skeletal muscles,* page 32.)

Muscle functions

Skeletal muscles move body parts or move the body as a whole. Responsible for both voluntary and reflex movements, they also generate body heat and maintain posture (through combined contraction of various skeletal muscles). Energy for muscle contraction comes from *adenosine triphosphate,* an enzyme released from cells.

Muscle structure

Skeletal muscle contains cell groups called muscle fibers, which have many nuclei and transverse striations. Because of these striations, skeletal muscle looks like long bands or strips when viewed through a microscope. (See *Muscle structure,* page 33.)

A sheath of connective tissue called the *perimysium* binds the muscle fibers into a bundle, or *fasciculus*. A stronger sheath, the *epimysium*, binds fasciculi together to form the fleshy part of the muscle.

Each muscle fiber is surrounded by a plasma membrane, the *sarcolemma.* Within the *sarcoplasm* (cytoplasm) of the muscle fiber lie tiny *myofibrils.* Arranged lengthwise, myofibrils contain still finer fibers — about 1,500 *myosin (thick) filaments* and about 3,000 *actin (thin) filaments.* These filaments are stacked in compartments called *sarcomeres,* the functional units of skeletal muscle. During muscle contraction, thin and thick filaments slide over each other, reducing sarcomere length.

Muscle attachment

Most skeletal muscles are attached to bones, either directly or indirectly. In a *direct attachment,* the epimysium of the muscle fuses to the periosteum of the bone. In an *indirect attachment,* the fascia extends past the muscle as a tendon or aponeurosis, which in turn attaches to the bone. In the human body, indirect attachments outnumber direct attachments.

Origin and insertion points

During contraction, one of the bones to which the muscle is attached stays relatively stationary while the other is pulled in the opposite direction. The point where the muscle attaches to the stationary or less movable bone is called the *origin;* where it attaches to

A structural view
Viewing the major skeletal muscles

The name of a skeletal muscle may come from its location, action, size, shape, attachment points, number of divisions, or direction of fibers. This illustration shows anterior and posterior views of some of the major muscles.

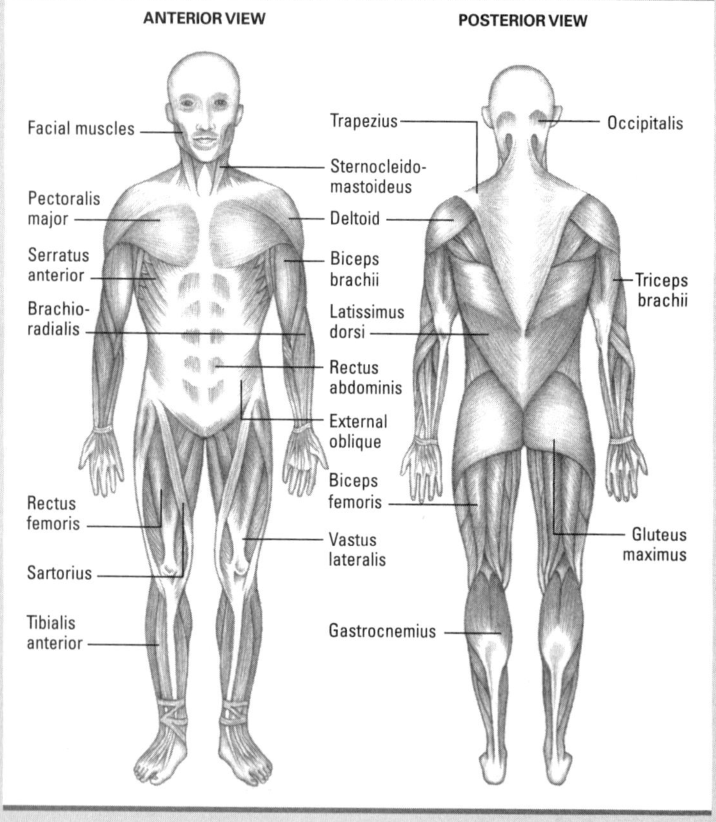

the more movable bone, the *insertion*. The origin usually lies on the proximal end of the bone and the insertion site on the distal end.

Muscle growth

Muscle develops when existing muscle fibers hypertrophy. Because of such factors as exercise, nutrition, gender, and genetic constitution, muscle strength and size vary among individuals. (See *Musculoskeletal system and exercise,* page 34.)

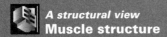

A structural view

Muscle structure

The perimysium—a sheath of connective tissue—binds muscle fibers together. The epimysium binds fasciculi together; beyond the muscle, it becomes a tendon.

A sarcolemma surrounds each muscle fiber. Tiny myofibrils within the muscle fibers contain even finer fibers called thick and thin fibers.

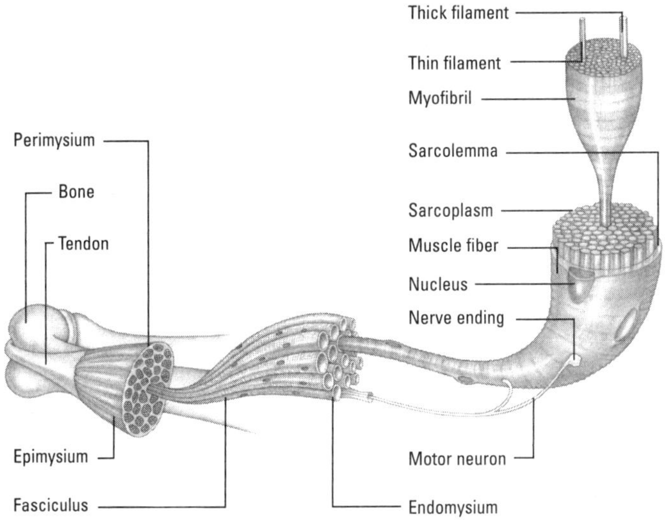

Muscle movements

Types of skeletal muscle movement include:

- *flexion*—decreasing the angle between two adjoining bones
- *extension*—increasing the angle between two adjoining bones
- *abduction*—moving a limb or other part away from the midline of the body
- *adduction*—moving a limb or other part toward the midline of the body
- *circumduction*—moving a limb in a circle (a combination of extension, flexion, abduction, and adduction)
- *internal (medial) rotation*—moving a body part toward the midline
- *external rotation*—moving a body part away from the midline
- *supination*—turning a body part upward
- *pronation*—turning a body part downward
- *inversion*—turning a body part inward
- *eversion*—turning a body part outward
- *retraction and protraction*—moving a body part backward and forward.

(See *Basics of body movement*, page 35.)

A muscle's functional name comes from the type of movement it permits. For example, a flexor muscle permits flexion, an adductor muscle permits adduction, and a circumductor muscle allows circumduction.

Musculoskeletal system and exercise

The musculoskeletal system undergoes different changes during different exercises. Aerobic exercise, also known as endurance exercise, causes the number of blood vessels in a muscle to increase, resulting in increased blood flow to the muscle. This increased blood flow efficiently delivers oxygen and glucose to the muscle fibers. The number of mitochondria in the muscle fibers also increases, allowing the production of adenosine triphosphate as a rapid energy source.

Strengthening exercises, such as isometric exercise and weight lifting, cause an increase in muscle size known as hypertrophy. Hypertrophy results as the number of myofilaments in each muscle fiber increases, resulting in increased muscle mass.

Bones are also affected by exercise. Scientists believe that when the bone is stressed by exercise, changes occur in the bone that stimulates the activity of bone-forming cells, leading to a buildup of calcium, which in turn leads to increased bone mass. The extent of increase in bone mass depends on the frequency and magnitude of exercise.

Muscles of the axial and appendicular skeleton

The *axial skeleton* includes the muscles of the head and neck, the vertebral column, and the thoracic muscles responsible for respiration. The muscles of the head and neck include those of the face, tongue, and neck and those of mastication.

Muscles of the vertebral column, situated along the spine, move the vertebral column. Muscles of the thorax promote movements necessary for breathing.

The *appendicular skeleton* includes the muscles of the shoulder, abdominopelvic cavity, and upper and lower extremities. Muscles of the upper extremities are classified according to the bones they move; those that move the arm are further categorized into those with an origin on the axial skeleton and those with an origin on the scapula. (See *Guide to skeletal muscles,* pages 36 to 48.)

Tendons

Tendons are bands of fibrous connective tissue that attach muscles to the *periosteum*, a fibrous membrane covering the bone. Tendons enable bones to move when skeletal muscles contract.

Ligaments

Ligaments are dense, strong, flexible bands of fibrous connective tissue that bind bones to other bones.

POINT TO REMEMBER

In patient care settings, the ligaments of greatest concern are those that connect the joint (articular) ends of bones. These ligaments either limit or promote movement; they also provide stability.

Bones

The human skeleton contains 206 bones: 80 form the axial skeleton and 126 form the appendicular skeleton. Bones of the axial skeleton include the facial and cranial bones, hyoid bone, vertebrae, ribs, and sternum. Bones of the appendicular skeleton include the clavicle, scapula, humerus, radius, ulna, metacarpals, pelvic bone, femur, patella, fibula, tibia, and metatarsals. (See *Viewing the major bones,* page 50.)

Bone classification

Bones are typically classified by shape. Thus, bones may be *long* (such as the humerus, radius, femur, and tibia), *short* (such as the carpals and tarsals), *flat* (such as the scapula, ribs, and skull), *irregular* (such as the vertebrae

(Text continues on page 49.)

Basics of body movement

Diarthrodial joints allow 13 angular and circular movements. The shoulder demonstrates circumduction; the elbow, flexion and extension; the hip, internal and external rotation; the arm, abduction and adduction; the hand, supination and pronation; the foot, eversion and inversion; and the jaw, retraction and protraction.

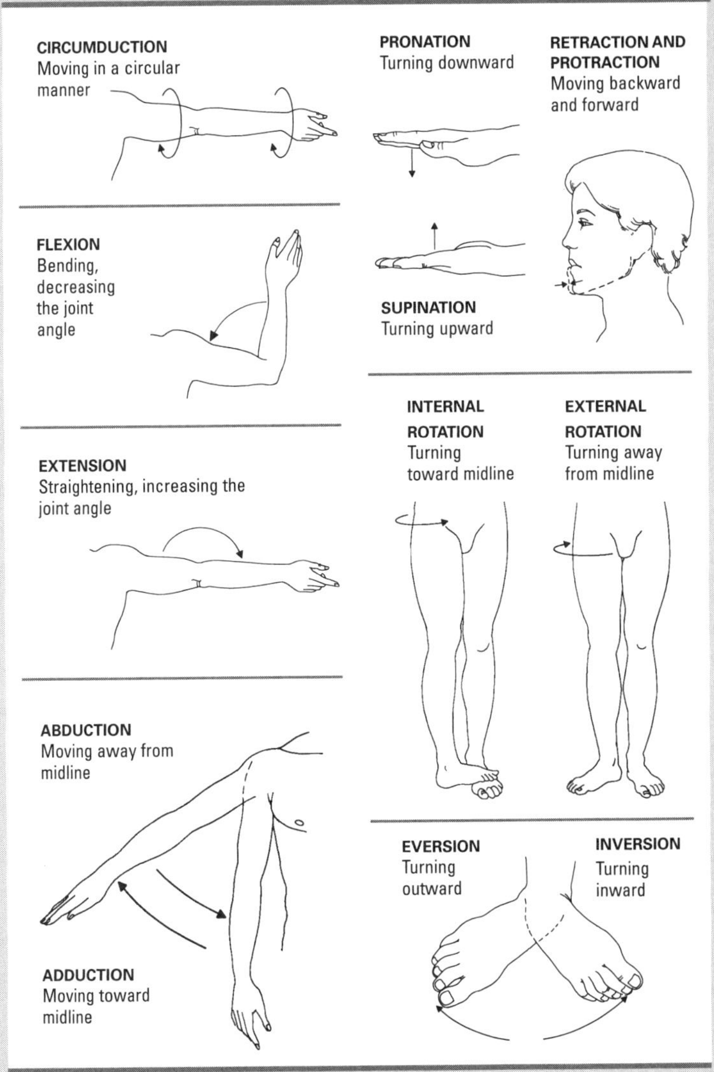

Guide to skeletal muscles

Muscle	Origin	Insertion
Muscles of the head and neck		
Muscles of the face		
Buccinator	▸ Mandible (alveolar process) ▸ Maxillary bone	▸ Orbicularis oris ▸ Skin at mouth angle
Corrugator supercilii	▸ Frontal bone	▸ Skin of eyebrows
Depressor anguli oris	▸ Mandible (below mental foramen)	▸ Skin and muscles at mouth angle
Depressor labii inferioris	▸ Mandible (between symphysis and mental foramen)	▸ Skin and muscles of lower lip
Epicranius frontalis	▸ Aponeurotic structure of scalp	▸ Skin and muscles of forehead
Epicranius occipitalis	▸ Occipital bone	▸ Aponeurotic structure of scalp
Levator labii superioris	▸ Eye orbit (lower margin)	▸ Skin and muscles of upper lip ▸ Wing of nose
Mentalis	▸ Mandible (near symphysis)	▸ Skin of chin
Orbicularis oculi	▸ Frontal and maxillary bones ▸ Medial palpebral ligament	▸ Skin around eye and eyelids
Orbicularis oris	▸ Muscles surrounding mouth	▸ Skin surrounding mouth
Platysma	▸ Fascia over pectoralis major and deltoid muscles	▸ Mandible (lower border) ▸ Skin of cheek and neck
Procerus	▸ Nasal bone (lower portion) ▸ Lateral nasal cartilage (upper part)	▸ Skin between eye brows

Guide to skeletal muscles *(continued)*

Muscle	Origin	Insertion
Muscles of the face *(continued)*		
Risorius	▸ Fascia of masseter muscle	▸ Skin at mouth angle
Zygomaticus major	▸ Zygomatic bone	▸ Skin and muscles above mouth angle
Zygomaticus minor	▸ Zygomatic bone	▸ Skin and muscles above mouth angle
Muscles of mastication		
Temporalis	▸ Temporal fossa	▸ Mandible (coronoid process and ramus)
Masseter	▸ Zygomatic arch	▸ Mandible (angle and ramus)
Medial pterygoid	▸ Sphenoid bone (lateral pterygoid plate)	▸ Mandible (inner surface)
Lateral pterygoid	▸ Lateral pterygoid plate (lateral surface) ▸ Sphenoid bone (great wing)	▸ Mandible (just below condyle)
Extrinsic muscles of the tongue		
Genioglossus	▸ Mandible (internal surface)	▸ Near symphysis
Hyoglossus	▸ Hyoid bone (body and greater projection)	▸ Tongue (sides)
Styloglossus	▸ Temporal bone (styloid process)	▸ Tongue (sides)
Muscles of the neck		
Sternocleidomastoid	▸ Sternum (manubrium) ▸ Clavicle (medial portion)	▸ Temporal bone (mastoid process)
Digastric	▸ Mandible (lower border) ▸ Temporal bone (mastoid notch)	▸ Intermediate tendon on hyoid bone
Stylohyoid	▸ Temporal bone (styloid process)	▸ Hyoid bone
Mylohyoid	▸ Mandible (inner surface, from symphysis to angle)	▸ Hyoid bone

(continued)

Guide to skeletal muscles *(continued)*

Muscle	Origin	Insertion
Muscles of the neck *(continued)*		
Geniohyoid	▸ Mandibular symphysis (inner surface)	▸ Hyoid bone
Sternohyoid	▸ Sternum (manubrium) and clavicle (medial end)	▸ Hyoid bone
Sternothyroid	▸ Manubrium	▸ Larynx (thyroid cartilage)
Thyrohyoid	▸ Larynx (thyroid cartilage)	▸ Hyoid bone
Omohyoid	▸ Scapula (superior border)	▸ Hyoid bone
Muscles of the vertebral column		
Semispinalis thoracis Semispinalis cervicis Semispinalis capitis	▸ Vertebrae (transverse processes of all thoracic and seventh cervical)	▸ Vertebrae (spinous processes of second cervical through fourth thoracic) ▸ Occipital bone
Multifidi	▸ Ilium and sacrum (posterior surface) ▸ Vertebrae (transverse processes of lumbar, thoracic, and lower cervical)	▸ Vertebrae (spinous processes of lumbar, thoracic, and cervical)
Rotatores	▸ Vertebrae (transverse processes)	▸ Next superior vertebra (base of spinous process)
Interspinales	▸ Vertebrae (superior surfaces of all spinous processes)	▸ Next superior vertebra (inferior surface of spinous process)
Scalene muscles	▸ Cervical vertebrae (transverse processes)	▸ Ribs (first and second)
Intertransversarii	▸ Vertebrae (transverse processes)	▸ Next superior vertebra (transverse process)
Splenius capitis Splenius cervicis	▸ Vertebrae (spinous processes of upper thoracic and seventh cervical, from ligamentum nuchae)	▸ Occipital bone ▸ Temporal bone (mastoid process) ▸ Vertebrae (tranverse processes of upper three cervical)

Guide to skeletal muscles *(continued)*

Muscle	Origin	Insertion
Erector spine group		
Iliocostalis lumborum Iliocostalis thoracis Iliocostalis cervicis	▸ Sacrum (crest) ▸ Vertebrae (spinous processes of lumbar and lower thoracic) ▸ Iliac crests ▸ Rib angles	▸ Rib angles ▸ Vertebrae (transverse processes of cervical)
Longissimus thoracis Longissimus cervicis Longissimus capitis	▸ Vertebrae (transverse processes of lumbar, thoracic, and lower cervical)	▸ Next superior vertebra (transverse process) ▸ Temporal bone (mastoid process)
Spinalis thoracis Spinalis cervicis	▸ Vertebrae (spinous process of upper lumbar, lower thoracic and seventh cervical)	▸ Vertebrae (spinous processes of upper thoracic, and cervical)
Muscles of respiration		
Diaphragm	▸ Rib cage (inferior border) ▸ Xiphoid process ▸ Costal cartilages ▸ Vertebrae (lumbar)	▸ Central tendon of diaphragm
External intercostal muscles	▸ Ribs (inferior border) ▸ Costal cartilages	▸ Next inferior rib (superior border)
Internal intercostal muscles	▸ Ribs (inner surface) ▸ Costal cartilages	▸ Next inferior rib (superior border)
Subcostales	▸ Ribs (inner surface, near angles)	▸ Second or third inferior rib (inner surface)
Transversus thoracis	▸ Sternum (inner surface) ▸ Xiphoid process	▸ Costal cartilages (inner surface)
Muscles of the shoulder		
Trapezius	▸ Occipital bone ▸ Ligamentum nuchae ▸ Vertebrae (spinous processes of seventh cervical and all thoracic)	▸ Clavicle (lateral third) ▸ Acromion process ▸ Scapula (spine)
Rhomboideus major	▸ Vertebrae (spinous processes of second through fifth thoracic)	▸ Scapula (vertebral border, below spine)

(continued)

Guide to skeletal muscles *(continued)*

Muscle	Origin	Insertion
Muscles of the shoulder *(continued)*		
Rhomboideus minor	▸ Vertebrae (spinous processes of seventh cervical and first thoracic)	▸ Scapula (vertebral border, at base of spine)
Levator scapulae	▸ Vertebrae (transverse processes of upper four cervical)	▸ Scapula (vertebral border, above spine)
Pectoralis minor	▸ Ribs (anterior surface of third through fifth)	▸ Scapula (coracoid process)
Serratus anterior	▸ Ribs (outer surface of first nine)	▸ Scapula (ventral surface of vertebral border)
Subclavius	▸ Rib (outer surface of first rib)	▸ Clavicle (inferior surface of lateral portion)
Muscles of the abdominopelvic cavity		
Muscles that move the abdominal wall		
External abdominal oblique	▸ Ribs (external surface of lower eight)	▸ Iliac crest (anterior half) ▸ Linea alba ▸ Pubic tubercle
Internal abdominal oblique	▸ Inguinal ligament ▸ Iliac crest ▸ Lumbodorsal fascia	▸ Linea alba ▸ Pubic crest ▸ Ribs (lower four)
Transversus abdominis	▸ Inguinal ligament ▸ Iliac crest ▸ Lumbodorsal fascia ▸ Ribs (costal cartilages of last six)	▸ Linea alba ▸ Pubic crest
Rectus abdominis	▸ Pubic crest	▸ Xiphoid process ▸ Ribs (costal cartilages of fifth through seventh)
Quadratus lumborum	▸ Iliac crest ▸ Iliolumbar ligament	▸ Rib (lower border of twelfth) ▸ Vertebrae (transverse processes of upper lumbar)

Guide to skeletal muscles *(continued)*

Muscle	Origin	Insertion
Muscles of the pelvic floor		
Levator ani	▸ Pubic bone (inner surface of superior ramus) ▸ Lateral pelvic wall ▸ Ischium (spine)	▸ Coccyx (inner surface)
Coccygeus	▸ Ischium (spine) ▸ Sacrospinous ligament	▸ Coccyx ▸ Sacrum
Muscles of the upper extremities		
Muscles that move the arm		
Pectoralis major	▸ Clavicle (medial half) ▸ Sternum ▸ Ribs (costal cartilages of upper six) ▸ External oblique (aponeurosis)	▸ Humerus (greater tubercle)
Latissimus dorsi	▸ Vertebrae (spinous processes of lower six thoracic and all lumbar) ▸ Sacrum ▸ Ilium (posterior crest)	▸ Humerus (medial margin of intertubercular groove)
Deltoid	▸ Clavicle (lateral third) ▸ Acromion process ▸ Scapula (spine)	▸ Humerus (deltoid tubercle)
Supraspinatus	▸ Scapula (supraspinatus fossa)	▸ Humerus (greater tubercle)
Infraspinatus	▸ Scapula (infraspinatus fossa)	▸ Humerus (greater tubercle)
Subscapularis	▸ Scapula (subscapular fossa)	▸ Humerus (lesser tubercle)
Teres major	▸ Scapula (dorsal surface of inferior angle)	▸ Humerus (lesser tubercle)
Teres minor	▸ Scapula (axillary border)	▸ Humerus (greater tubercle)
Coracobrachialis	▸ Scapula (coracoid process)	▸ Humerus (medial surface of medial third)

(continued)

Guide to skeletal muscles *(continued)*

Muscle	Origin	Insertion
Muscles that move the forearm		
Biceps brachii	▸ Long head: scapula (supraglenoid tubercle) ▸ Short head: scapula (coracoid process)	▸ Radius (tubercle)
Brachialis	▸ Humerus (anterior surface of distal half)	▸ Ulna (coronoid process)
Triceps brachii	▸ Long head: scapula (infraglenoid tubercle) ▸ Lateral head: humerus (posterior surface, above radial groove) ▸ Medial head: humerus (posterior surface, below radial groove)	▸ Ulna (olecranon process)
Anconeus	▸ Humerus (lateral epicondyle)	▸ Ulna (lateral surface, olecranon process)
Brachioradialis	▸ Humerus (lateral supracondylar ridge)	▸ Radius (styloid process)
Muscles that move the wrist, hand, and fingers		
Anterior superficial muscles		
Pronator teres	▸ Humerus (medial epicondyle) ▸ Ulna (coronoid process)	▸ Radius (shaft, middle of lateral surface)
Flexor carpi radialis	▸ Humerus (medial epicondyle)	▸ Second and third metacarpals (ventral surface)
Palmaris longus	▸ Humerus (medial epicondyle)	▸ Palmar aponeurosis
Flexor carpi ulnaris	▸ Humerus (medial epicondyle) ▸ Olecranon process ▸ Ulna (posterior surface of proximal two-thirds)	▸ Fifth metacarpal ▸ Pisiform
Flexor digitorum superficialis	▸ Humerus (medial eipcondyle) ▸ Ulna coronoid process ▸ Radius (anterior surface)	▸ Second through fifth fingers (ventral surface of middle phalanges)

Guide to skeletal muscles *(continued)*

Muscle	Origin	Insertion
Anterior deep muscles		
Flexor digitorum profundus	▸ Interosseous membrane ▸ Ulna (upper three-fourths of shaft)	▸ Second through fifth fingers (distal, phalanges, ventral surface of base)
Flexor pollicis longus	▸ Radius (ventral surface) ▸ Interosseous membrane	▸ Thumb (distal phalange, ventral surface of base)
Pronator quadratus	▸ Ulna (distal ventral surface)	▸ Radius (distal ventral surface)
Posterior superficial muscles		
Extensor carpi radialis longus	▸ Humerus (lateral supracondylar ridge)	▸ Second metacarpal (dorsal surface of base)
Extensor carpi radialis brevis	▸ Humerus (lateral epicondyle)	▸ Third metacarpal (dorsal surface of base)
Extensor digitorum communis	▸ Humerus (lateral epicondyle)	▸ Second through fifth fingers (dorsal surface of phalanges)
Extensor digiti minimi	▸ Tendon of extensor digitorum communis	▸ Fifth finger (tendon of extensor digitorum communis, on dorsum)
Extensor carpi ulnaris	▸ Humerus (lateral epicondyle)	▸ Fifth metacarpal (base)
Posterior deep muscles		
Supinator	▸ Humerus (lateral epicondyle)	▸ Radius (proximal end, lateral surface of shaft)
Abductor pollicis longus	▸ Radius and ulna (posterior surface of middle portions) ▸ Interosseous membrane	▸ First metacarpal (base)
Extensor pollicis brevis	▸ Radius (posterior surface of middle portion) ▸ Interosseous membrane	▸ Thumb (base of first phalange)

(continued)

Guide to skeletal muscles *(continued)*

Muscle	Origin	Insertion
Posterior deep muscles *(continued)*		
Extensor pollicis longus	▸ Ulna (posterior surface of middle portion) ▸ Interosseous membrane	▸ Thumb (base of last phalange)
Extensor indicis	▸ Ulna (posterior surface of distal end) ▸ Interosseous membrane	▸ Second finger (tendon of extensor digitorum communis)
Intrinsic muscles of the hand		
Abductor pollicis brevis	▸ Flexor retinaculum ▸ Scaphoid ▸ Trapezium	▸ Thumb (proximal phalange)
Opponens pollicis	▸ Flexor retinaculum ▸ Trapezium	▸ Thumb (metacarpal, lower border)
Flexor pollicis brevis	▸ Flexor retinaculum ▸ Trapezium ▸ First metacarpal	▸ Thumb (base of proximal phalange)
Palmaris brevis	▸ Flexor retinaculum	▸ Hand (skin on ulnar border)
Adductor pollicis	▸ Capitate ▸ Second and third metacarpals	▸ Thumb (inner side of base of first phalange)
Abductor digiti minimi	▸ Pisiform ▸ Flexor carpi ulnaris (tendon)	▸ Fifth finger (base of proximal phalange)
Flexor digiti minimi brevis	▸ Flexor retinaculum ▸ Hamate	▸ Fifth finger (base of proximal phalange)
Opponens digiti minimi	▸ Flexor retinaculum ▸ Hamate	▸ Fifth finger (metacarpal)
Lumbricales	▸ Tendons of flexor digitorum profundus	▸ Tendons of extensor digitorum communis
Dorsal interossei	▸ Metacarpals (adjacent sides)	▸ Second through fourth fingers (proximal phalange)
Palmar interossei	▸ Second metacarpal (medial side) ▸ Fourth and fifth metacarpals (lateral side)	▸ Same finger (proximal phalange)

Guide to skeletal muscles *(continued)*

Muscle	Origin	Insertion
Muscles of the lower extremities		
Muscles that move the femur (thigh)		
Iliopsoas	▸ Psoas major vertebrae (transverse processes and bodies of last thoracic and all lumbar) ▸ Iliacus: iliac crest and fossa	▸ Femur (lesser trochanter)
Gluteus maximus	▸ Ilium (posterior gluteal line) ▸ Sacrum and coccyx (posterior surfaces)	▸ Femur (gluteal tubercle) ▸ Iliotibial band
Gluteus medius	▸ Ilium (outer surface, between posterior and anterior gluteal lines)	▸ Femur (lateral surface of greater trochanter)
Gluteus minimus	▸ Ilium (outer surface, between anterior and inferior gluteal lines)	▸ Femur (anterior surface of greater trochanter)
Tensor fasciae latae	▸ Iliac crest (anterior portion) ▸ Anterior superior iliac spine	▸ Fascia latae (iliotibial band)
Piriformis	▸ Sacrum (anterior surface)	▸ Femur (superior border of greater trochanter)
Obturator internus	▸ Obturator membrane (inner surface) ▸ Obturator foramen (bony margins)	▸ Femur (trochanteric fossa)
Obturator externus	▸ Obturator membrane (outer surface) ▸ Obturator foramen (bony margins)	▸ Femur (trochanteric fossa)
Gemellus superior	▸ Ischial spine	▸ Femur (greater trochanter)
Gemellus inferior	▸ Ischial tubercle	▸ Femur (greater trochanter)
Quadratus femoris	▸ Ischial tubercle	▸ Femur (shaft, just below greater trochanter)

(continued)

Guide to skeletal muscles *(continued)*

Muscle	Origin	Insertion
Muscles that move the femur (thigh) *(continued)*		
Adductor magnus	▸ Pubis and ischium (inferior rami) ▸ Ischial tubercle	▸ Femur (linea aspera, adductor tubercle)
Adductor longus	▸ Pubis (crest and symphysis)	▸ Femur (linea aspera)
Adductor brevis	▸ Pubis (inferior ramus)	▸ Femur (linea aspera)
Pectineus	▸ Pubis (superior ramus)	▸ Femur (posterior surface, just below lesser trochanter
Gracilis	▸ Symphysis pubis ▸ Pubic arch	▸ Tibia (medial surface, just below condyle)
Anterior compartment		
Sartorius	▸ Anterior superior iliac spine	▸ Tibia (proximal medial surface, below tubercle)
Quadriceps femoris	▸ Rectus femoris: ilium (anterior inferior spine) ▸ Vastus lateralis: femur (linea aspera, greater trochanter) ▸ Vastus medialis: femur (linea aspera) ▸ Vastus intermedias: femur (anterior surface of shaft)	▸ Tibia (via patella and patellar ligament)
Hamstring group		
Biceps femoris	▸ Long head: ischial tubercle ▸ Short head: linea aspera	▸ Fibula (lateral surface of head) ▸ Tibia (lateral condyle)
Semitendinosus	▸ Ischial tubercle	▸ Tibia (medial surface of proximal end)
Semimembranosus	▸ Ischial tubercle	▸ Tibia (medial surface of proximal end)

Guide to skeletal muscles *(continued)*

Muscle	Origin	Insertion
Muscles that move the foot and toes		
Anterior compartment		
Tibialis anterior	▸ Tibia (lateral condyle, proximal two-thirds of shaft) ▸ Interosseous membrane	▸ Tarsal (first cuneiform) ▸ Metatarsal (first)
Extensor hallucis longus	▸ Fibula (anterior surface of middle portion) ▸ Interosseous membrane	▸ Great toe (dorsal surface of distal phalange)
Extensor digitorum longus	▸ Tibia (lateral condyle) ▸ Fibula (proximal three-fourths of anterior surface) ▸ Interosseous membrane	▸ Second through fifth toes (dorsal surface of phalanges)
Peroneus tertius	▸ Fibula (distal one-third of anterior surface) ▸ Interosseous membrane	▸ Fifth metatarsal (dorsal surface)
Lateral compartment		
Peroneus longus	▸ Fibula (proximal two-thirds of lateral surface)	▸ First metatarsal ▸ Medial cuneiform
Peroneus brevis	▸ Fibula (distal two-thirds)	▸ Fifth metatarsal (lateral side)
Posterior compartment		
Gastrocnemius	▸ Femur (medial and lateral condyles	▸ Calcaneus (via Achilles tendon)
Soleus	▸ Fibula (posterior surface of proximal one-third) ▸ Tibia (middle one-third)	▸ Calcaneus (via Achilles tendon)
Plantaris	▸ Femur (lower surface, above lateral condyle)	▸ Calcaneus (via Achilles tendon)
Popliteus	▸ Femur (lateral condyle)	▸ Tibia (proximal portion)
Flexor hallucis longus	▸ Fibula (lower two-thirds)	▸ Great toe (distal phalange)
Flexor digitorum longus	▸ Tibia (posterior surface)	▸ Second through fifth toes (distal phalanges)

(continued)

Guide to skeletal muscles *(continued)*

Muscle	Origin	Insertion
Posterior compartment *(continued)*		
Tibialis posterior	▸ Tibia (posterior surface) ▸ Fibula (posterior surface) ▸ Interosseous membrane (posterior surface)	▸ Navicular bone ▸ All three cuneiforms ▸ Cuboid bone ▸ Second through fourth metatarsals
Intrinsic muscles of the foot		
Dorsal muscle		
Extensor digitorum brevis	▸ Calcaneus (lateral surface)	▸ Tendon of extensor digitorum longus
Plantar muscles		
Abductor hallucis	▸ Calcaneus	▸ Great toe (proximal phalange), with tendon of flexor hallucis brevis
Flexor digitorum brevis	▸ Calcaneus ▸ Plantar aponeurosis	▸ Second through fifth toes (middle phlanges)
Abductor digiti minimi	▸ Calcaneus ▸ Plantar aponeurosis	▸ Fifth toe (proximal phalanges)
Quadratus plantae	▸ Calcaneus	▸ Into tendons of flexor digitorum longus
Lumbricales	▸ From tendons of flexor digitorum longus	▸ Into tendons of extensor digitorum longus
Flexor hallucis brevis	▸ Cuboid bone ▸ Lateral cuneiform	▸ Great toe (proximal phalange)
Adductor hallucis	▸ Oblique head: second, third, and fourth metatarsals ▸ Transverse head: ligaments of metatarsophalangeal joints	▸ Great toe (proximal phalange)
Flexor digiti minimi brevis	▸ Fifth metatarsal	▸ Fifth toe (proximal phalange)
Plantar interossei	▸ Third through fifth metatarsals	▸ Same toe (proximal phalange)
Dorsal interossei	▸ Adjacent metatarsal (bases) ▸ Second toe (both sides) ▸ Third and fourth toes (lateral side)	▸ Proximal phalanges

and mandible), or *sesamoid* (such as the patella).

Bone functions

Bones perform various anatomic (mechanical) and physiologic functions:

- They protect internal tissues and organs; for example, the 33 vertebrae surround and protect the spinal cord.
- They stabilize and support the body.
- They provide a surface for muscle, ligament, and tendon attachment.
- They move through "lever" action when contracted.
- They produce red blood cells in the bone marrow (a process called *hematopoiesis*).
- They store mineral salts — for example, approximately 99% of the body's calcium.

Bone structure

Bone consists of layers of calcified *matrix* containing spaces occupied by *osteocytes* (bone cells). Bone layers (*lamellae*) are arranged around central canals (*haversian canals*). Small cavities called *lacunae,* which lie between the lamellae, contain osteocytes. Tiny canals (*canaliculi*) connect the lacunae, forming the structural units of the bone. Canaliculi also provide nutrients to bone tissue.

A typical long bone has a *diaphysis* (main shaft) and an *epiphysis* (end). The epiphyses are separated from the diaphysis with cartilage at the *epiphyseal line.* Articular cartilage, which cushions the joint, lies beneath the epiphyseal articular surface.

The *periosteum,* a tough fibrous membrane sheath, surrounds the diaphysis. It consists of an outer fibrous layer and an inner bone-forming layer. In children, the periosteum is thicker than in adults and has an increased blood supply to assist new bone formation around the shaft. The *endosteum,* a thin layer of cells, lines the medullary cavity — the inner surface of bone that contains the marrow. (See *Structure of a long bone,* page 51.)

Types of bone tissue

Each bone consists of an outer layer of dense, smooth *compact bone,* which contains haversian systems (made up of lamellae, lacunae, canaliculi, and a haversian canal), and an inner layer of spongy *cancellous* bone, which lacks these systems. Cancellous bone consists of thin plates called *trabeculae* that interlace to form a latticework. Red marrow fills the spaces between the trabeculae of some bones.

Compact bone is found in the diaphyses of long bones and the outer layers of short, flat, and irregular bones. Cancellous bone fills the central regions of the epiphyses and the inner portions of short, flat, and irregular bones.

Blood supply

Blood reaches bone by way of arterioles in haversian canals; through vessels in Volkmann's canals, which enter bone matrix from the periosteum; and through vessels in the bone ends and within the marrow.

Bone formation

Cartilage composes the fetal skeleton at 3 months in utero. By about 6 months, the fetal cartilage has been transformed into bony skeleton. After birth, some bones — most notably the carpals and tarsals — harden (ossify). The change results from *endochondral ossification,* a process by which *osteoblasts* (bone-forming cells) produce *osteoid,* a collagenous material that ossifies.

Bone remodeling

Two types of osteocytes, osteoblasts and *osteoclasts,* are responsible for remodeling — the continuous process whereby bone is created and destroyed. Osteoblasts deposit new bone, while osteoclasts increase long-bone diameter through reabsorption of previously deposited bone. These activities promote longitudinal bone growth, which continues until the *epiphyseal growth plates,* located at the bone ends, close during adolescence.

A person's age, race, and gender affect bone mass, structural integrity

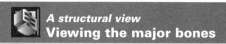

A structural view
Viewing the major bones

These illustrations show anterior and posterior views of some of the major bones.

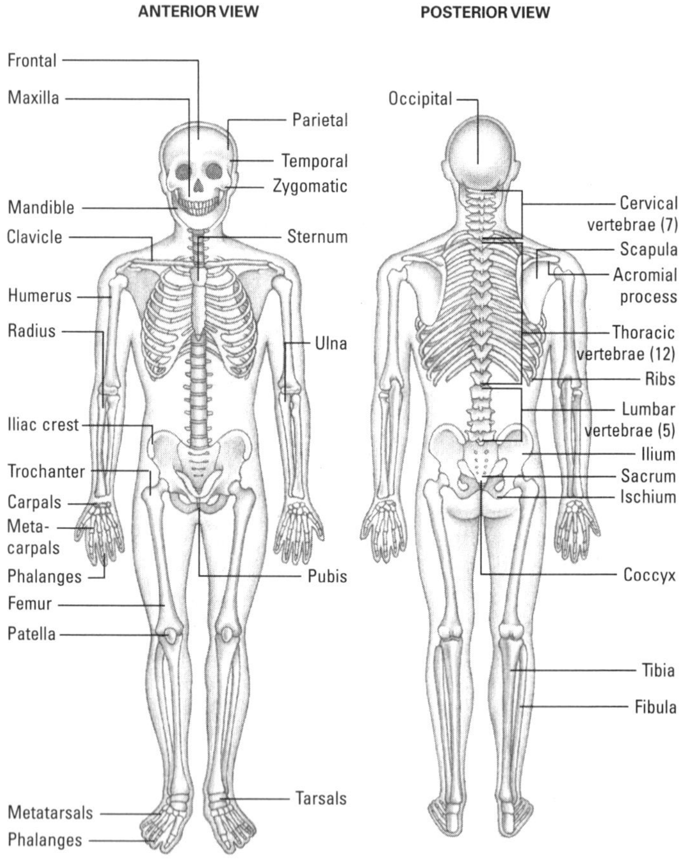

(ability to withstand stress), and bone loss. For example, blacks commonly have denser bones than whites, and men commonly have denser bones than women.

POINT TO REMEMBER
Bone density and structural integrity decrease after age 30 in women and after age 45 in men. Thereafter, a relatively steady quantitative loss of bone matrix occurs.

Cartilage

Cartilage is a dense connective tissue that consists of fibers embedded in a strong, gel-like substance. Unlike rigid bone, cartilage has the flexibility of firm plastic.

Cartilage supports and shapes various structures, such as the auditory canal and the intervertebral disks. It also cushions and absorbs shock, preventing direct transmission to the bone. Cartilage has no blood supply or innervation.

Types of cartilage

Cartilage may be fibrous, hyaline, or elastic. *Fibrous* cartilage forms the symphysis pubis and the intervertebral disks. *Hyaline* cartilage covers the articular bone surfaces (where one or more bones meet at a joint), connects the ribs to the sternum, and appears in the trachea, bronchi, and nasal septum. *Elastic* cartilage is located in the auditory canal, external ear, and epiglottis.

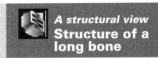

A structural view

Structure of a long bone

The main parts of a long bone are the diaphysis (shaft) and the epiphyses (ends). Periosteum surrounds the diaphysis; endosteum lines the medullary cavity. At the epiphyseal line, cartilage separates the epiphyses from the diaphysis.

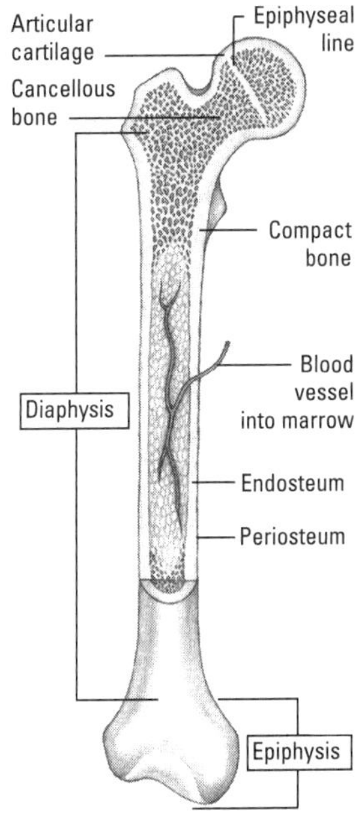

Joints

Joints (articulations) are points of contact between two bones that hold the bones together. Many joints also allow flexibility and movement.

Joints can be classified by function (extent of movement) or by structure (what they're made of). The body has three major types of joints classified by function and three major types classified by structure.

Functional classification

By function, a joint may be classified as *synarthrosis* (immovable), an *amphiarthrosis* (slightly movable), or a *diarthrosis* (freely movable).

Structural classification

By structure, a joint may be classified as fibrous, cartilaginous, or synovial.

Fibrous joints

In fibrous joints, the articular surfaces of the two bones are bound closely by fibrous connective tissue, and little movement is possible. Fibrous joints include *sutures, syndesmoses* (such as the radioulnar joints), and *gomphoses* (such as the dental alveoli).

Cartilaginous joints

In cartilaginous joints (also called *amphiarthroses)*, cartilage connects one bone to another. Cartilaginous joints allow slight movement. They occur in two types:

- *synchondroses* — typically, temporary joints in which the intervening hyaline cartilage converts to bone by adulthood (examples include the epiphyseal plates of long bones)
- *symphyses* — joints with an intervening pad of fibrocartilage (an example is the symphysis pubis).

Synovial joints

Contiguous bony surfaces in the synovial joints are covered by articular cartilage and joined by ligaments lined with synovial membrane. Freely movable, synovial joints include most joints of the arms and legs.

Other features of synovial joints include:

- *joint cavity* — a potential space that separates the articulating surfaces of the two bones
- *articular capsule* — a saclike envelope whose outer layer is lined with a vascular synovial membrane
- *synovial fluid* — a viscid fluid, produced by the synovial membrane, that lubricates the joint
- reinforcing ligaments consisting of fibrous connective tissue, which connect bones within the joint and reinforce the joint capsule.

Based on their structure and the type of movement they allow, synovial joints fall into various subdivisions — gliding, hinge, pivot, condylar, saddle, and ball-and-socket.

Gliding joints

Gliding joints, which have flat or slightly curved articular surfaces, allow gliding movements. However, because they're bound by ligaments, they may not allow movement in all directions. Examples of gliding joints are the intertarsal and intercarpal joints of the hands and feet.

Hinge joints

In hinge joints, a convex portion of one bone fits into a concave portion of another. The movement of a hinge joint resembles that of a metal hinge and is limited to flexion and extension. Hinge joints include the elbow and knee.

Pivot joints

A rounded portion of one bone in a pivot joint fits into a groove in another bone. Pivot joints allow only uniaxial rotation of the first bone around the second. An example of a pivot joint is the head of the radius, which rotates within a groove of the ulna.

Condylar joints

In condylar joints, an oval surface of one bone fits into a concavity in another bone. Condylar joints allow flexion, extension, abduction, adduction, and circumduction. Examples include the radiocarpal and metacarpophalangeal joints of the hand.

Saddle joints

Saddle joints resemble condylar joints but allow greater freedom of movement. The only saddle joints in the body are the carpometacarpal joints of the thumb.

Ball-and-socket joints

The ball-and-socket joint gets its name from the way its bones connect: The spherical head of one bone fits into a concave "socket" of another bone.

POINT TO REMEMBER

The body's only ball-and-socket joints are the shoulder and hip joints. These joints allow more freedom of movement than any other synovial joints.

Bursae

Bursae are small synovial fluid sacs located at friction points around joints between tendons, ligaments, and bones. Acting as cushions, bursae decrease stress on adjacent structures. Examples of bursae include the subacromial bursa (located in the shoulder) and the prepatellar bursa (located in the knee).

How the body moves

The various parts of the musculoskeletal system work with the nervous system to produce voluntary movements. Muscles contract when stimulated by impulses from the nervous system. During contraction, the muscle shortens, pulling on the bones to which it's attached. Force is applied to the tendon; then one bone is pulled toward, moved away from, or rotated around a second bone, depending on the type of muscle that has contracted. Most movement involves groups of muscles rather than one muscle.

5 Nervous system

The nervous system coordinates all body functions, enabling a person to adapt to changes in internal and external environments. It has two main types of cells — neurons and neuroglia — and two main divisions — central nervous system (CNS) and peripheral nervous system.

Cells of the nervous system

The nervous system is packed with densely intertwined cells.

Neurons

The conducting cells of the nervous system, *neurons* detect and transmit stimuli by means of electromechanical messages. These highly specialized cells don't reproduce themselves.

The main parts of a neuron are the *cell body* and its cytoplasmic processes — *axons* and *dendrites*. In a typical neuron, one axon and many dendrites extend from the cell body. (See *Parts of a neuron.*) The axon conducts nerve impulses away from the cell body; dendrites conduct impulses toward the cell body.

The axon may vary from quite short to very long — up to 3¼′ (1 m). A typical axon has terminal branches and is wrapped in a *myelin sheath,* a white, fatty segmented covering. In the peripheral nervous system, the myelin sheath is produced by *Schwann cells.*

Dendrites are short, thick, diffusely branched extensions that receive impulses arriving at the neuron from other cells.

Nerve impulse transmission

The action of neurons is responsible for *neurotransmission* — conduction of electrochemical impulses throughout the nervous system. Neuron activity may be provoked by mechanical stimuli, such as touch or pressure; thermal stimuli, such as heat or cold; or chemical stimuli, such as external chemicals or a chemical released by the body such as histamine. (See *How neurotransmission occurs,* page 56.)

Neuroglia

The supportive cells of the nervous system, *neuroglia,* are also called *glial cells* (derived from the Greek word for *glue* because these cells hold neurons together).

Four types of neuroglia exist. *Astroglia,* or astrocytes, exist throughout the nervous system. They supply nutrients to neurons and help them maintain their electrical potential. Astrocytes also form part of the *blood-brain barrier.*

POINT TO REMEMBER
The blood-brain barrier, a feature of the brain that separates CNS tissue from the bloodstream, guards against invasion by disease-causing organisms and other substances.

A second type of neuroglia, *ependymal cells,* line the four small cavities in the brain called *ventricles* as well as the choroid plexuses. These cells help produce cerebrospinal fluid (CSF). *Microglia* are phagocytic cells that ingest and digest microorganisms and waste products from injured neurons. *Oligodendroglia* support and electrically insulate CNS axons by forming protective myelin sheaths.

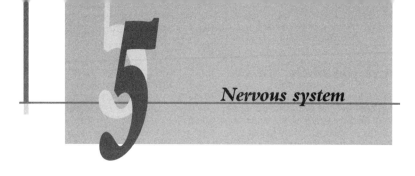

Central nervous system

The CNS includes the brain and spinal cord.

Brain

The brain consists of the cerebrum, cerebellum, brain stem, and diencephalon. (See *Major structures in the brain,* page 57.)

Cerebrum

The cerebrum has right and left hemispheres. The *corpus callosum,* a mass of nerve fibers, bridges the hemispheres, allowing communication between corresponding centers in each. The rolling surface of the cerebrum is made up of convolutions (*gyri*) and creases or fissures (*sulci*). The thin surface layer, the *cerebral cortex,* consists of *gray matter* (neuronal cell bodies and unmyelinated nerve fibers). Within the cerebrum lie *white matter* (myelinated nerve fibers) and islands of internal gray matter.

Each cerebral hemisphere is divided into four lobes, based on anatomic landmarks and functional differences. The lobes are named for the cranial bones that lie over them — frontal, temporal, parietal, and occipital.

The *frontal lobe* influences personality, judgment, abstract reasoning, social behavior, language expression, and movement (in the motor portion). The *temporal lobe* controls hearing, language comprehension, and storage and recall of memories (although memories are stored throughout the entire brain). The limbic system is a primitive brain area deep within the temporal lobe. Besides initiating basic drives — hunger, aggression, and emotional and sexual arousal — the limbic system screens all sensory messages traveling to the cerebral cortex. (See *The limbic system,* page 58.) The *parietal lobe* interprets and integrates sensations, including pain, temperature, and touch. It also interprets size, shape, distance, and texture. The parietal lobe of the nondominant hemisphere is especially important for awareness of body shape. The *occipital lobe* functions mainly to interpret visual stimuli.

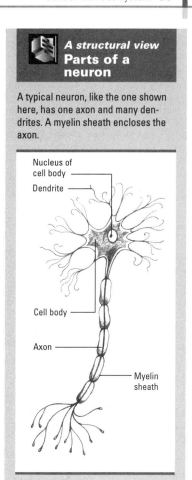

A structural view

Parts of a neuron

A typical neuron, like the one shown here, has one axon and many dendrites. A myelin sheath encloses the axon.

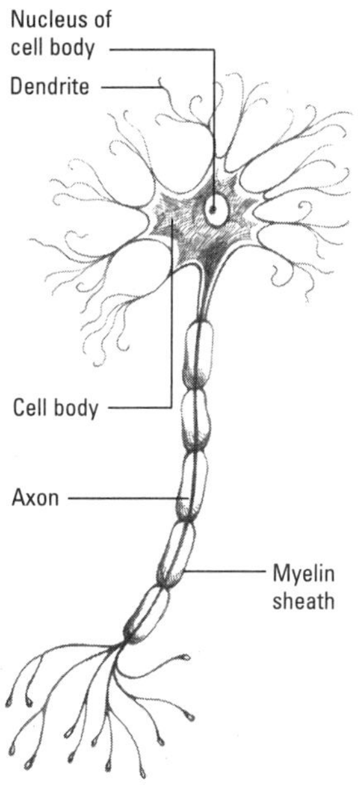

Cerebellum

The second largest brain region, the *cerebellum* lies posterior to the brain stem and inferior to the occipital lobe of the cerebrum. Like the cerebrum, it has two hemispheres, an outer cortex of gray matter and an inner core of white matter. The cerebellum functions to maintain muscle tone, coordinate muscle movement, and control balance.

Focus on function
How neurotransmission occurs

Neurons detect and transmit stimuli by electrochemical messages. Dendrites on the neuron receive an impulse arriving from other cells and conduct it toward the cell body. The axon then conducts the impulse away from the cell.

When the impulse reaches the end of the axon, it stimulates synaptic vesicles in the presynaptic axon terminal to release a neurotransmitter substance into the synaptic cleft between neurons. The neurotransmitter diffuses across the cleft and binds to special receptors on the cell membrane of the postsynaptic neuron. This stimulates or inhibits stimulation of the postsynaptic neuron.

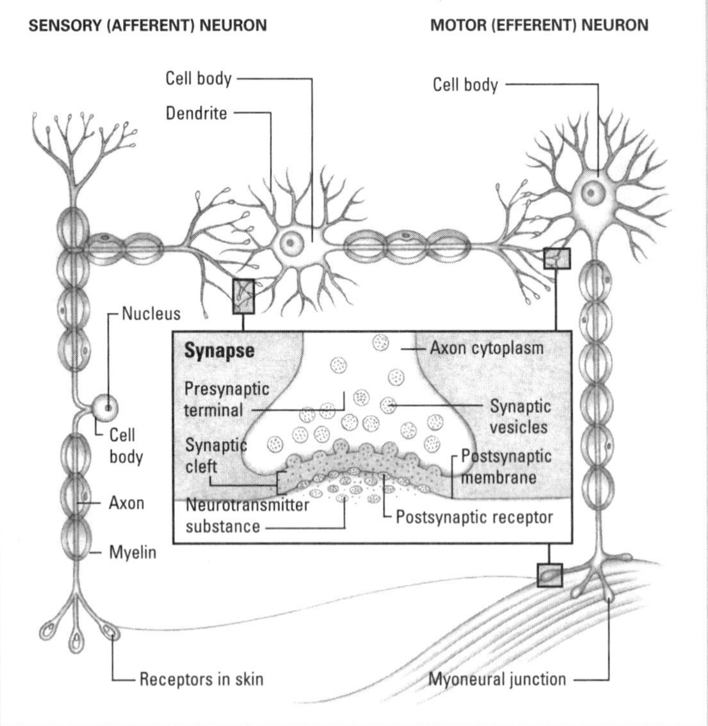

Brain stem

The *brain stem* lies immediately inferior to the cerebrum, just anterior to the cerebellum. It's continuous with the cerebrum superiorly and with the spinal cord inferiorly.

Composed of the midbrain, pons, and medulla oblongata, the brain stem relays messages between the parts of the nervous system. It has three main functions:

- It produces the rigid autonomic behaviors necessary for survival, such as

A structural view
Major structures in the brain

This illustration shows the two largest structures of the brain—the cerebrum and cerebellum. Note the locations of the four cerebral lobes and of the sensory cortex and motor cortex.

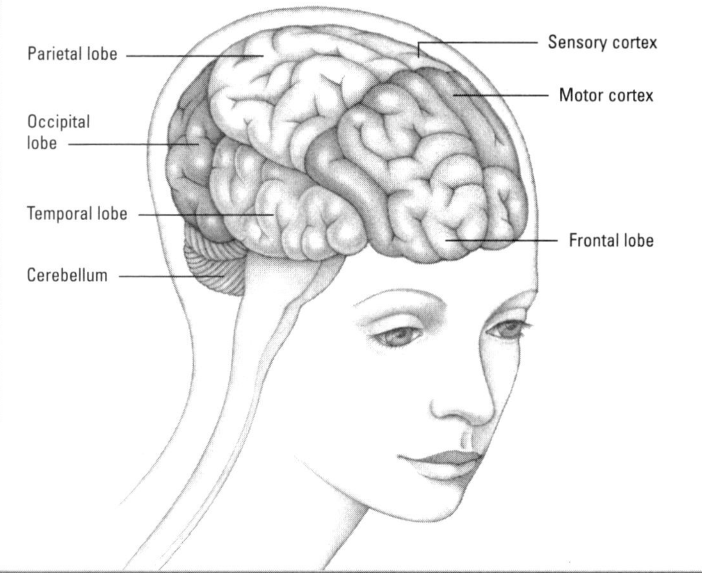

The illustration below reveals a cross section of the brain, from its outermost portion (cerebrum) to its innermost (diencephalon).

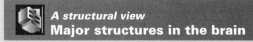

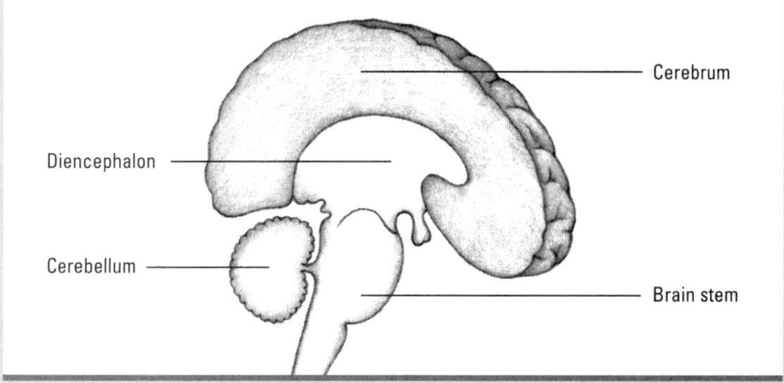

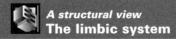

A structural view
The limbic system

The major structures of the limbic system, represented by the shaded area, are associated with such emotions as anger, fear, and sexual arousal. The hippocampus and amygdala also help convert new information into long-term memories.

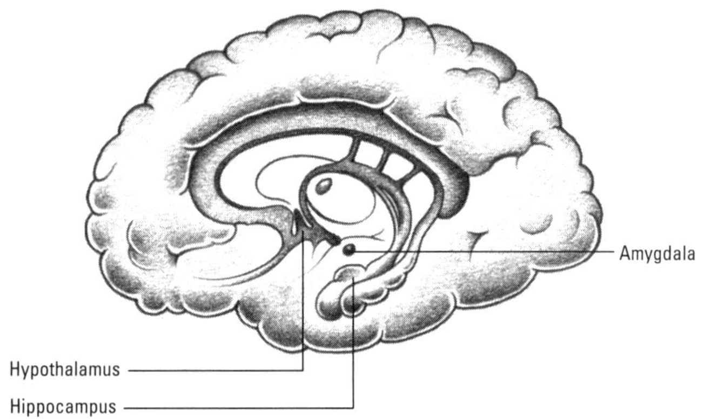

increasing the heart rate and stimulating the adrenal medulla to produce epinephrine.

- It provides pathways for nerve fibers between higher and lower neural centers.
- It serves as the origin for 10 of the 12 pairs of cranial nerves.

A diffuse network of hyperexcitable neurons, the *reticular activating system* (RAS) fans out from the brain stem through the cerebral cortex. After screening all incoming sensory information, the RAS channels it to appropriate areas of the brain for interpretation.

POINT TO REMEMBER

RAS activity stimulates wakefulness. When such activity declines, the person falls asleep. (See *The nervous system and exercise.*)

Midbrain

The *midbrain* connects superiorly with the cerebellum. It contains large voluntary motor nerve tracts running between the brain and spinal cord. The midbrain also contains ascending sensory tracts and houses cranial nerves III and IV.

Pons

The *pons* connects the cerebellum with the cerebrum and links the midbrain to the medulla oblongata. Besides housing one of the brain's respiratory centers, the pons acts as a pathway for conduction tracts between brain centers and the spinal cord and serves as the exit point for cranial nerves V, VI, and VII.

Medulla oblongata

The most inferior portion of the brain stem, the *medulla oblongata* is a small, cone-shaped structure. It joins the spinal cord at the level of the *foramen magnum,* an opening in the occipital portion of the skull. The medulla oblongata serves as an autonomic reflex center to maintain homeostasis, regulating respiratory, vasomotor, and cardiac functions. The medulla oblongata is also associated with cranial nerves IX, X, XI, and XII.

Diencephalon

The *diencephalon* consists of the thalamus and hypothalamus, which lie beneath the surface of the cerebral hemispheres. The *thalamus* relays all sensory stimuli (except olfactory) as they ascend to the cerebral cortex. Its functions include primitive awareness of pain, screening of incoming stimuli, and focusing of attention. The *hypothalamus* controls or affects body temperature, appetite, water balance, pituitary secretions, emotions, and autonomic functions (including sleep and wake cycles).

Circulation within the brain

Four major arteries — two vertebral and two carotid — supply the brain with oxygenated blood. The two *vertebral arteries* (branches of the subclavian veins) converge to become the *basilar artery,* which supplies the posterior brain (pons, midbrain, cerebellum, and posterior cerebrum). The common carotids branch into the two *internal carotids,* which divide further to supply the anterior brain and the middle brain. These arteries interconnect through the *circle of Willis,* an anastomosis at the base of the brain that ensures continual circulation to the brain despite interruption of any of the brain's major vessels. (See *Arteries of the brain,* page 60.)

Spinal cord

A cylindrical structure in the vertebral canal, the *spinal cord* extends from the foramen magnum at the base of the skull to the upper lumbar region of the vertebral column. The spinal nerves arise from the cord. At the cord's inferior end, nerve roots cluster in the *cauda equina.* (See *Spinal cord and spinal nerves,* page 61, and *Inside the spinal cord,* page 62.)

Within the spinal cord, the H-shaped mass of gray matter is divided into horns, which consist mainly of neuron cell bodies. Cell bodies in the *posterior (dorsal) horn* primarily relay sensations; those in the *anterior (ventral) horn* play a part in voluntary and reflex motor activity. White matter surrounding the outer part of these horns consists of myelinated nerve fibers grouped functionally in vertical columns, or *tracts.*

The spinal cord conducts sensory nerve impulses to the brain and conducts motor impulses from the brain. It also controls reflexes such as the knee-jerk (patellar) reaction to a reflex hammer.

The nervous system and exercise

During exercise, the entire nervous system is stimulated. The nervous system coordinates the body's activities, and neurons send signals to the muscles that cause them to contract. Sensory receptors located throughout the body provide the brain with information about the body's movement and activities. The brain processes this information and modifies movements and activities as needed. As exercise progresses, the body's core temperature rises, causing the interaction between the nerves and muscles to become more efficient.

Hormonal changes also occur during exercise. As exercise progresses, hormones that act on a specific area of the brain are released. These hormones stimulate the area of the brain that controls pleasure, causing the euphoria that people commonly report during exercise. People also experience increased alertness during exercise. Studies have shown that mental agility scores improve during exercise treadmill testing.

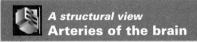

A structural view
Arteries of the brain

As this illustration of the inferior surface of the brain shows, the anterior and posterior arteries join with smaller arteries to form the circle of Willis.

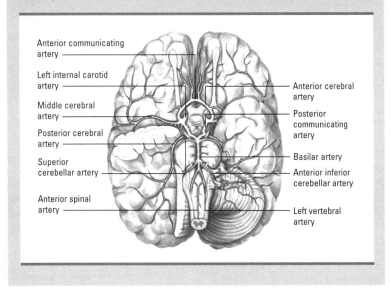

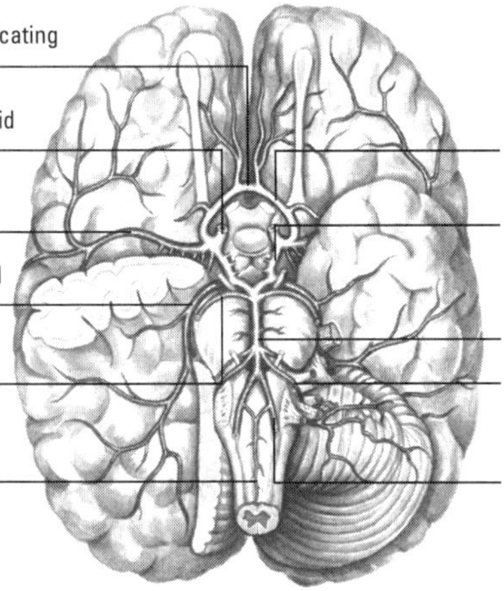

Sensory pathways
Sensory impulses travel via the sensory (*afferent,* or ascending) neural pathways to the sensory cortex in the parietal lobe of the brain where they're interpreted. These impulses use two major parallel pathways:

- Pain and temperature sensations enter the spinal cord through the dorsal horn. After immediately crossing over to the opposite side of the cord, these stimuli then travel to the thalamus through the *spinothalamic tract.*
- Tactile, pressure, and vibration sensations enter the cord through relay stations called *ganglia,* knotlike masses of nerve cell bodies on the dorsal roots of spinal nerves. These stimuli then travel up the cord in the dorsal column to the medulla, where they cross to the opposite side and enter the thalamus. The thalamus relays all incoming sensory impulses (except olfactory impulses) to the sensory cortex for interpretation.

Motor pathways
Motor impulses travel from the brain to the muscles via the motor (*efferent,* or descending) pathways. Originating in the motor cortex of the frontal lobe, these impulses reach the lower motor neurons of the peripheral nervous system via *upper motor neurons.*

Upper motor neurons originate in the brain and form two major systems:

- The *pyramidal system (corticospinal tract)* is responsible for fine, skilled movements of the extremities. Impulses in this system travel from the motor cortex through the internal capsule to the medulla, where they cross to the opposite side and continue down the spinal cord.
- The *extrapyramidal system (extracor-*

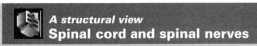

A structural view
Spinal cord and spinal nerves

The illustration below shows the spinal cord and its relationship to the spinal nerves and major parts of the brain.

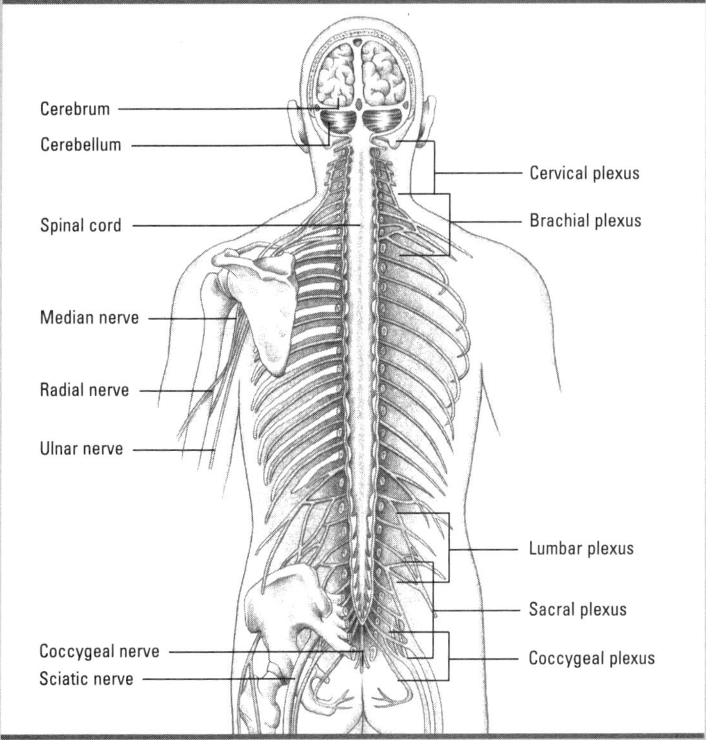

ticospinal tract) controls gross motor movements. Impulses originate in the premotor area of the frontal lobe and travel to the brain stem, where they cross to the opposite side. Then the impulses travel down the spinal cord to the anterior horn, where they're relayed to the lower motor neurons. These neurons, in turn, carry the impulses to the muscles. (See *Major neural pathways*, page 63.)

Reflex responses

Reflex responses occur automatically, without any brain involvement, to protect the body. Spinal nerves, which have both sensory and motor portions, mediate *deep tendon reflexes* (involuntary contractions of a muscle after brief stretching caused by tendon percussion) and *superficial reflexes* (withdrawal reflexes elicited by noxious or tactile stimulation of the skin, cornea, or mucous membranes).

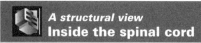

A structural view
Inside the spinal cord

This cross section of the spinal cord shows a central H-shaped mass of gray matter, divided into dorsal and ventral horns. Gray matter in the dorsal horn relays sensory impulses; gray matter in the ventral horn transmits motor impulses. White matter surrounding these horns forms the ascending and descending tracts.

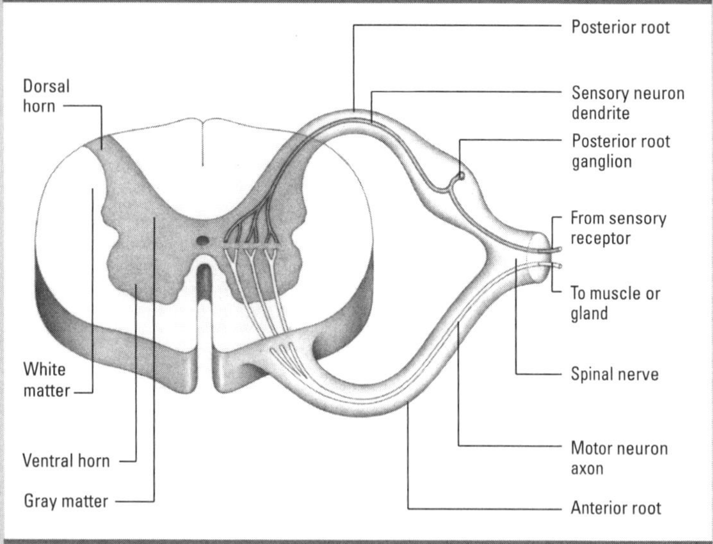

A simple reflex like the *knee-jerk (patellar) reflex* requires a sensory (afferent) neuron and a motor (efferent) neuron. In this reflex, the following events occur:

- A sensory receptor detects the mechanical stimulus produced by the reflex hammer striking the patellar tendon.
- The sensory neuron carries the impulse along its axon via a spinal nerve to the dorsal root, where it enters the spinal cord.
- In the anterior horn of the cord, the sensory neuron synapses with a motor neuron, which carries the impulse along its axon via a spinal nerve to the muscle.
- The motor neuron transmits the impulse to muscle fibers via stimulation of the *motor end plate,* a band of terminal fibers of the motor nerves of skeletal muscles. In response, the muscle contracts and the leg extends.

POINT TO REMEMBER
If the brain can't send a message to a patient's leg after a severe spinal cord injury, a stimulus can still cause the knee-jerk reflex as long as the spinal cord remains intact at the level of this reflex.

Protective structures
The brain and spinal cord are protected from shock and infection by bones, the

Focus on function

Major neural pathways

Sensory and motor impulses travel through different pathways to the brain for interpretation. Sensory impulses travel through two major sensory (afferent, or ascending) pathways to the sensory cortex in the cerebrum. Motor impulses travel from the motor cortex in the cerebrum to the muscles via motor (efferent, or descending) pathways.

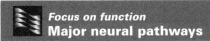

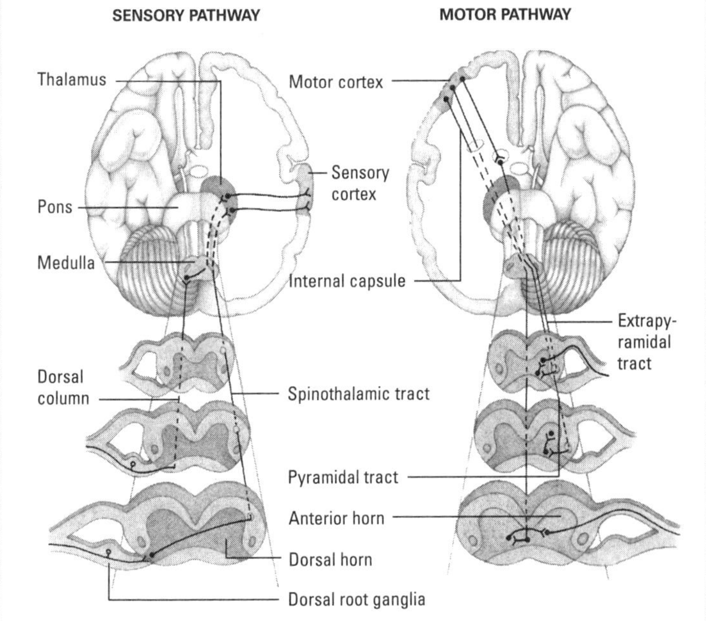

meninges, several additional cushioning layers, and CSF.

Bones

The *skull,* formed of cranial bones, completely surrounds the brain. It opens at the foramen magnum, where the spinal cord exits.

The *vertebral column* protects the spinal cord. Its 30 vertebrae are separated from each other by an intervertebral disk that allows flexibility.

Meninges

The *meninges* cover and protect the cerebral cortex and spinal column. They consist of three layers of connective tissue — *dura mater, arachnoid membrane,* and *pia mater*. (See *Protective membranes of the CNS,* page 64.)

Dura mater

The dura mater is a fibrous membrane that lines the skull and forms folds, or reflections, that descend into the brain's fissures and provide stability. The dural folds include:

A structural view
Protective membranes of the CNS

Three membranes—dura mater, arachnoid membrane, and pia mater—help protect the central nervous system (CNS). Among the dural folds are the falx cerebri, a membrane that separates the cerebral hemispheres. The arachnoid villi project through the dura mater into the superior sagittal and transverse sinuses. The subarachnoid space, filled with cerebrospinal fluid, separates the arachnoid membrane and the pia mater.

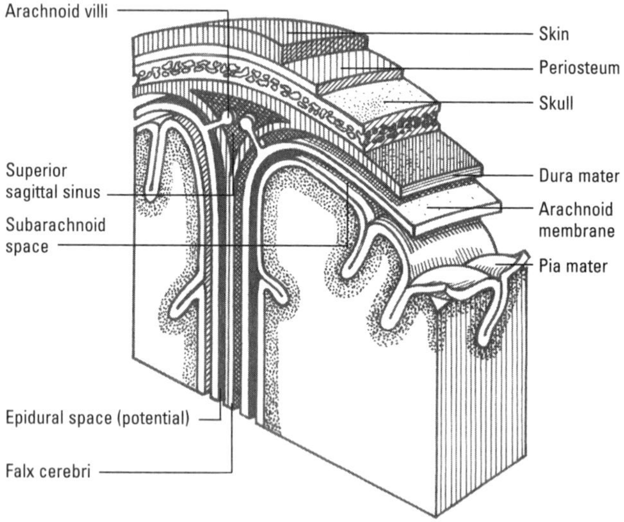

- *falx cerebri,* which lies in the longitudinal fissure and separates the cerebral hemispheres
- *tentorium cerebelli,* which separates the cerebrum from the cerebellum
- *falx cerebelli,* which separates the two lobes of the cerebellum.

The *arachnoid villi*—projections of the arachnoid protrude through the overlying dura mater and into the superior sagittal and transverse sinuses—serve as the exit points for CSF drainage into the venous circulation.

Arachnoid membrane
A fragile, fibrous layer of moderate vascularity, the arachnoid membrane lies between the dura mater and the pia mater. Injury to its blood vessels during lumbar or cisternal puncture may cause hemorrhage.

Pia mater
Extremely thin, the pia mater has a rich blood supply. It closely covers the brain's surface and extends into its fissures.

Cushioning layers

Three layers of space further cushion the brain and spinal cord against injury. The *epidural space* (actually, a potential space) lies over the dura mater. The *subdural space* is situated between the dura mater and arachnoid membrane. This closed area — commonly the site of hemorrhage after head trauma — offers no escape route for blood accumulation. The *subarachnoid space,* filled with CSF, separates the arachnoid membrane and pia mater.

Cerebrospinal fluid

CSF is a colorless fluid that arises from blood plasma and has a similar composition. However, CSF contains less protein than plasma, fewer calcium and potassium ions, and more sodium, magnesium, chloride, and hydrogen ions. Besides cushioning the brain and spinal cord, CSF nourishes cells and transports metabolic waste.

CSF forms continuously in clusters of capillaries called the *choroid plexuses*, located in the roof of each ventricle. The choroid plexuses produce approximately 500 ml (17 oz) of CSF per day.

From the lateral ventricles, CSF flows through the *interventricular foramen (foramen of Monro)* to the third ventricle of the brain. From there, it reaches the subarachnoid space, then by diffusing through foramen that are located in the fourth ventricle, it passes under the base of the brain, upward over the brain's upper surfaces, and down around the spinal cord. Eventually, it reaches the arachnoid villi, where it's reabsorbed into venous blood at the venous sinuses on top of the brain.

Peripheral nervous system

The peripheral nervous system consists of the cranial nerves, spinal nerves, and autonomic nervous system (ANS).

Cranial nerves

The 12 pairs of *cranial nerves* transmit motor or sensory messages or both, primarily between the brain or brain stem and the head and neck. All cranial nerves except the olfactory and optic nerves exit from the midbrain, pons, or medulla oblongata of the brain stem. (See *Exit points for the cranial nerves,* page 66.)

Spinal nerves

The 31 pairs of *spinal nerves* are named for the vertebra from which they exit. The first 8 pairs of spinal nerves travel above their respective vertebrae, while the remaining 23 pair travel below their respective vertebrae. Thus, they're designated from top to bottom as C1 through S5, plus the coccygeal nerve. Each spinal nerve consists of afferent (sensory) and efferent (motor) neurons, which carry messages to and from particular body regions.

Autonomic nervous system

The vast ANS innervates all internal organs. Sometimes known as visceral efferent nerves, the nerves of the ANS carry messages to the viscera from the brain stem and neuroendocrine regulatory centers. The ANS has two major subdivisions: the *sympathetic (thoracolumbar)* nervous system and *parasympathetic (craniosacral)* nervous system.

Sympathetic nervous system

Sympathetic nerves called *preganglionic neurons* exit the spinal cord between the levels of the first thoracic and second lumbar vertebrae. After they leave the spinal cord, these nerves enter small ganglia near the cord. The ganglia form a chain that spreads the impulse to *postganglionic neurons,* which reach many organs and glands and can produce widespread, generalized physiologic responses. These responses include:

- vasoconstriction
- elevated blood pressure
- enhanced blood flow to skeletal muscles

A structural view

Exit points for the cranial nerves

As this illustration shows, 10 of the 12 pairs of cranial nerves (CNs) exit from the brain stem. The remaining two pairs—the olfactory and optic nerves—exit from the forebrain.

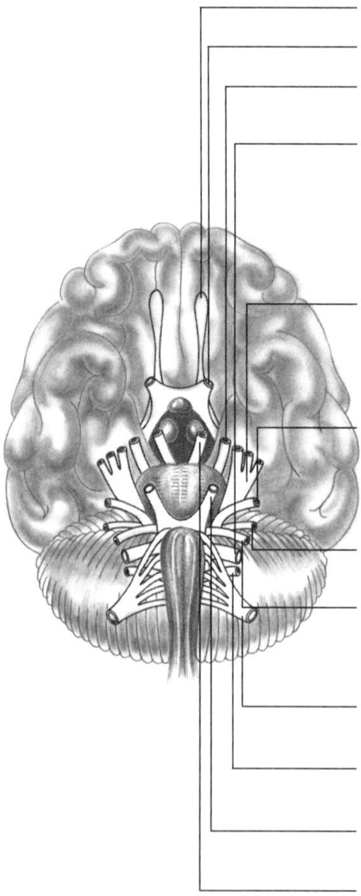
Olfactory (CN I). Sensory: smell
Optic (CN II). Sensory: vision
Trochlear (CN IV). Motor: extraocular eye movement (inferior medial)
Vagus (CN X). Motor: movement of palate, swallowing, gag reflex; activity of the thoracic and abdominal viscera, such as heart rate and peristalsis. Sensory: sensations of throat, larynx, and thoracic and abdominal viscera (heart, lungs, bronchi, and GI tract)
Trigeminal (CN V). Sensory: transmitting stimuli from face and head, corneal reflex. Motor: chewing, biting, and lateral jaw movements
Facial (CN VII). Sensory: taste receptors (anterior two-thirds of tongue). Motor: facial muscle movement, including muscles of expression (those in the forehead and around the eyes and mouth)
Acoustic (CN VIII). Sensory: hearing, sense of balance
Glossopharyngeal (CN IX). Motor: swallowing movements. Sensory: sensations of throat; taste receptors (posterior one-third of tongue)
Hypoglossal (CN XII). Motor: tongue movement
Spinal accessory (CN XI). Motor: shoulder movement, head rotation
Abducens (CN VI). Motor: extraocular eye movement (lateral)
Oculomotor (CN III). Motor: extraocular eye movement (superior, medial, and inferior lateral), pupillary constriction, and upper eyelid elevation

- increased heart rate and contractility
- increased respiratory rate
- smooth-muscle relaxation of the bronchioles, GI tract, and urinary tract
- sphincter contraction
- pupillary dilation and ciliary muscle relaxation
- increased sweat gland secretion
- reduced pancreatic secretion.

Parasympathetic nervous system

Fibers of the parasympathetic nervous system leave the CNS by way of the cranial nerves from the midbrain and medulla and the spinal nerves between the second and fourth sacral vertebrae (S2 to S4).

After leaving the CNS, the long preganglionic fiber of each parasympathetic nerve travels to a ganglion near a particular organ or gland; the short postganglionic fiber enters the organ or gland. This creates a more specific response involving only one organ or gland.

Although the parasympathetic system has little effect on mental or metabolic activity, its effects on other body activities are myriad and include:

- reductions in heart rate, contractility, and conduction velocity
- bronchial smooth-muscle constriction
- increased GI tract tone and peristalsis, with sphincter relaxation
- increased bladder tone and urinary system sphincter relaxation
- vasodilation of external genitalia, causing erection
- pupil constriction
- increased pancreatic, salivary, and lacrimal secretions.

Special sense organs

Sensory stimulation allows the body to interact with the environment. The distal ends of the dendrites of sensory neurons serve as *sensory receptors*, sending messages to the brain. Thus, the body has millions of sensory receptors. The brain also receives stimulation from the special sense organs — the eyes, the ears, and the gustatory and olfactory organs located in the nose and mouth.

Eyes

The organ of vision, the eye contains about 70% of the body's sensory receptors. Although the eye measures about 1″ (2.5 cm) in diameter, only its anterior surface is visible.

Extraocular muscles

Extraocular muscles hold the eyes in place and control their movement. Their coordinated action keeps both eyes parallel and creates binocular vision.

These muscles have mutually antagonistic actions: As one muscle contracts, its opposing muscle relaxes. Each muscle has specific actions:

- The *superior rectus* rotates the eye upward and adducts and rotates the eye inward.
- The *inferior rectus* rotates the eye downward and adducts and rotates the eye outward.
- The *lateral rectus* turns the eye outward (laterally).
- The *medial rectus* turns the eye inward (medially).
- The *superior oblique* turns the eye downward and abducts and rotates the eye inward.
- The *inferior oblique* turns the eye upward and adducts and turns the eye outward.

Extraocular structures

Extraocular structures include the eyelids, conjunctivae, and lacrimal apparatus. Together with the extraocular muscles, these structures support and protect the eyes.

Eyelids

Also called the *palpebrae*, the eyelids are loose folds of skin that cover the anterior portion of eye. The lid margins contain hair follicles, which in turn contain eyelashes and sebaceous glands.

When closed, the upper and lower eyelids cover the eye completely. When open, the upper eyelid extends beyond the *limbus* (the junction of the cornea and the sclera) and covers a small portion of the iris.

The *palpebral fissure* is the opening between the margins of the upper and lower lids; it should be equal in both eyes. The juncture of the upper and lower lids is called the *canthus.*

The eyelids contain three types of glands:

- *meibomian glands* — sebaceous glands that secrete *sebum,* an oily substance that prevents evaporation of tears and keeps the eye lubricated
- *glands of Zeis* — modified sebaceous glands connected to the follicles of the eyelashes
- *Moll's glands* — ordinary sweat glands.

POINT TO REMEMBER
The eyelids protect the eye from foreign bodies, regulate the entrance of light, and distribute tears over the eye by blinking.

Conjunctivae

Conjunctivae are thin mucous membranes that line the inner surface of each eyelid and the anterior portion of the sclera, guarding the eye from invasion by foreign matter. The *palpebral conjunctiva* — the portion that lines the inner surface of the eyelids — appears shiny pink or red. The *bulbar conjunctiva,* which joins the palpebral portion, contains many small, normally visible blood vessels.

Lacrimal apparatus

The structures of the *lacrimal apparatus* — lacrimal glands, punctum, lacrimal sac, and nasolacrimal duct — lubricate and protect the cornea and conjunctivae by producing and absorbing tears.

The *lacrimal gland,* located in a shallow fossa beneath the superior temporal orbital rim, secretes tears, which flow through excretory ducts. In addition to keeping the cornea and conjunctiva moist, tears contain lysozyme, an enzyme that protects against bacterial invasion.

As the eyelids blink, they direct the flow of tears to the inner canthus, where the tears pool and then drain through the *punctum,* a tiny opening at the medial junction of the upper and lower eyelids. From there, tears flow through the lacrimal canals into the *lacrimal sac* and then drain through the *nasolacrimal duct* and into the nose.

Intraocular structures

Intraocular structures within the eyeball are directly involved with vision. They include the sclera, cornea, iris, pupil, anterior chamber, lens, ciliary body, posterior chamber, vitreous humor, choroid, and retina. (See *Intraocular structures.*)

The white *sclera* coats four-fifths of the outside of the eyeball, maintaining its size and form. The *cornea* is continuous with the sclera at the limbus, revealing the pupil and iris. A smooth, transparent tissue, the cornea has no blood supply. The corneal epithelium merges with the bulbar conjunctiva at the limbus. Kept moist by tears, the cornea is highly sensitive to touch.

The *iris* is a circular contractile disk containing smooth and radial muscles. It has an opening in the center for the pupil. Eye color depends on the amount of pigment in the endothelial layers of the iris.

Pupils should be equal and round; depending on the patient's age, they should measure 1/8" to 1/4" (3 to 7 mm) in diameter. Pupil size is controlled by involuntary dilatory and sphincter muscles in the posterior portion of the iris that regulate light entry.

The *anterior chamber,* a cavity bounded anteriorly by the cornea and posteriorly by the lens and iris, is filled with a clear, watery fluid called *aqueous humor.* This fluid flows from the posterior chamber to the anterior chamber through the pupil. From there, it flows peripherally and filters through bundles of connective tissue called the *trabecular meshwork* to *Schlemm's canal,* a venous sinus deep within the

A structural view
Intraocular structures

Some intraocular structures, such as the sclera, cornea, iris, pupil, and anterior chamber, are visible to the naked eye. Others, such as the retina, are visible only with an ophthalmoscope. These illustrations feature the major structures within the eye.

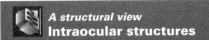

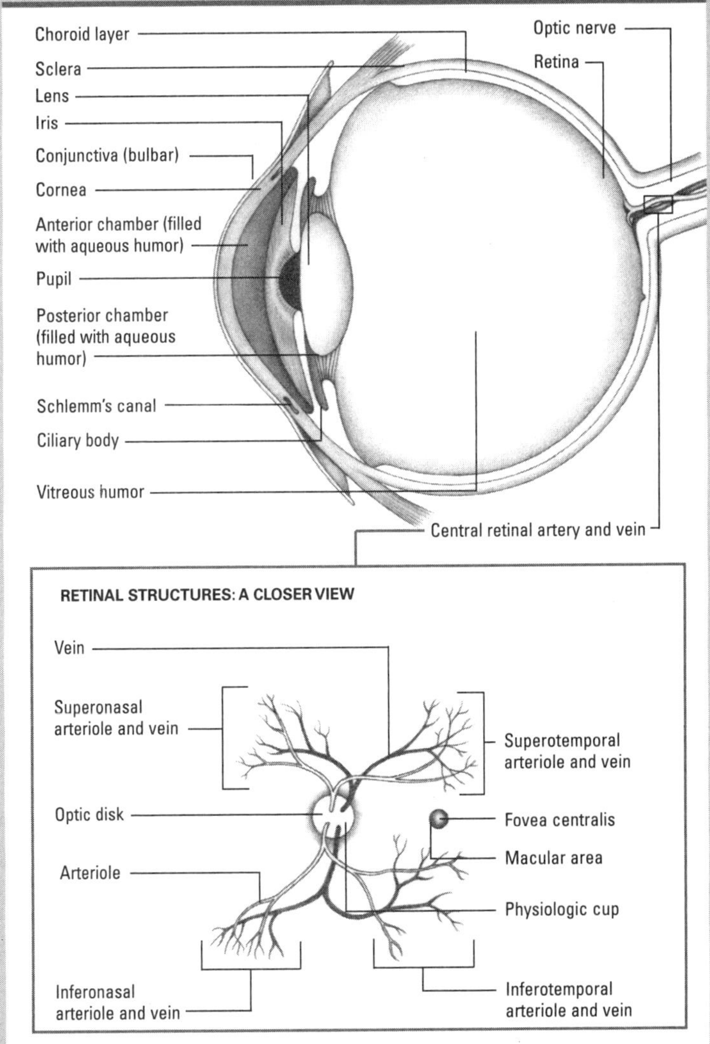

sclera. From this canal, the fluid ultimately enters the venous circulation.

The *lens,* situated directly behind the iris at the pupillary opening, acts like a camera lens, refracting and focusing light onto the retina. It's composed of transparent fibers in an elastic membrane called the *lens capsule.*

The *ciliary body* (three muscles and the iris that make up the anterior part of the vascular uveal tract) controls the lens thickness. Together with the coordinated action of muscles in the iris, the ciliary body regulates the light focused through the lens onto the retina.

The *posterior chamber,* a small space directly posterior to the iris but anterior to the lens, is filled with aqueous humor.

Consisting of a thick, gelatinous material, the *vitreous humor* fills the area behind the lens. There, it maintains placement of the retina and the spherical shape of the eyeball.

The *posterior sclera,* a white, opaque, fibrous layer, covers the posterior portion of the eyeball, continuing back to the dural sheath and covering the optic nerve. The *choroid* lines the inner aspect of the eyeball beneath the retina (adjacent to the sclera); it contains many small arteries and veins.

Retina

The retina, the innermost coat of the eyeball, receives visual stimuli and sends them to the brain. Each of the four sets of retinal vessels contains a transparent arteriole and vein.

Arterioles and veins become progressively thinner as they leave the *optic disk,* a well-defined, 1.5-mm (less than $\frac{1}{8}$") round or oval area within the nasal portion of the retina. Creamy yellow to pink, the optic disk allows the optic nerve to enter the retina at a point called the nerve head. A whitish to grayish crescent of scleral tissue may be present on the lateral side of the disk.

The *physiologic cup* is a light-colored depression within the optic disk on the temporal side. It covers one-third of the center of the disk.

Photoreceptor neurons called *rods* and *cones* compose the visual receptors of the retina. These receptors are responsible for vision. Rods, concentrated toward the periphery of the retina, respond to low-intensity light and shades of gray. Cones, concentrated in the central fovea of the retina, respond to bright light and color.

The *macula,* lateral to the optic disk, is slightly darker than the rest of the retina and without visible retinal vessels. The *central fovea,* a slight depression in the center of the macula, contains the heaviest concentration of cones and is a main receptor for vision and color.

Vision pathway

Intraocular structures perceive and form images and then send them to the brain for interpretation. To interpret these images properly, the brain relies on structures along the vision pathway, including the optic nerve, optic chiasm, and retina, to create the proper visual fields.

In the *optic chiasm,* fibers from the nasal aspects of both retinas cross to opposite sides, and fibers from the temporal portions remain uncrossed. Both crossed and uncrossed fibers form the *optic tracts.* Injury to one of the optic nerves can cause blindness in the corresponding eye; an injury or lesion in the optic chiasm can cause partial vision loss (for example, loss of the two temporal visual fields).

POINT TO REMEMBER

Even though fewer people today lose their sight from infections or injuries, the incidence of blindness is rising. The main causes of new blindness in the United States include macular degeneration among elderly patients, glaucoma, diabetic retinopathy, cataracts, and optic atrophy.

Image perception and formation

Image formation begins when eye structures refract light rays from an object. Normally, the cornea, aqueous humor, lens, and vitreous humor refract light rays from an object, focusing them on the central fovea where an inverted and reversed image clearly forms. Within the retina, rods and cones turn the projected image into an impulse and transmit it to the optic nerve.

The impulse travels to the optic chiasm where the two optic nerves unite, split again into two optic tracts, and then continue into the optic section of the cerebral cortex. There the inverted and reversed image on the retina changes back to its original form.

Ears

The ears are the organs of hearing; they also maintain the body's equilibrium. The ear is divided into three main parts: external, middle, and inner. (See *Ear structures,* page 72.)

External ear

The external ear consists of the auricle (pinna) and the external auditory canal. The *auricle* consists of the cartilaginous anthelix, crux of the helix, lobule, tragus, and concha. Although not part of the external ear, the mastoid process is an important bony landmark behind the lower part of the auricle. This structure is an anchoring site for some of the neck muscles.

The *external auditory canal* is a narrow chamber measuring about 1″ (2.5 cm) long. In the adult, this canal leads inward, downward, and forward to the middle ear, connecting the auricle with the tympanic membrane in the middle ear. Thin, sensitive skin covers the cartilage that forms the outer one-third of the external auditory canal; bone covered by thin skin forms the inner two-thirds. Modified apocrine sweat glands in this thin skin secrete *cerumen,* brown earwax.

Middle ear

Also called the *tympanic cavity,* the middle ear is an air-filled cavity within the hard portion of the temporal bone. Lined with mucosa, it's bounded distally by the tympanic membrane and medially by the oval and round windows.

The *tympanic membrane,* consisting of layers of skin, fibrous tissue, and mucous membrane, transmits sound vibrations to the internal ear. It appears pearly gray, shiny, and translucent.

The *oval window (fenestra ovalis)* is an opening in the wall behind the middle and inner ears into which part of the stapes (a tiny bone of the middle ear) fits; it transmits vibrations to the inner ear. The *round window (fenestra cochleae),* another opening in the same wall, is enclosed by the *secondary tympanic membrane.* Like the oval window, the round window transmits vibrations to the inner ear.

The middle ear contains three small bones called *ossicles* — the malleus (hammer), incus (anvil), and stapes (stirrup) — which link together to transmit sounds. The *malleus* attaches to the tympanic membrane; the *stapes,* to the oval window. The *incus* articulates with these structures during transmission of vibratory motion from the eardrum to the inner ear, where the vibration excites receptor nerve endings.

The center of the tympanic membrane, called the *umbo,* covers the long process of the malleus. Around the outer border of the membrane is a pale white, fibrous ring called the *annulus.*

Inner ear

A *bony labyrinth* and a *membranous labyrinth* combine to form the inner ear. The inner ear contains the vestibule, the cochlea, and the semicircular canals.

The *vestibule,* located posterior to the cochlea and anterior to the semicircular canals, serves as the entrance to the inner ear. It houses two membranous sacs, the *saccule* and *utricle.* Suspended in a fluid called *perilymph,* the saccule and utricle sense gravity changes and linear and angular acceleration.

The *cochlea,* a bony, spiraling cone, extends from the anterior part of the vestibule. Within it lies the *cochlear duct,* a triangular, membranous structure housing the *organ of Corti.* The receptor organ for hearing, the organ of

A structural view
Ear structures

The organ of hearing, the ear has three divisions—external, middle, and inner—shown here with their anatomic structures.

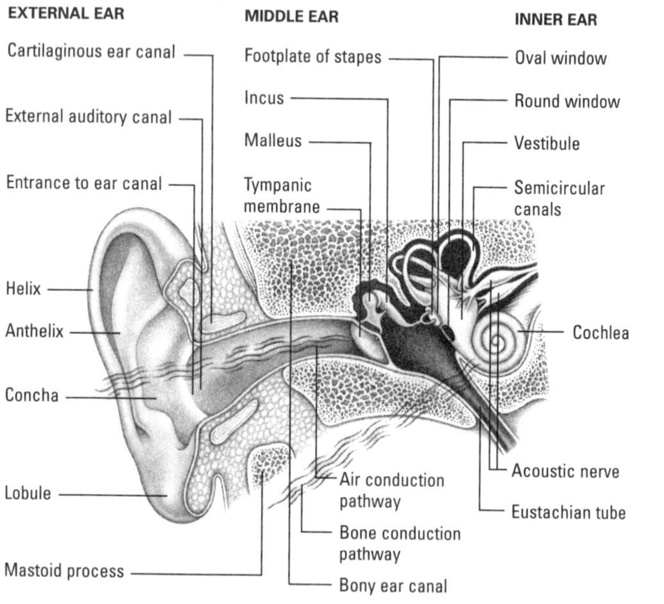

Corti transmits sound to the cochlear branch of the acoustic (eighth) cranial nerve.

The three *semicircular canals* project from the posterior aspect of the vestibule. Each canal is oriented in one of three planes—superior, posterior, or lateral. The semicircular duct, which traverses the canals, is continuous with the utricle anteriorly. The *crista ampullaris,* which sits at the end of each canal, contains hair cells and support cells. It's stimulated by sudden movements or changes in the rate or direction of movement.

Hearing pathways

For hearing to occur, sound waves travel through the ear by two pathways — air conduction and bone conduction. *Air conduction* occurs when sound waves travel in the air through the external and middle ear to the inner ear. *Bone conduction* occurs when sound waves travel through bone to the inner ear.

Vibrations transmitted through air and bone stimulate nerve impulses in the inner ear. The cochlear branch of the acoustic nerve transmits these vibrations to the auditory area of the cerebral cortex, which then interprets the sound.

Nose and mouth

The nose is the sense organ for smell. The mucosal epithelium that lines the uppermost portion of the nasal cavity houses receptors for fibers of the olfactory (first) cranial nerves. Called *olfactory (smell) receptors,* these organs consist of hair cells. Highly sensitive but easily fatigued, hair cells are stimulated by the slightest odors but stop sensing even the strongest smells after a short time.

The tongue and the roof of the mouth contain most of the receptors for the taste nerve fibers (located in branches of the seventh and ninth cranial nerves). Called *taste buds,* these receptors are stimulated by chemicals. They respond to four taste sensations: sweet, sour, bitter, and salty. All the other flavors a person senses result from a combination of olfactory receptor and taste bud stimulation.

6 Endocrine system

Along with the nervous system, the endocrine system regulates and integrates the body's metabolic activities. The three major components of the endocrine system are glands, hormones, and receptors.

- *Glands* are specialized cell clusters or organs.
- *Hormones* are chemical substances secreted by glands in response to stimulation.
- *Receptors* are protein molecules that trigger specific physiologic changes in a target cell in response to hormonal stimulation.

Glands

The major glands of the endocrine system include:

- pituitary gland
- thyroid gland
- parathyroid glands
- adrenal glands
- thymus
- pineal gland

Several organs of the body contain areas comprised of endocrine tissue that produce hormones. These include the pancreas and gonads (ovaries and testes). The hypothalamus also produces and releases hormones and is therefore an important component of the endocrine system. (See *Components of the endocrine system.*)

Pituitary gland

Also called the *hypophysis* or master gland, the pituitary gland rests in the *sella turcica*, a depression in the sphenoid bone at the base of the brain. This pea-sized gland, which weighs less than 1/8 oz (less than 0.75 g), connects with the hypothalamus via the infundibulum, from which it receives chemical and nervous stimulation. (See *How the hypothalamus affects endocrine activities,* page 76.)

The pituitary has two main regions. The larger region, the *anterior pituitary* (*adenohypophysis*), produces at least six hormones:

- growth hormone (GH), or somatotropin
- thyrotropin, or thyroid-stimulating hormone (TSH)
- corticotropin
- follicle-stimulating hormone (FSH)
- luteinizing hormone (LH)
- prolactin.

The *posterior pituitary,* which makes up about 25% of the gland, serves as a storage area for antidiuretic hormone (ADH) and oxytocin, which are produced by the hypothalamus.

Thyroid gland

The thyroid lies directly below the larynx, partially in front of the trachea. Its two lateral lobes — one on either side of the trachea — join with a narrow tissue bridge, called the *isthmus,* to give the gland its butterfly shape.

The two lobes of the thyroid function as one unit to produce the hormones triiodothyronine (T_3), thyroxine (T_4), and calcitonin. Collectively referred to as thyroid hormone, T_3 and T_4 are the body's major metabolic hormones, regulating metabolism by speeding cellular respiration. T_3 has several times the biologic activity of T_4.

Calcitonin maintains the blood calcium level by inhibiting the release of calcium from bone. Its secretion is con-

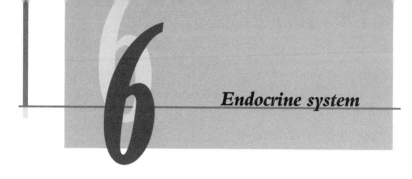

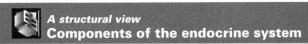

A structural view
Components of the endocrine system

Endocrine glands secrete hormones directly into the bloodstream to regulate body function. This illustration shows the location of the endocrine glands and other organs that have endocrine function.

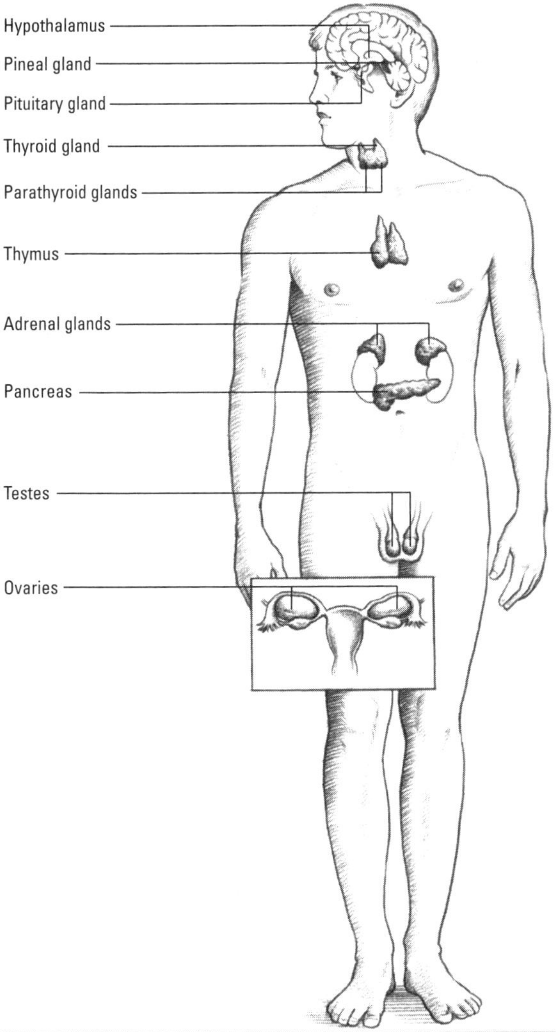

> *Focus on function*
> **How the hypothalamus affects endocrine activities**
>
> The hypothalamus, which forms the floor and part of the lateral wall of the brain's third ventricle, is the main integrative center for the endocrine system. It controls the function of endocrine organs by neural and hormonal pathways.
>
> **Prime activator**
>
> The hypothalamus activates endocrine activities by controlling the release of hormones produced by the anterior pituitary lobe and by producing two hormones—antidiuretic hormone (ADH, or vasopressin) and oxytocin. ADH and oxytocin are transmitted along axons to the posterior pituitary lobe, where they're stored.
>
> The hypothalamus also produces many releasing and inhibiting hormones and other factors, with which it regulates functions of the anterior pituitary lobe.

trolled by the calcium concentration of the fluid surrounding thyroid cells.

Parathyroid glands

The body's smallest known endocrine glands, the parathyroid glands are embedded on the posterior surface of the thyroid, one in each corner.

POINT TO REMEMBER
Most people have four parathyroid glands.

Working together as a single gland, the parathyroid glands produce parathyroid hormone (PTH). The main function of PTH is to help regulate the blood's calcium balance. This hormone adjusts the rate at which calcium and magnesium ions are removed from the urine and increases the movement of phosphate ions from the blood to urine for excretion.

Adrenal glands

The two adrenal glands (sometimes called the *suprarenal glands*) each lie atop a kidney. These almond-shaped glands contain two distinct structures that function as separate endocrine glands.

The *adrenal medulla,* or inner layer of the adrenal gland, functions as an extension of the sympathetic nervous system, producing two catecholamines, epinephrine and norepinephrine. Because these substances play important roles in the autonomic nervous system (ANS), the adrenal medulla is considered a neuroendocrine structure.

The much larger outer layer, the *adrenal cortex,* forms the bulk of the adrenal gland. It has three zones, or cell layers. The outermost zone, the *zona glomerulosa,* produces mineralocorticoids, primarily aldosterone. The middle and largest zone, the *zona fasciculata,* produces the glucocorticoids cortisol (hydrocortisone), cortisone, and corticosterone as well as small amounts of the sex hormones androgen and estrogen. The innermost zone, the *zona reticularis,* produces mainly glucocorticoids and some sex hormones.

Pancreas

A triangular organ, the pancreas lies across the posterior abdominal wall. Its head and neck nestle in the curve of the duodenum, its body stretches horizontally behind the stomach, and its tail extends to the spleen.

The pancreas performs both endocrine and exocrine functions. *Acinar cells,* which make up most of the gland, regulate pancreatic exocrine function.

The endocrine cells of the pancreas are called the *islet cells,* or *islets of Langerhans.* Existing in clusters found scattered among the acinar cells, the islets contain alpha, beta, and delta cells. These three cell types produce important hormones:

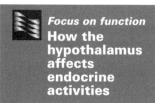

- *Alpha cells* produce glucagon, a hormone that raises the blood glucose level by triggering the breakdown of glycogen to glucose.

- *Beta cells* produce insulin, which lowers the blood glucose level by stimulating the conversion of glucose to glycogen.
- *Delta cells* produce somatostatin, which inhibits the release of GH, corticotropin, and certain other hormones.

Thymus

Located below the sternum, the thymus contains lymphatic tissue. It reaches maximal size at puberty and then starts to atrophy.

Because the thymus produces T cells, important in cell-mediated immunity, its major role seems related to the immune system. However, the thymus also produces the peptide hormones thymosin and thymopoietin. Active in immunity, these hormones promote growth of peripheral lymphoid tissue. (For more information on the thymus, see chapter 9, Immune system.)

Pineal gland

The tiny pineal gland — only about 1/4″ (8 mm) in diameter — lies at the back of the third ventricle within the diencephalon of the brain. It produces the hormone melatonin. Melatonin levels peak during the night, causing drowsiness, and are at their lowest levels around noon.

Gonads

The gonads consist of the ovaries in females and the testes in males.

Ovaries

The *ovaries* are paired, oval glands situated on either side of the uterus. They produce ova (eggs) and the steroidal hormones estrogen and progesterone. These hormones have several functions:

- They promote development and maintenance of female sex characteristics.
- They regulate the menstrual cycle.
- They maintain the uterus for pregnancy.
- Along with other hormones, they prepare the mammary glands for lactation.

Testes

The testes are paired structures that lie in an extra-abdominal pouch (scrotum) in the male. They produce spermatozoa and the male sex hormone testosterone, which stimulates and maintains male sex characteristics.

Hormones

Hormones are complex chemical substances that trigger or regulate the activity of an organ or a group of cells.

Types of hormones

Structurally, hormones are classified as polypeptides, steroids, or amines.

Polypeptides are proteins with a defined, genetically coded structure. They include:

- anterior pituitary hormones (GH, TSH, FSH, LH, and prolactin)
- posterior pituitary hormones (ADH and oxytocin)
- PTH
- pancreatic hormones (insulin and glucagon).

Steroids are derived from cholesterol. They include:

- the adrenocortical hormones secreted by the adrenal cortex (aldosterone and cortisol)
- the sex hormones secreted by the gonads (estrogen and progesterone in females and testosterone in males).

Amines are derived from tyrosine, an essential amino acid found in most proteins. They include:

- thyroid hormones (T_3 and T_4)
- catecholamines (epinephrine, norepinephrine, and dopamine).

Hormone release and transport

Although all hormone release results from endocrine gland stimulation, release patterns of hormones vary greatly. (See *Hormone storage and release,* page 78.) For example:

- Corticotropin (secreted by the anteri-

Focus on function
Hormone storage and release

Endocrine cells manufacture and release their hormones in several ways, as described here.

Pancreas

Many endocrine cells possess receptors on their membranes that respond to stimuli:

- Stimulation of the pancreatic beta cell (shown below) by neurons causes it to produce the hormone precursor *preproinsulin.*
- Preproinsulin is converted to *proinsulin* in beadlike ribosomes located on the endoplasmic reticulum.
- Proinsulin is transferred to the Golgi complex, which collects it into secretory granules and converts it to *insulin.*
- Secretory granules fuse with the plasma membrane and disperse insulin into the bloodstream.
- Hormonal release by membrane fusion is called *exocytosis.*

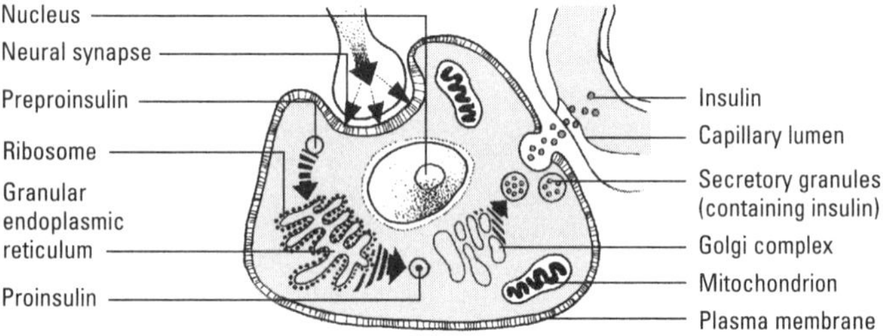

Thyroid

Thyroid cells store a hormone precursor, colloidal iodinated thyroglobulin, which contains iodine and thyroglobulin. When stimulated by thyroid-stimulating hormone (TSH), a follicular cell (shown below) takes up some stored thyroglobulin by *endocytosis*—the reverse of exocytosis.

- The cell membrane extends fingerlike projections into the colloid, and then pulls portions of it back into the cell.
- Lysosomes fuse with the colloid, which is then degraded into triiodothyronine (T_3) and thyroxine (T_4).
- These thyroid hormones are released into the circulation and lymphatic system by exocytosis.

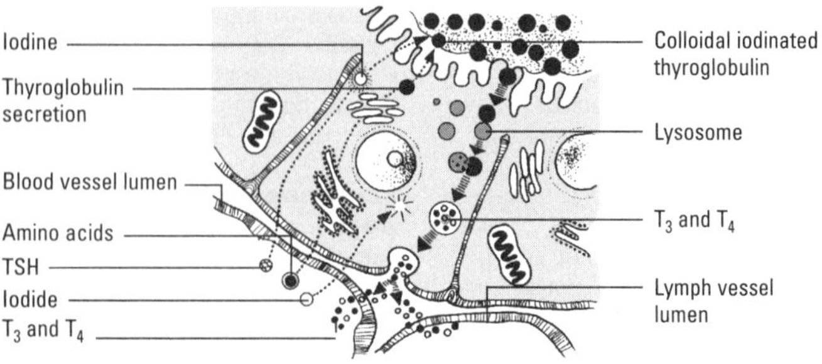

Hormone storage and release *(continued)*

Hypothalamus and pituitary

Anterior and posterior pituitary secretions are controlled by signals from the hypothalamus:

- As shown on the left side of the illustration below, the hypothalamic neuron produces antidiuretic hormone (ADH), which travels down the axon and is stored in secretory granules in nerve endings in the posterior pituitary for later release.
- As shown on the right side of the illustration below, the hypothalamus stimulates the anterior pituitary to produce its many hormones. A hypothalamic neuron manufactures inhibitory and stimulatory hormones and secretes them into a capillary of the portal system. The hormones travel down the pituitary stalk to the anterior pituitary. There, they cause inhibition or release of many pituitary hormones, including corticotropin, TSH, growth hormone, follicle-stimulating hormone, luteinizing hormone, and prolactin.

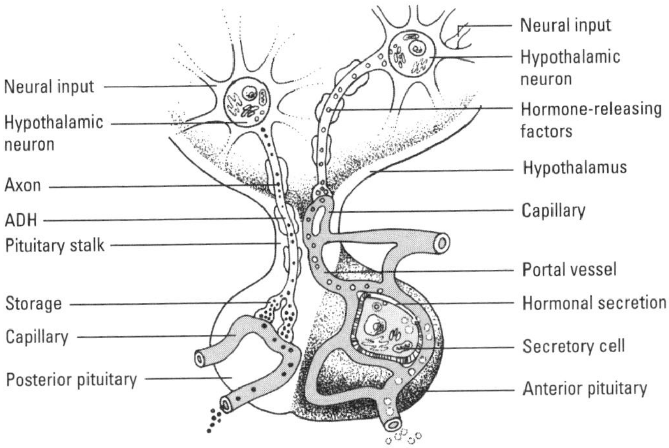

or pituitary) and cortisol (secreted by the adrenal cortex) are released in irregular spurts in response to body rhythm cycles, with levels peaking in the morning.

- Secretion of PTH (by the parathyroid gland) and prolactin (by the anterior pituitary) occurs fairly evenly throughout the day.
- Insulin, secreted by the pancreas, has both steady and sporadic release patterns.

POINT TO REMEMBER

Pancreatic beta cells secrete small amounts of insulin continuously — but secrete additional insulin in response to food intake.

After release into the bloodstream, thyroid and steroid hormones circulate bound to plasma proteins, whereas catecholamines and most polypeptides circulate “free” (not protein-bound).

Hormonal action

When a hormone reaches its target site, it binds to a specific receptor on the cell membrane or within the cell. Polypeptides and some amines bind to membrane receptor sites. The smaller, more lipid-soluble steroids and thyroid hormones diffuse through the cell membrane and bind to intracellular receptors.

After binding occurs, each hormone produces unique physiologic changes, depending on its target site and its specific action at that site. A particular hormone may have different effects at different target sites.

Hormonal regulation

Hormone secretion ebbs and flows according to biological need. To maintain the body's delicate equilibrium, a feedback mechanism regulates hormone production and secretion. The mechanism involves hormones, blood chemicals and metabolites, and the nervous system. (See *Biological need: Key to endocrine function.*)

POINT TO REMEMBER

Feedback refers to information sent to endocrine glands that signals the need for changes in hormone levels, either increasing or decreasing hormone production and release.

For normal function, each gland must contain enough appropriately programmed secretory cells to release active hormone on demand. A secretory cell can't sense on its own when to release the hormone — or how much to release. It gets this information from sensing and signaling systems that integrate many messages.

Although experts formerly considered hormone release (stimulation) an active process and lack of release (inhibition) passive, studies show that both are active. Thus, stimulatory and inhibitory signals together actively control the rate and duration of hormone release.

When released, the hormone travels to target cells, where a receptor molecule recognizes it and binds to it. The receptor-hormone complex then initiates target cell changes, resulting in biological effects specific to the target cell. In this way, the hormone serves as a signal molecule that interacts with its target cell to stimulate or inhibit the cell's programmed processes.

After the desired biological effects take place, two other processes occur:

- The secretory cell recognizes that the biological need has been fulfilled — a task requiring feedback inhibition.
- All biochemical messages from the secretory cell, plasma, and target cell deteriorate fast enough so that the sensing cell can obtain and act on new information.

Mechanisms that control hormone release

Four basic mechanisms control hormone release: the pituitary-target gland axis, the hypothalamic-pituitary-target gland axis, chemical regulation, and nervous system regulation.

Pituitary-target gland axis

The pituitary gland regulates other endocrine glands — and their hormones — through secretion of trophic hormones, including corticotropin, TSH, and LH. Corticotropin regulates adrenocortical hormones, TSH regulates T_3 and T_4, and LH regulates gonadal hormones.

The pituitary gets feedback about target glands by continuously monitoring the levels of the hormones produced by these glands. If a change occurs, the pituitary corrects it in one of two ways:

- by increasing the trophic hormones, which stimulate the target gland to cause an increase in target gland hormones
- by decreasing the trophic hormones, thereby decreasing target gland stimulation and target gland hormones.

The pituitary increases or decreases its trophic hormones from moment to moment by continuously monitoring its target gland hormone and changing its own level in the opposite direction. For instance, if the cortisol level rises, corticotropin levels decline and so reduce adrenal cortex stimulation; this, in turn, decreases cortisol secretion. However, if the cortisol level drops, corticotropin levels rise, stimulating the adrenal cortex to produce and secrete more cortisol.

Focus on function
Biological need: Key to endocrine function

Hormone secretion depends on the body's needs. For recognition of these needs, each endocrine gland depends on a feedback mechanism. The flowchart below shows the chain of events from the recognition of a need and hormone release through deterioration of the biochemical message that triggered the release.

ENDOCRINE GLAND FUNCTION

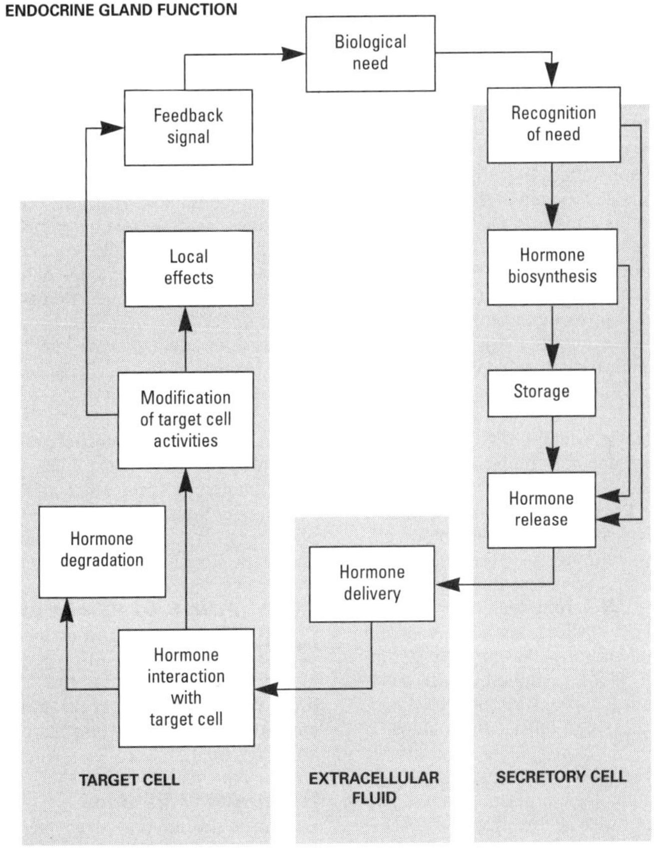

Hypothalamic-pituitary-target gland axis
The hypothalamus also produces trophic hormones — releasing and inhibiting hormones that regulate anterior pituitary hormones. By controlling anterior pituitary hormones, which regulate the target gland hormones, the hypothalamus affects target glands as well.

Exercise and the endocrine system

Hormones play an essential role during exercise. Insulin, a small protein hormone secreted by the pancreas, helps maintain a therapeutic blood glucose level. When exercise intensity increases or is prolonged, blood glucose levels fall, causing insulin secretion to fall. As glucose levels continue to fall, glucagon and cortisol are released in an attempt to increase glucose levels.

Epinephrine and growth hormone also provide fuel during exercise after glycogen stores become depleted. Epinephrine works by stimulating lipolysis in adipose tissue. Growth hormone stimulates lipolysis when exercise duration progresses beyond 15 minutes.

Chemical regulation

Endocrine glands not controlled by the pituitary gland may be controlled by specific substances that trigger gland secretions. For example, the blood glucose level is a major regulator of glucagon and insulin release. When the blood glucose level rises, the pancreas is stimulated to increase insulin secretion and suppress glucagon secretion. A depressed level of blood glucose, on the other hand, triggers increased glucagon secretion and suppresses insulin secretion.

Similarly, calcium regulates PTH secretion. A decreased blood calcium level stimulates the parathyroid glands to increase PTH secretion, making the calcium level rise. An increased blood calcium level suppresses PTH secretion.

Sodium and potassium indirectly regulate aldosterone secretion. Decreased extracellular sodium levels and increased serum potassium levels stimulate formation of angiotensin II, a polypeptide that in turn induces the adrenal cortex to release more aldosterone.

ADH regulation occurs mainly through changes in plasma osmolality, although other factors also affect ADH levels. Elevated plasma osmolality (indicating dehydration) stimulates ADH to promote water retention; diminished osmolality (indicating fluid overload) suppresses ADH secretion to promote *diuresis* (excretion of water).

Nervous system regulation

The central nervous system (CNS) helps to regulate hormone secretion in several ways:

- The hypothalamus controls pituitary hormones, as described earlier. Because hypothalamic nerve cells produce the posterior pituitary hormones ADH and oxytocin, these hormones are controlled directly by the CNS.
- Nervous system stimuli — such as *hypoxia* (oxygen deficiency), nausea, pain, stress, and certain drugs — also affect ADH levels.
- The ANS controls catecholamine secretion by the adrenal medulla.

The nervous system also affects other endocrine hormones. For example, stress, which leads to sympathetic stimulation, causes the pituitary to release corticotropin.

POINT TO REMEMBER

The nervous and endocrine systems share other regulatory mechanisms as part of the fight-or-flight reaction and other stress responses. (See *Exercise and the endocrine system.*)

Hormonal imbalance

Endocrine dysfunction takes one of two forms: *hyperfunction,* resulting in excessive hormone effects, or *hypofunction,* caused by relative or absolute hormone deficiency. (See *Endocrine function: Too little or too much?*)

Hormonal imbalance also may be classified according to disease site:

- *Primary dysfunction* results from disease within an endocrine gland — for

Endocrine function: Too little or too much?

The flowchart below describes what happens when endocrine function becomes abnormal.

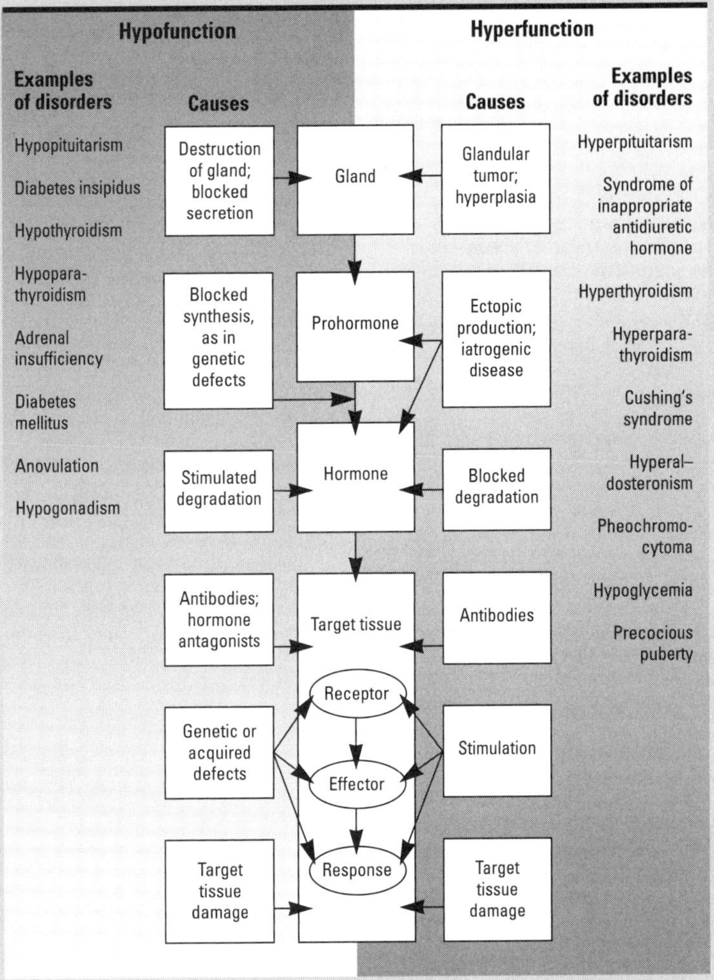

example, Addison's disease (adrenal hypofunction).

- *Secondary dysfunction* occurs when a disease in a tissue that secretes hormones affects the target tissue.
- *Hyperfunction* or *hypofunction* results from disease in a nonendocrine tissue or organ that affects hormone balance.

7 Cardiovascular system

The cardiovascular system (sometimes called the *circulatory system*) consists of the heart, blood vessels, and lymphatics. This network brings life-sustaining oxygen and nutrients to the body's cells, removes metabolic waste products, and carries hormones from one part of the body to another. The cardiovascular system is so vital that its activity defines the presence of life.

Heart

The heart is a physiologic pump that moves the body's entire volume of blood to and from the lungs and tissues. Actually, it acts as two separate pumps, the right side serving as a pulmonary pump and the left side as a systemic pump.

About the size of a closed fist, the heart is roughly cone-shaped. It weighs approximately $10\frac{1}{4}$ to $12\frac{1}{4}$ oz (290 to 350 g) in an adult male and 9 to $10\frac{1}{2}$ oz (255 to 300 g) in an adult female.

The heart lies beneath the sternum in the mediastinum, between the second and sixth ribs. About one-third of the organ lies to the right of the midsternal line; the remainder, to the left.

In most people, the heart rests obliquely, its right side almost in front of the left, the broad part at the top, and the pointed end (apex) at the bottom.

POINT TO REMEMBER
The position of the heart varies with body build. In a tall, thin person, it's positioned more vertically than in a short, stocky person.

The heart's structure consists of the pericardium, three layers of the heart wall, four chambers, and four valves. (See *Inside the heart.*)

Pericardium

The *pericardium* is a fibroserous sac that surrounds the heart and the roots of the great vessels. It consists of the serous pericardium and the fibrous pericardium.

The *serous pericardium,* the thin, smooth inner portion, has two layers. The *parietal layer* lines the inside of the fibrous pericardium. The *visceral layer* adheres to the surface of the heart.

The *fibrous pericardium,* composed of tough, white fibrous tissue, fits loosely around the heart, protecting the heart and serous membrane.

Between the two layers is the *pericardial space,* containing a few milliliters of *pericardial fluid*. This fluid lubricates the surfaces of the space and allows the heart to move easily during contraction.

Heart wall

The wall of the heart consists of three layers — epicardium, myocardium, and endocardium. The *epicardium*, the outer layer (and the visceral layer of the pericardium), is made up of squamous epithelial cells overlying connective tissue.

The *myocardium*, the middle layer, is composed of interlacing bundles of cardiac muscle fibers. Forming most of the heart wall, the myocardium has striated muscle fibers that cause the heart to contract.

The *endocardium*, the heart's smooth inner layer, consists of endothelial tissue with small blood vessels and bundles of smooth muscle.

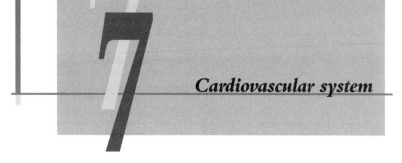

A structural view
Inside the heart

Within the heart lie four chambers (two atria and two ventricles) and four valves (two atrioventricular and two semilunar valves). Surrounded by a sac called the pericardium, the heart has a wall made up of three layers: myocardium, endocardium, and epicardium (see the inset). A system of blood vessels carries blood to and from the heart.

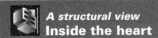

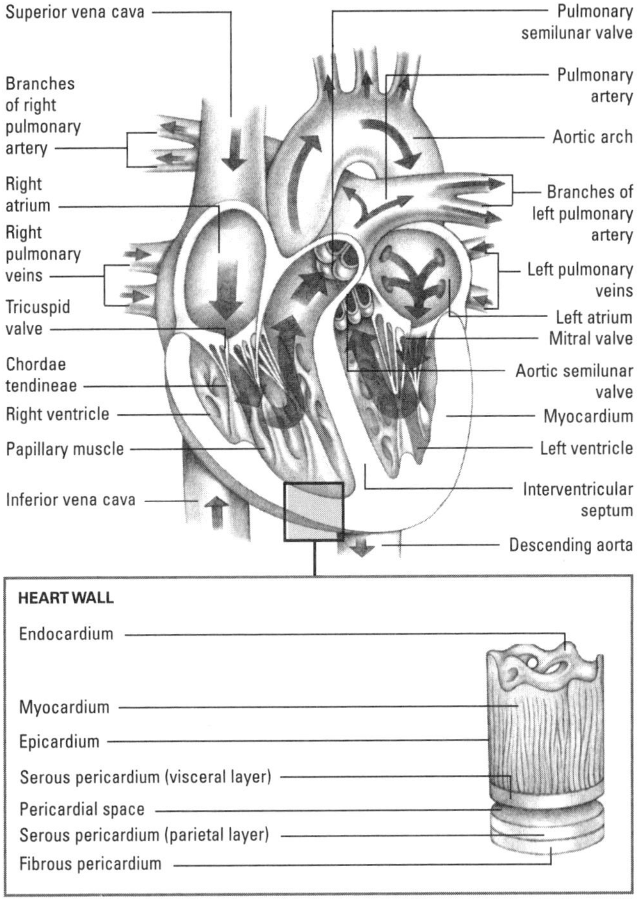

Chambers

The heart contains four hollow chambers: two *atria* (singular: *atrium*) and two ventricles. The atria, the upper chambers, are separated by the *interatrial septum.* They receive blood returning to the heart and pump blood only to the ventricles. The *right atrium* lies in front and to the right of the left atrium. It receives blood from the superior and inferior venae cavae. The *left atrium*, smaller but with thicker walls than the right atrium, forms the uppermost part of the heart's left border, extending to the left of and behind the right atrium.

The right and left ventricles, separated by the *interventricular septum,* make up the two lower chambers. Composed of highly developed musculature, the ventricles are larger and have thicker walls than the atria. The *right ventricle* pumps blood to and from the lungs. The *left ventricle,* which is larger than the right, pumps blood through all other vessels of the body. The ventricles receive blood from the atria.

Valves

Four valves keep blood flowing in one direction through the heart: two atrioventricular (AV) valves and two semilunar valves.

The *AV valves* separate the atria from the ventricles. The right AV valve, also called the *tricuspid valve*, has three triangular cusps, or leaflets. It controls the flow of blood through the right AV opening. Thin but strong *chordae tendineae* attach the cusps of the tricuspid valve to the papillary muscles in the right ventricle.

The left AV valve guards the left AV opening. Called the *mitral* or *bicuspid* valve, the left AV valve contains two cusps, a large anterior and a smaller posterior. Chordae tendineae attach these cusps to papillary muscles in the left ventricle.

The *semilunar valves* — the *pulmonary valve* and the *aortic valve* — have three cusps shaped like halfmoons. Both valves open and close in response to pressure changes brought on by ventricular contraction and blood ejection. The *pulmonary valve* guards the opening between the right ventricle and the pulmonary artery. The *aortic valve* guards the opening between the left ventricle and the aorta.

Cardiac conduction system

An electrical conduction system regulates the heartbeat, or contractions of the myocardium. This system includes the nerve fibers of the autonomic nervous system and specialized nerves and fibers in the heart. These fibers spread an impulse rapidly throughout the heart's network of muscle cells, causing a generalized, coordinated heart contraction. (See *Cardiac conduction system.*)

POINT TO REMEMBER

The autonomic nervous system increases or decreases heart activity to meet the body's metabolic needs.

Both sympathetic and parasympathetic nerves participate in the control of cardiac function. With the body at rest, the parasympathetic nervous system controls the heart through branches of the vagus nerve (cranial nerve X). Heart rate and electrical impulse propagation are slow.

In times of activity or stress, the sympathetic nervous system takes control. It stimulates the heart's nerves and fibers to fire and conduct more rapidly and makes the ventricles contract more forcefully.

Pacemaker cells

Specialized *pacemaker cells* in the myocardium allow electrical impulse conduction. Pacemaker cells control the heart rate and rhythm (a property known as *automaticity*). However, under certain circumstances, any myocardial muscle cell can control the rate and rhythm of contractions.

Normally, the *sinoatrial (SA) node* (located on the endocardial surface of the right atrium, near the superior vena cava) paces the heart. SA node firing spreads an impulse throughout the

Focus on function
Cardiac conduction system

Specialized fibers propagate electrical impulses throughout the heart's cells, causing the heart to contract. An impulse normally originates in the sinoatrial (SA) node and travels throughout the right and left atrium, causing atrial contraction. The atrioventricular (AV) node picks up the impulse before it travels through the bundle of His to the Purkinje fibers, causing the ventricles to contract.

This illustration shows the elements of the cardiac conduction system.

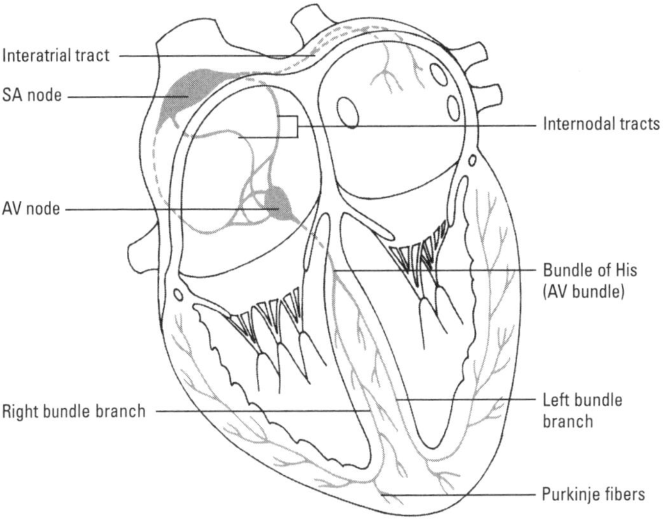

right and left atria, resulting in atrial contraction.

The *AV node* (situated low in the septal wall of the right atrium) then takes up impulse conduction. Normally, the AV node forms the only electrical connection between the atria and ventricles. Initially, it slows the impulse, delaying ventricular activity and allowing blood to fill from the atria. Then conduction speeds through the AV node and a network of fibers called the *bundle of His*, or AV bundle.

The bundle of His arises in the AV node and continues along the right interventricular septum, dividing in the ventricular septum to form the right and left bundle branches. Fibers from the bundle of His rapidly spread the impulse throughout both ventricles.

Purkinje fibers, the distal portions of the left and right bundle branches, fan across the subendocardial surface of the ventricles, from the endocardium through the myocardium. As the impulse spreads, it causes the ventricles to contract.

Cardiac cycle

The *cardiac cycle* is the period from the beginning of one heartbeat to the beginning of the next. During this cycle, electrical and mechanical events must occur in the proper sequence and to the proper degree to provide adequate blood flow to all body parts. The cardiac cycle has two phases — *systole* and *diastole*. (See *Phases of the cardiac cycle*.)

POINT TO REMEMBER
Many heart dysfunctions cause abnormal signs and symptoms that correlate with specific events in the cardiac cycle.

Systole

At the beginning of systole, the ventricles contract, increasing pressure and forcing the mitral and tricuspid valves to close. This valvular closing prevents blood from flowing backward into the atria and coincides with the first heart sound, known as S_1 (the *lub* of *lub-dub*).

As the ventricles contract, ventricular pressure builds until it exceeds the pressure in the pulmonary artery and the aorta. Then the aortic and pulmonary semilunar valves open, and the ventricles eject blood into the aorta and the pulmonary artery.

Diastole

When the ventricles empty and relax, ventricular pressure falls below that in the pulmonary artery and the aorta. At the beginning of diastole, the semilunar valves close to prevent the backflow of blood into the ventricles. This coincides with the second heart sound, known as S_2 (the *dub* of *lub-dub*).

Also during the diastole phase, the mitral and tricuspid valves open and blood starts to flow into the ventricles from the atria. When the ventricles become full near the end of this phase, the atria contract to send the remaining blood to the ventricles. This is known as the *atrial kick*. The atrial kick contributes 20% to 30% of the cardiac output. Then a new cardiac cycle begins as the heart enters systole.

Cardiac output and stroke volume

Cardiac output refers to the amount of blood the heart pumps in 1 minute. Normal cardiac output for an average-sized adult is 5 to 7 L. It's determined by the *stroke volume* — the amount of blood ejected with each heart beat multiplied by the number of beats per minute. Stroke volume, in turn, depends on three major factors — contractility, preload, and afterload.

- *Contractility* refers to the inherent ability of the myocardium to contract normally.
- *Preload* is the stretching of muscle fibers in the ventricles. This stretching results from blood volume in the ventricles at end diastole. According to *Starling's law*, the more the heart muscles stretch during diastole, the more forcefully they contract during systole.
- *Afterload* refers to the pressure the ventricular muscles must generate to overcome the higher pressure in the aorta. Normally, pressure at end diastole (end-diastolic pressure) in the left ventricle measures 5 to 10 mm Hg; in the aorta, it measures 70 to 80 mm Hg.

Blood vessels

As blood courses through the vascular system, it travels through five distinct types of blood vessels: arteries, arterioles, capillaries, venules, and veins. The structure of each type of vessel differs with its function in the cardiovascular system and the pressure exerted by the volume of blood at various sites in the system.

Blood pressure

In the aorta, vascular resistance to blood flow is almost nil and mean arterial pressure remains almost constant at 100 mm Hg. When blood reaches the arterioles, which have much smaller diameters, vascular resistance has risen enough to reduce mean blood pressure to 85 mm Hg.

When blood crosses the arterioles to the capillaries, vascular resistance causes the mean blood pressure to fall to 35 mm Hg. Blood pressure measures only about 15 mm Hg when blood begins its return to the heart. Because many veins are collapsed by pressure from the surrounding tissues, venous

Focus on function

Phases of the cardiac cycle

The cardiac cycle has two phases: systole and diastole. In the top illustration, which shows systolic events, the arrows indicate ventricular contraction, opening of the aortic and pulmonary valves, and ejection of blood into the aorta and pulmonary artery.

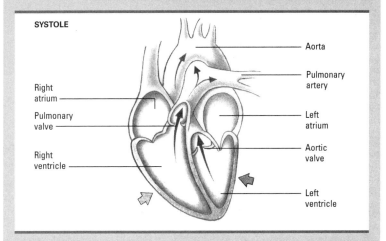

In the illustration below, which depicts diastolic events, the arrows indicate ventricular relaxation, opening of the tricuspid and mitral valves, and the flow of blood into the ventricles.

Events on the right side of the heart occur a fraction of a second after events on the left side because right-sided pressure is lower.

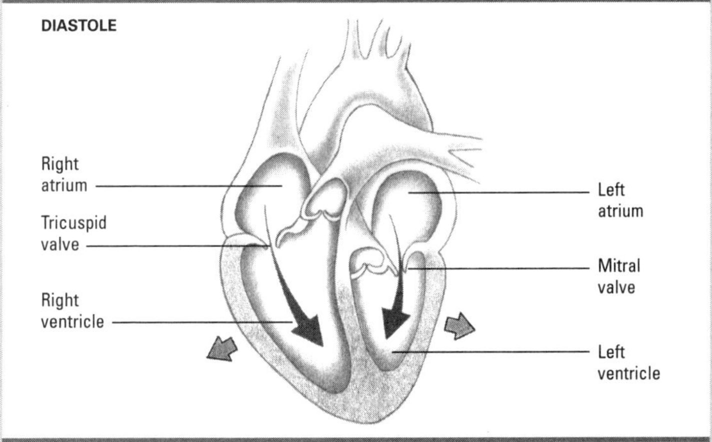

pressure continues to decline to 0 to 6 mm Hg when blood reaches the right atrium, despite a steady increase in venous diameter.

Vessel structure

Differences in blood pressure are reflected in vessel structure. Thus, *arteries* have thick, muscular walls to accommodate the flow of blood at high speeds and pressures. *Arterioles* have thinner walls than arteries; they can constrict or dilate as needed to control blood flow to the capillaries. *Capillaries,* which are microscopic, have walls composed of only a single layer of endothelial cells. *Venules* gather blood from the capillaries; their walls are thinner than those of arterioles. *Veins* have thinner walls than arteries but have larger diameters because of the low blood pressures required for venous return to the heart. (See *Blood vessels: Form follows function.*)

Blood circulation

About 60,000 miles of arteries, arterioles, capillaries, venules, and veins keep blood circulating to and from every functioning cell in the body. (See *Major blood vessels,* page 92.) This network has two branches: pulmonary circulation and systemic circulation.

In the heart itself, blood flowing through the chambers doesn't exchange oxygen and other nutrients with myocardial cells. Instead, a specialized part of the systemic circulation, the coronary circulation, supplies blood to the heart.

Pulmonary circulation

Blood travels to the lungs to pick up oxygen and release carbon dioxide as follows:

- Unoxygenated blood travels from the right ventricle through the pulmonary semilunar valve into the pulmonary arteries.
- Blood passes through progressively smaller arteries and arterioles into the capillaries of the lungs.
- Blood reaches the alveoli and exchanges carbon dioxide for oxygen.
- Oxygenated blood then returns through venules and veins to the pulmonary veins, which carry it back to the heart's left atrium.

Systemic circulation

Through the systemic circulation, blood carries oxygen and other nutrients to body cells and transports waste products for excretion.

POINT TO REMEMBER
The pumping action of the heart that forces blood through the arteries can be felt (or becomes palpable) at certain sites. This regular expansion and contraction of arteries is called the *pulse*.

The major artery — the aorta — branches into vessels that supply specific organs and areas of the body. The *left common carotid artery, left subclavian artery,* and *innominate artery* arise from the arch of the aorta and supply blood to the brain, arms, and upper chest.

As the aorta descends through the thorax and abdomen, its branches supply the organs of the GI and genitourinary systems, spinal column, and lower chest and abdominal muscles. Then the aorta divides into the *iliac arteries,* which further divide into *femoral arteries.*

As the arteries divide into smaller units, the number of vessels increases dramatically, thereby increasing the area of tissue to which blood flows (also called the *area of perfusion*).

At the end of the arterioles and the beginning of the capillaries, strong sphincters control blood flow into the tissues. These sphincters dilate to permit more flow when needed, close to shunt blood to other areas, or constrict to increase blood pressure.

Although the capillary bed contains the smallest vessels, it supplies blood to the largest area. Capillary pressure is extremely low to allow for the exchange of nutrients, oxygen, and carbon dioxide with body cells. From the capillar-

Blood vessels: Form follows function

The structure of a blood vessel depends on its function:

- An *artery's* thick, highly muscled walls allow high-speed, high-pressure flow of blood.
- An *arteriole's* thinner walls can narrow or expand to regulate blood flow to the capillaries.
- *Capillary* walls consist of one layer of endothelial cells, allowing for exchange of substances between blood and tissue cells.
- The walls of *venules,* which collect blood from the capillaries, are thinner than those of arterioles.
- *Veins* have larger diameters than arteries because they return blood to the heart. However, their walls are thinner. Valves in the veins of the neck, arms, and legs prevent venous backflow.

Three-layered walls

The walls of blood vessels have three layers, shown in the illustrations below. The *tunica adventitia,* the outermost layer, is made up of elastic fibers and connective tissue. The *tunica media,* the middle layer, consists of transverse elastic fibers and muscle fibers. The *tunica intima,* the innermost layer, is made up of endothelial cells surrounded by elastic fibers and connective tissue.

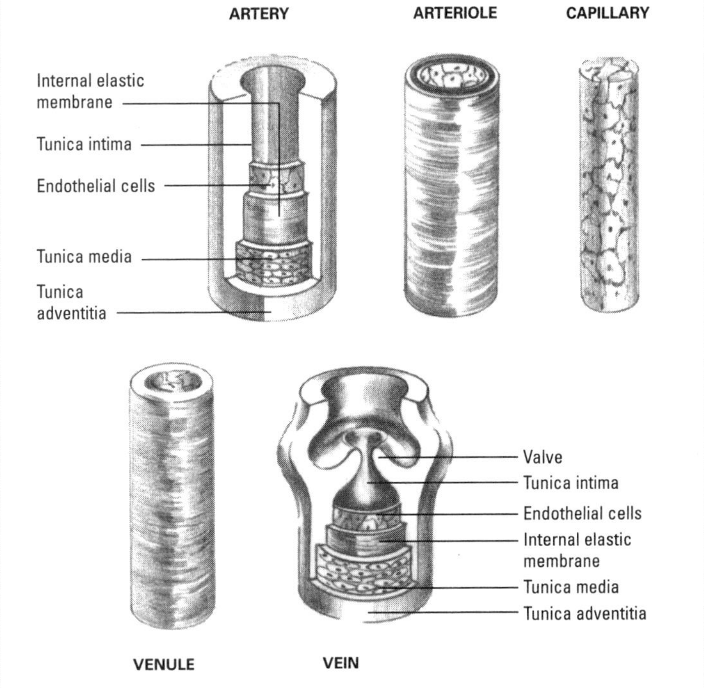

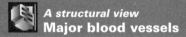

A structural view
Major blood vessels

Arteries carry blood away from the heart to the body's cells. Veins return unoxygenated blood back to the heart.

This illustration shows the body's major arteries and veins.

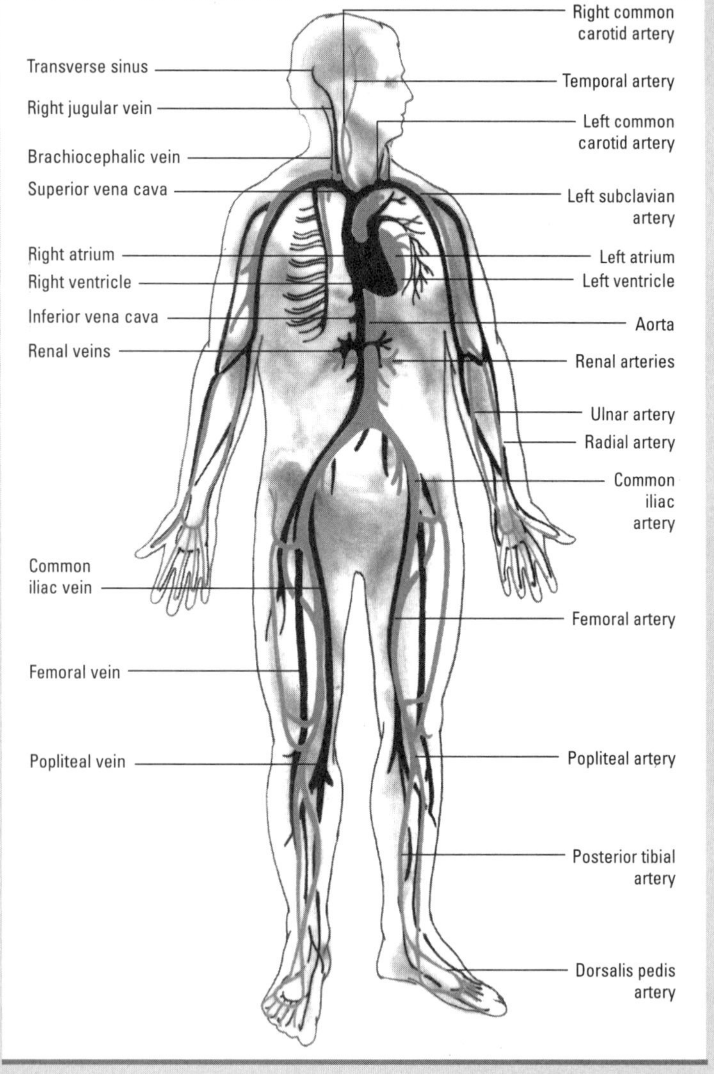

A structural view
Vessels that supply the heart

The coronary circulation involves the arterial system of blood vessels that supply oxygenated blood to the heart and the venous system that removes oxygen-depleted blood from it.

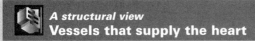

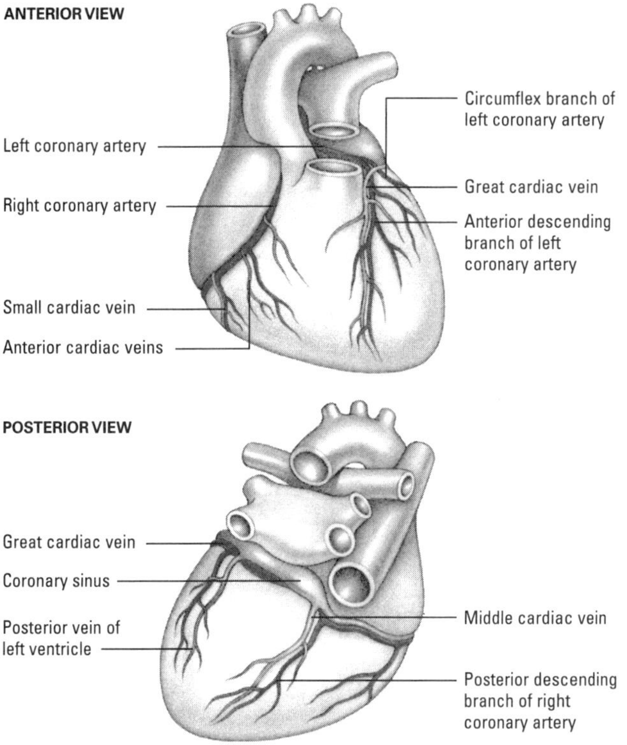

ies, blood flows into venules and, eventually, into veins.

Valves in the veins prevent blood backflow, and the pumping action of skeletal muscles aids return of blood to the heart. The veins merge until they form two main branches — the *superior vena cava* and *inferior vena cava* — that return blood to the right atrium. (See *How exercise affects the cardiovascular system*, page 94.)

Coronary circulation

The heart relies on the coronary arteries and their branches for its supply of oxygenated blood; it depends on the cardiac veins to remove oxygen-depleted blood. (See *Vessels that supply the heart.*)

How exercise affects the cardiovascular system

The cardiovascular system provides functions essential to life. The continuously pumping heart propels blood through the vessels of the body, bringing life-sustaining oxygen and nutrients to the cells and carrying away metabolic waste.

The control of blood flow is critical during exercise. The ability to sustain effort in long-distance running, for example, depends on a strong oxygen transport system. Blood must be rapidly directed to working muscles to meet the demands for oxygen and fuel. This is accomplished by increasing cardiac output from 5 L per minute to as much as 25 L per minute. This is primarily due to an increase in heart rate. The heart rate, however, can only increase up to a maximum value, which is determined mainly by the person's age.

Endurance training can reduce a person's resting heart rate. It isn't unusual to see a resting heart rate of less that 40 beats/minute in a champion endurance runner. Training, along with a reduction in one's resting heart rate, is an important sign of fitness. Endurance training also results in increased maximum cardiac output, stroke volume, and blood volume.

During left ventricular systole, blood is ejected into the aorta. During diastole, blood flows through the coronary arteries to nourish the heart muscle.

The *right coronary artery* supplies blood to the right atrium (including the SA and AV nodes), part of the left atrium, most of the right ventricle, and the inferior part of the left ventricle.

The *left coronary artery*, which splits into the *anterior descending artery* and *circumflex artery*, supplies blood to the left atrium, most of the left ventricle, and most of the interventricular septum. Many collateral arteries connect the branches of the right and left coronary arteries.

The *cardiac veins* lie superficial to the arteries. The largest vein, the *coronary sinus*, opens into the right atrium.

Most of the major cardiac veins empty into the coronary sinus, except for the anterior cardiac veins, which empty into the right atrium.

8 Hematologic system

The hematologic system consists of the blood and the bone marrow, which manufactures new blood cells through a process called *hematopoiesis*. (See *Tracing blood cell formation,* pages 96 and 97.) Blood delivers oxygen and nutrients to all tissues, removes wastes, and performs many other functions.

Blood

The body's major fluid tissue, blood consists of various formed elements, or blood cells, suspended in a fluid called *plasma*. Blood transports gases, nutrients, metabolic wastes, blood cells, immune cells, and hormones throughout the body. Although confined to the vascular system, blood constantly interacts with the body's extracellular fluid for exchange and transfer.

Formed elements in the blood include red blood cells (RBCs, or *erythrocytes*), platelets, and white blood cells (WBCs, or *leukocytes*). RBCs and platelets function entirely within blood vessels; WBCs act mainly in the tissues outside the blood vessels. (For more information on how WBCs function, see chapter 9, Immune system.)

Red blood cells

RBCs transport oxygen and carbon dioxide to and from body tissues. These minute cells lose their nuclei during maturation, developing a biconcave shape and the flexibility to travel through blood vessels of different sizes.

RBCs contain *hemoglobin*, the oxygen-carrying substance that gives blood its red color. The RBC surface carries *antigens,* which determine a person's blood group, or blood type. (See *Exercise and the hematologic system*, page 98.)

RBC replenishment

Constant circulation wears out RBCs, which have an average life span of 120 days. To maintain normal levels of RBCs, the body must manufacture billions of new cells each day.

Bone marrow releases RBCs into circulation in immature form as *reticulocytes*. The reticulocytes mature into RBCs in about 1 day. The spleen *sequesters,* or isolates, old, worn-out RBCs, removing them from circulation. The rate of reticulocyte release usually equals the rate of old RBC removal. When RBC depletion occurs (for example, with hemorrhage) the bone marrow increases reticulocyte production to maintain normal RBC levels.

Platelets

Platelets are small (2 to 4 microns in diameter), colorless, disk-shaped cytoplasmic fragments split from cells in bone marrow called megakaryocytes. These fragments, which have a life span of approximately 10 days, perform three vital functions:

- They initiate contraction of damaged blood vessels to minimize blood loss.
- They form hemostatic plugs in injured blood vessels.
- With plasma, they provide materials that accelerate blood coagulation — notably coagulation factor 3.

Coagulation factors

Designated by name and Roman numeral, *coagulation factors* circulate in

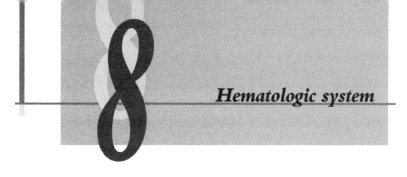

Focus on function

Tracing blood cell formation

Blood cells form and develop in the bone marrow in a process called *hematopoiesis.* This chart illustrates how five unipotential stem cells originate from a multipotential stem cell and then mature into fully formed cells that can be erythrocytes, granulocytes, agranulocytes, or platelets.

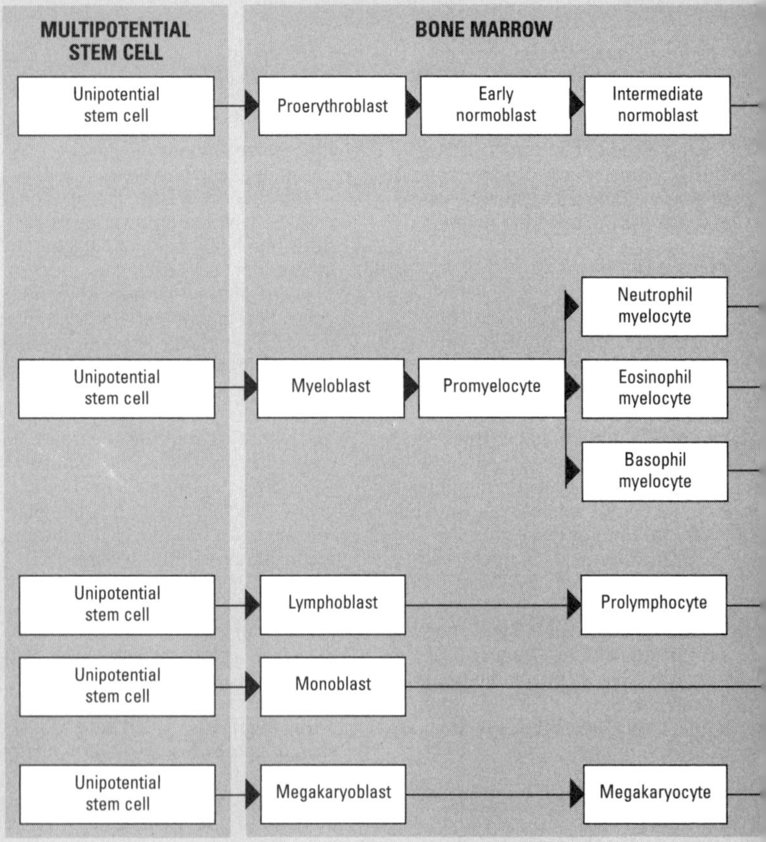

the bloodstream as precursor compounds. During coagulation, these factors are activated in a chain reaction, each one in turn activating the next coagulation factor in the chain.

- *Factor I* (also called *fibrinogen*) is a high-molecular-weight protein synthesized in the liver and converted to fibrin during the coagulation cascade.
- *Factor II* (also called *prothrombin*) is

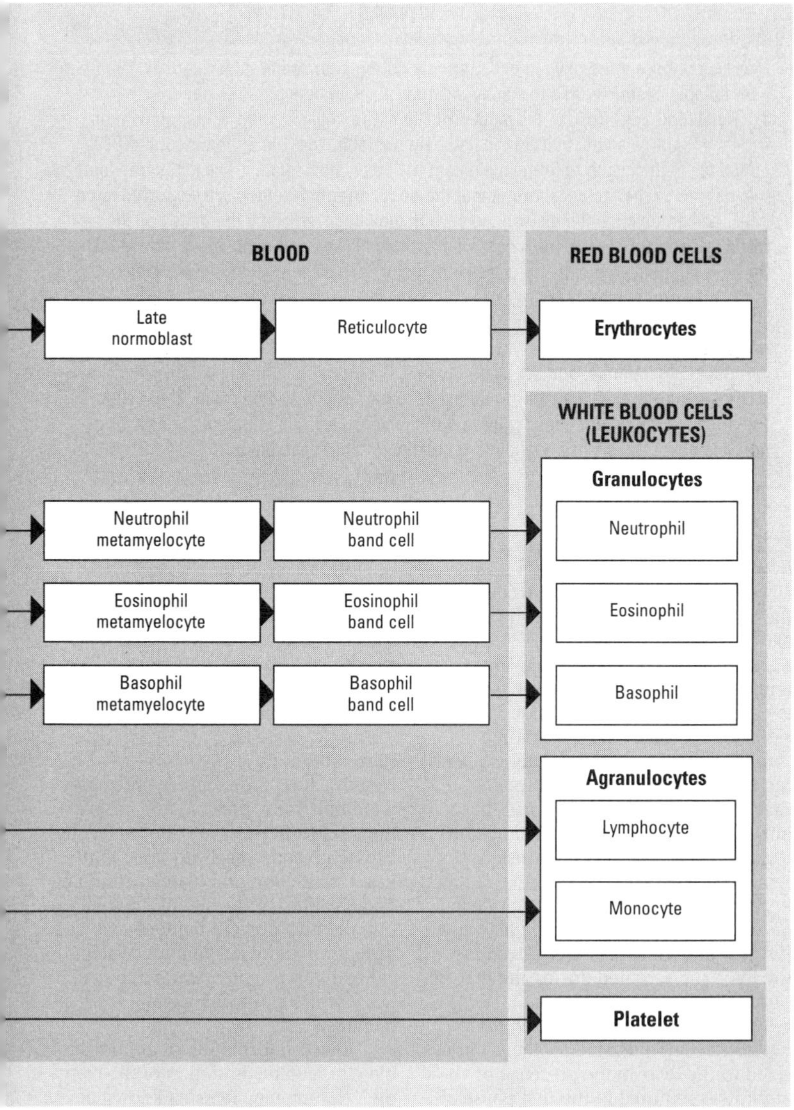

a protein synthesized in the liver in the presence of vitamin K and converted to thrombin during coagulation.

- *Factor III* (also called *tissue thromboplastin*) is released from damaged tissue; it's required in the first phase of the extrinsic cascade system.
- *Factor IV* (consisting of calcium ions) is required through the entire clotting sequence.

Exercise and the hematologic system

Muscles require more oxygen and nutrients during exercise than during rest. The hematologic system works to supply the muscles with both of these needs.

Red blood cells (RBCs), the most prevalent type of blood cells, transport oxygen from the lungs to all the cells in the body. Hemoglobin, the primary element of RBCs, combines with oxygen to form an element called oxyhemoglobin. The RBCs transport this form of oxygen to cells throughout the body. After the oxygen is transferred to the cells, hemoglobin combines with the carbon dioxide given off by the cells and the RBCs transport it back to the lungs, where some of the carbon dioxide is exhaled. This process is completed with increased efficiency during exercise because cellular demand for oxygen increases.

Plasma, the liquid portion of blood, contains nutrients, hormones, plasma proteins, and various waste materials. Plasma proteins produced by the liver aid clotting, help maintain fluid balance, and act as antibodies. Plasma also contains electrolytes, such as potassium, sodium, calcium, magnesium, bicarbonate, and chloride. These electrolytes are vital to functions required during exercise, such as muscle contraction, nerve impulse transmission, and the regulation of acid-base balance.

- *Factor V* (also called *proaccelerin,* or *labile factor*) is a protein that's synthesized in the liver and functions during the first two phases of the intrinsic and extrinsic systems.
- *Factor VI* is no longer used. The protein it was previously used to describe is now thought to be identical to factor V.
- *Factor VII* (also called *serum prothrombin conversion accelerator, stable factor,* or *proconvertin*) is a protein that's synthesized in the liver in the presence of vitamin K; it functions during the first phase of the extrinsic system.
- *Factor VIII* (also known as *antihemophilic factor* or *antihemophilic globulin*) is a protein that's synthesized in the liver and required during the first phase of the intrinsic system.
- *Factor IX* (also called *plasma thromboplastin component*), a protein synthesized in the liver in the presence of vitamin K, is required in the first phase of the intrinsic system.
- *Factor X* (also called *Stuart factor* or *Stuart-Prower factor*) is a protein that's synthesized in the liver in the presence of vitamin K; it's required in phase 1 of the intrinsic and extrinsic systems.
- *Factor XI* (plasma thromboplastin antecedent) is a protein that's synthesized in the liver and required in phase 1 of the intrinsic system.
- *Factor XII* (Hageman factor) is a protein that's required in phase 1 of the intrinsic system.
- *Factor XIII* (fibrin stabilizing factor) is a protein that's required to stabilize the fibrin strands in phase 3.

Hemostasis

Hemostasis is the complex process by which platelets, plasma, and coagulation factors interact to control bleeding. When a blood vessel ruptures, local vasoconstriction and platelet clumping (aggregation) at the site of the injury initially help prevent hemorrhage. This activation of the coagulation system, called the *extrinsic cascade,* requires release of tissue thromboplastin from the damaged cells.

However, formation of a more stable clot requires initiation of the complex clotting mechanisms known as the *intrinsic cascade system.* When this system becomes activated by endothelial vessel injury or a foreign body in the bloodstream, clotting is triggered by activating factor XII. In the final common pathway, prothrombin is converted to thrombin and fibrinogen to fibrin,

How blood clots

Through a three-part process, the circulatory system guards against excessive blood loss. In this process, vascular injury activates a complex chain of events — vasoconstriction, platelet aggregation, and coagulation — that leads to clotting. This process stops bleeding without hindering blood flow through the injured vessel.

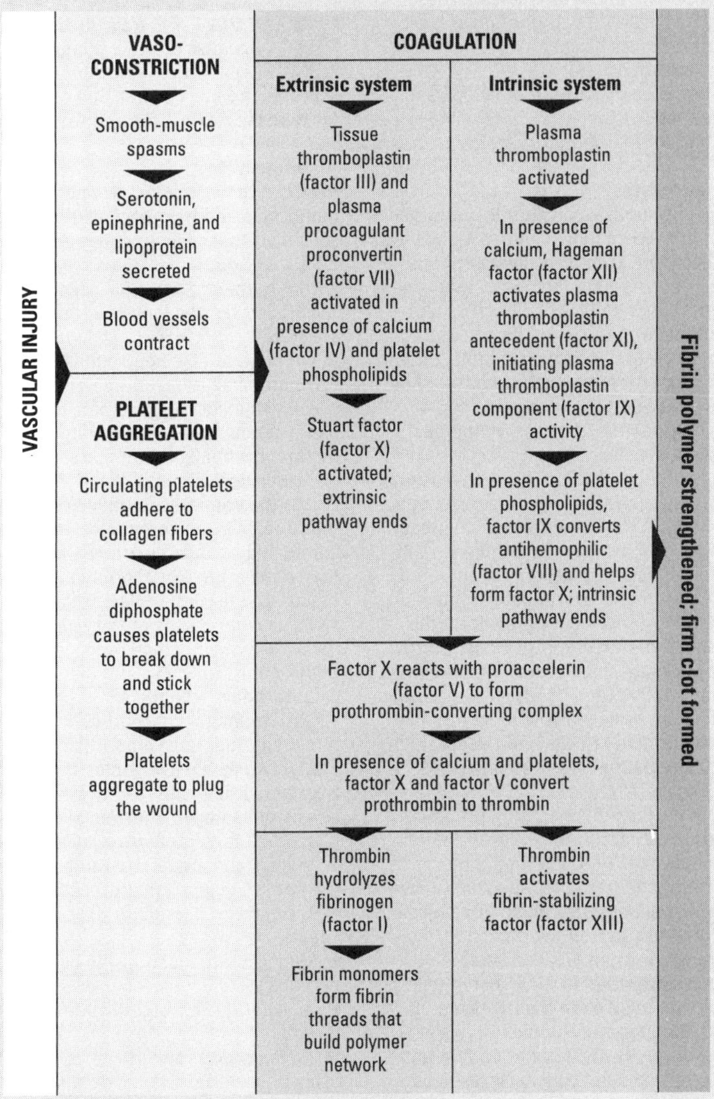
VASCULAR INJURY
VASO-CONSTRICTION
Smooth-muscle spasms
Serotonin, epinephrine, and lipoprotein secreted
Blood vessels contract
PLATELET AGGREGATION
Circulating platelets adhere to collagen fibers
Adenosine diphosphate causes platelets to break down and stick together
Platelets aggregate to plug the wound
COAGULATION
Extrinsic system
Tissue thromboplastin (factor III) and plasma procoagulant proconvertin (factor VII) activated in presence of calcium (factor IV) and platelet phospholipids
Stuart factor (factor X) activated; extrinsic pathway ends
Intrinsic system
Plasma thromboplastin activated
In presence of calcium, Hageman factor (factor XII) activates plasma thromboplastin antecedent (factor XI), initiating plasma thromboplastin component (factor IX) activity
In presence of platelet phospholipids, factor IX converts antihemophilic (factor VIII) and helps form factor X; intrinsic pathway ends
Factor X reacts with proaccelerin (factor V) to form prothrombin-converting complex
In presence of calcium and platelets, factor X and factor V convert prothrombin to thrombin
Thrombin hydrolyzes fibrinogen (factor I)
Fibrin monomers form fibrin threads that build polymer network
Thrombin activates fibrin-stabilizing factor (factor XIII)
Fibrin polymer strenghthened; firm clot formed

which is necessary for creation of a fibrin clot. (See *How blood clots,* page 99.)

White blood cells

Five types of WBCs participate in the body's defense and immune systems: neutrophils, eosinophils, basophils, monocytes, and lymphocytes. These cells are classified as *granulocytes* or *agranulocytes* based on:

- nuclear shape
- presence or absence of cytoplasmic granules
- affinity for laboratory stains or dyes.

Granulocytes

The granulocyte category includes neutrophils, eosinophils, and basophils — collectively known as *polymorphonuclear leukocytes*. All granulocytes contain a single multilobed nucleus and prominent granules in the cytoplasm. However, each cell type exhibits different properties and each is activated by different stimuli.

Neutrophils, the most numerous granulocytes, account for 55% to 70% of circulating WBCs. These phagocytic cells engulf, ingest, and digest foreign materials. They leave the bloodstream by passing through the capillary walls into the tissues (*diapedesis*) and then migrate to and accumulate at infection sites. Worn-out neutrophils form the main component of pus. Bone marrow produces their replacements, immature neutrophils called *bands*. In response to infection, bone marrow must produce many immature cells and release them into circulation, elevating the band count.

Less numerous than neutrophils, *eosinophils* account for 1% to 3% of circulating WBCs. These granulocytes also migrate from the bloodstream by diapedesis, but they do so in response to different stimuli. During allergic responses, eosinophils accumulate in loose connective tissue, where they become involved in the ingestion of antigen-antibody complexes.

Basophils, the least abundant granulocytes, usually constitute less than 1% of circulating WBCs. They possess little or no phagocytic ability. However, their cytoplasmic granules secrete *histamine* in response to certain inflammatory and immune stimuli. Histamine makes the blood vessels more permeable and eases the passage of fluids from the capillaries into body tissues.

POINT TO REMEMBER

Because of their phagocytic capabilities, granulocytes serve as the body's first line of cellular defense against foreign organisms.

Agranulocytes

WBCs in the agranulocyte category — monocytes and lymphocytes — lack specific cytoplasmic granules and have nuclei without lobes. (See *Comparing granulocytes and agranulocytes.*)

Monocytes, the largest of the WBCs, constitute only 0.6% to 9.6% of WBCs in circulation. Like neutrophils, monocytes are phagocytic and enter the tissues by diapedesis. Once outside the bloodstream, monocytes enlarge and mature, becoming tissue macrophages, or histiocytes.

As macrophages, monocytes may roam freely through the body when stimulated by inflammation. Usually, they remain immobile, populating most organs and tissues. Collectively, they serve as components of the *reticuloendothelial system*, which defends the body against infection and disposes of cell breakdown products.

Macrophages concentrate in structures that filter large amounts of body fluid, such as the liver, spleen, and lymph nodes, where they defend against invading organisms. Macrophages exhibit different physical characteristics and are referred to by different names, depending on their location:

- *Kupffer's cells* reside in the hepatic sinuses.
- *Microglia* are found in the central nervous system.
- *Alveolar macrophages* reside the lung alveoli.

Macrophages are efficient phagocytes of bacteria, cellular debris (in-

Comparing granulocytes and agranulocytes

Granulocytes—the most numerous white blood cells—include basophils, which contain cytoplasmic granules that stain readily with alkaline dyes; eosinophils, which stain with acidic dyes; and neutrophils, which are finely granular and recognizable by their multinucleated appearance.

GRANULOCYTES

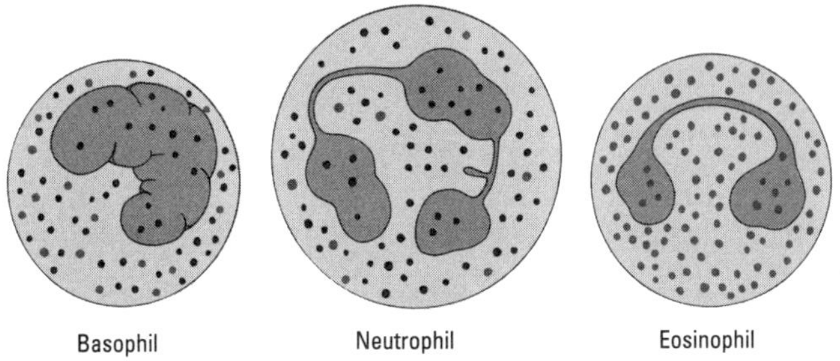

In contrast, *agranulocytes* have few, if any, granulated particles in their cytoplasm.

AGRANULOCYTES

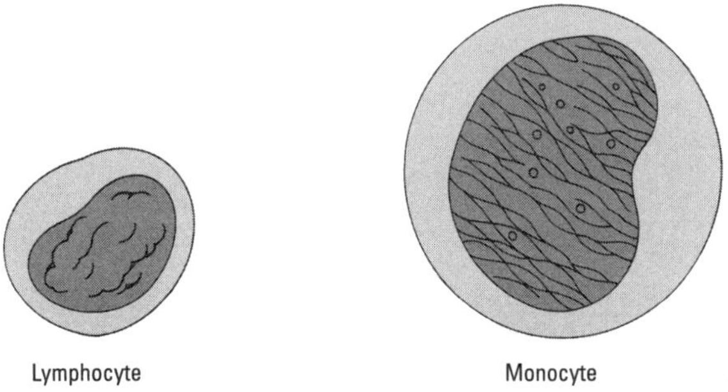

cluding worn-out neutrophils), and necrotic tissue. When mobilized at an infection site, they phagocytize cellular remnants and promote wound healing.

Lymphocytes, the smallest of the WBCs and the second most numerous (16.2% to 43%), derive from stem cells in the bone marrow. Unlike other blood cells, they mature in two different locations:

- T lymphocytes (T cells) mature in the thymus.
- B lymphocytes (B cells) usually mature in the bone marrow.

Blood groups

Blood groups are determined by the presence or absence of genetically determined antigens or agglutinogens (glycoproteins) on the surface of RBCs.

Reviewing blood type compatibility

Precise blood typing and crossmatching can prevent the transfusion of incompatible blood, which can be fatal. Usually, typing the recipient's blood and crossmatching it with available donor blood takes less than 1 hour.

Agglutinogen (antigen in red blood cells [RBCs]) and agglutinin (antibody in plasma) distinguish the four ABO blood groups. This chart shows ABO compatibility at a glance from the perspective of the recipient and the donor.

Blood group	Antibodies present in plasma	Compatible RBCs	Compatible plasma
Recipient			
O	Anti-A and Anti-B	O	O, A, B, AB
A	Anti-B	A, O	A, AB
B	Anti-A	B, O	B, AB
AB	Neither Anti-A nor Anti-B	AB, A, B, O	AB
Donor			
O	Anti-A and Anti-B	O, A, B, AB	O
A	Anti-B	A, AB	A, O
B	Anti-A	B, AB	B, O
AB	Neither Anti-A nor Anti-B	AB	AB, A, B, O

A, B, and Rh are the most clinically significant blood antigens; ABO blood groups are the most important system for classifying blood.

ABO groups

The ABO group is identified by testing for A and B antigens on the RBC surface. Each person's blood falls into one of four types:

- *Type A* blood has A antigen on its surface.
- *Type B* blood has B antigen.
- *Type AB* blood has both A and B antigens.
- *Type O* blood has neither A nor B antigen.

Plasma may contain antibodies that interact with these antigens, causing the cells to agglutinate, or combine into a mass. However, plasma can't contain antibodies to its own cell antigen, or it would destroy itself. Thus, type A blood has A antigen but no anti-A antibodies; however, it does have anti-B antibodies.

POINT TO REMEMBER

Precise blood typing and crossmatching (mixing and observing for agglutination of donor cells) are essential. This is especially crucial with blood transfusions: A donor's blood must be compatible with a recipient's or the result can be

fatal. The following blood groups are compatible:

- **type A with type A or O**
- **type B with type B or O**
- **type AB with type A, B, AB, or O**
- **type O with type O only. (See *Reviewing blood type compatibility.*)**

Rh typing

Rh typing determines whether the Rh factor is present or absent in the blood. Of the eight types of Rh antigens, only C, D, and E are common.

Normally, blood contains the Rh antigen. Blood with the Rh antigen is Rh-positive (Rh+); blood without the Rh antigen is Rh-negative (Rh–).

Anti-Rh antibodies can appear only in a person who has become sensitized. Anti-RH antibodies can appear in the blood of an Rh– person after entry of RH+ RBCs in the bloodstream—for example, from transfusion of Rh+ blood. An Rh– female who carries an Rh+ fetus may also acquire anti-RH antibodies.

9 Immune system

The immune system consists of specialized cells and structures that defend the body against invasion by harmful organisms or chemical toxins. The blood is an important part of this protective system. Although the immune system and blood are distinct entities, they're closely related. For example, their cells share a common origin in the bone marrow, and the immune system uses the bloodstream to transport its components. (For more information on blood, see chapter 8, Hematologic system.)

Components

The components of the immune system fall into three categories:

- central lymphoid organs and tissues
- peripheral lymphoid organs and tissues
- accessory lymphoid organs and tissues. (See *Organs and tissues of the immune system.*)

POINT TO REMEMBER

The term *lymphoid* is used to refer to immune system organs and tissues because these are all involved in some way in the growth, development, and dissemination of lymphocytes (white blood cells [WBCs]).

Central lymphoid organs and tissues

The *bone marrow* and *thymus* play a role in the development of B cells and T cells — the two major types of lymphocytes.

Bone marrow

The bone marrow contains *stem cells,* which may develop into any of several different cell types. Such cells are called *pluripotent*, meaning that they are capable of taking many forms. The immune system and blood cells develop from stem cells in a process called *hematopoiesis*.

Some stem cells destined to produce immune system cells serve as sources for lymphocytes, whereas others develop into phagocytes. Those that become lymphocytes are differentiated to become either *B cells* (which mature in the bone marrow) or *T cells* (which travel to the thymus and mature there). Almost all cells in the body carry a unique molecule that identifies them as coming from the same body.

B cells and T cells are distributed throughout the lymphoid organs, especially the lymph nodes and spleen. They travel through the blood system and the body's network of *lymphatic vessels*.

Thymus

In the thymus, T cells undergo a process called *T-cell education*, in which the cells are "trained" to recognize other cells from the same body (*self cells*) and distinguish them from all other cells (*nonself cells*).

Peripheral lymphoid organs and tissues

Peripheral structures include the lymph nodes, lymph, lymphatic vessels, and spleen.

Lymph nodes

The lymph nodes are small, oval-shaped structures located along a network of lymph channels. Most abundant in the head, neck, axillae, ab-

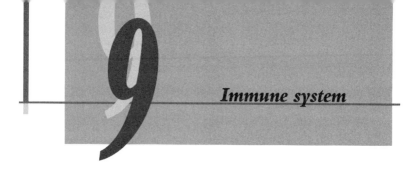

A structural view

Organs and tissues of the immune system

The immune system includes organs and tissues in which lymphocytes predominate as well as cells that circulate in peripheral blood. This illustration shows central, peripheral, and accessory lymphoid organs and tissues.

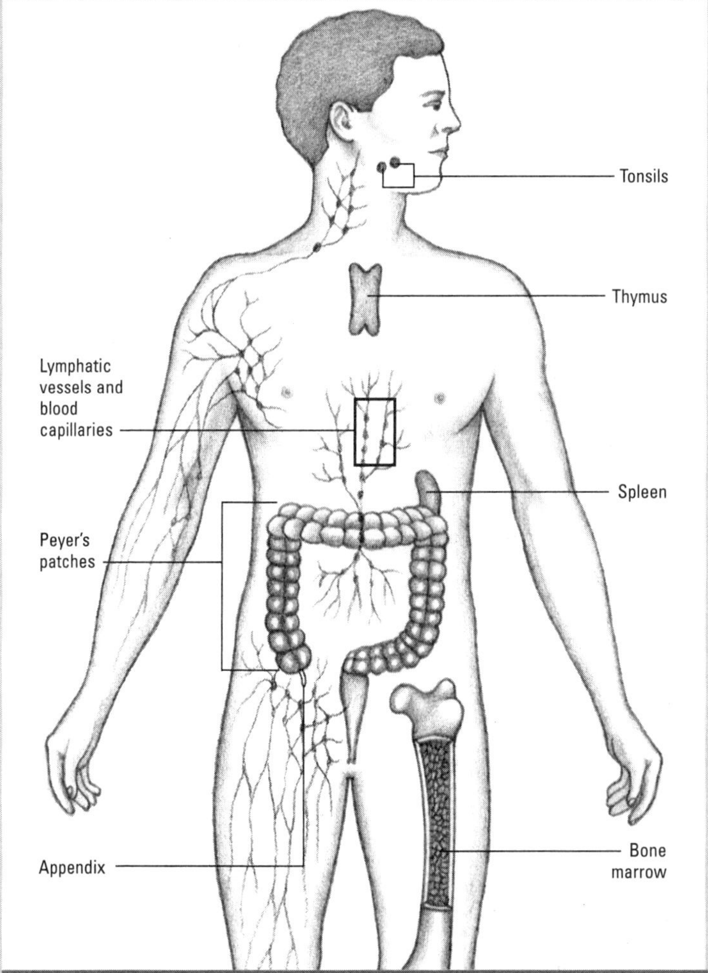

domen, pelvis, and groin, they help remove and destroy *antigens* (substances capable of triggering an immune response) that circulate in the blood and lymph.

Each lymph node is enclosed by a fibrous capsule whose bands of connective tissue extend into the node and divide it into three compartments: superficial cortex, deep cortex, and medulla:

- The *superficial cortex* contains follicles made up predominantly of B cells.
- The deep cortex and interfollicular areas consist mostly of T cells.
- The medulla contains numerous plasma cells that actively secrete *immunoglobulins*. Also called *antibodies*, immunoglobulins are large protein molecules that bind to antigens; they consist of 82% to 96% polypeptides and 4% to 18% carbohydrates.

Lymph and lymphatic vessels

Lymph is a clear fluid that bathes the body tissues. It contains a liquid portion that resembles blood plasma as well as WBCs (mostly lymphocytes and macrophages) and antigens. Collected from body tissues, lymph seeps into lymphatic vessels across the vessels' thin walls. (See *Lymphatic vessels and lymph nodes.*)

Afferent lymphatic vessels carry lymph into the subcapsular sinus of the lymph node. From there, lymph flows through cortical sinuses and smaller radial medullary sinuses. Phagocytic cells in the deep cortex and medullary sinuses attack the antigen carried in lymph. The antigen also may be trapped in the follicles of the superficial cortex.

Cleansed lymph leaves the node through *efferent* lymphatic vessels at the hilum of the node. These vessels drain into lymph node chains which, in turn, empty into large lymph vessels, or trunks, that drain into the subclavian vein of the vascular system. In most parts of the body, lymphatic vessels and lymphatic capillaries aid the function of veins and blood capillaries by draining many body tissues and enhancing blood return to the heart.

Usually, lymph travels through more than one lymph node because numerous nodes line the lymphatic channels that drain a particular region. For example, axillary nodes (located under the arm) filter drainage from the arms, and femoral nodes (in the inguinal region) filter drainage from the legs. This arrangement prevents organisms that enter peripheral areas from migrating unchallenged to central areas. Lymph nodes also serve as primary sources of circulating lymphocytes, which provide specific immune responses.

Spleen

Located in the left upper quadrant of the abdomen beneath the diaphragm, the *spleen* is a dark red, oval structure roughly the size of a fist. It's posterior and inferior to the stomach. Bands of connective tissue from the dense fibrous capsule surrounding the spleen extend into the spleen's interior.

The interior, called the *splenic pulp,* contains white and red pulp. White pulp contains compact masses of lymphocytes surrounding branches of the splenic artery. Red pulp consists of a network of blood-filled sinusoids, supported by a framework of reticular fibers and mononuclear phagocytes along with some lymphocytes, plasma cells, and monocytes.

The spleen has several functions:

- Its phagocytes engulf and break down worn-out red blood cells (RBCs), causing release of hemoglobin, which then breaks down into its components. These phagocytes also selectively retain and destroy damaged or abnormal RBCs and cells with large amounts of abnormal hemoglobin.
- The spleen filters and removes bacteria and other foreign substances that enter the bloodstream; these substances are promptly removed by splenic phagocytes.
- Splenic phagocytes interact with lymphocytes to initiate an immune response.
- The spleen stores blood and 20% to 30% of platelets.

Lymphatic vessels and lymph nodes

Lymphatic tissues are connected by a network of thin-walled drainage channels called lymphatic vessels. Resembling veins, the lymphatic vessels carry lymph into the lymph node. Lymph filters slowly through the node and is collected into efferent lymphatic channels.

Lymphatic capillaries are located throughout most of the body. Wider than blood capillaries, they permit interstitial fluid to flow in but not out.

The bottom illustration provides an inside view of a lymph node.

LYMPHATIC VESSELS AND CAPILLARIES

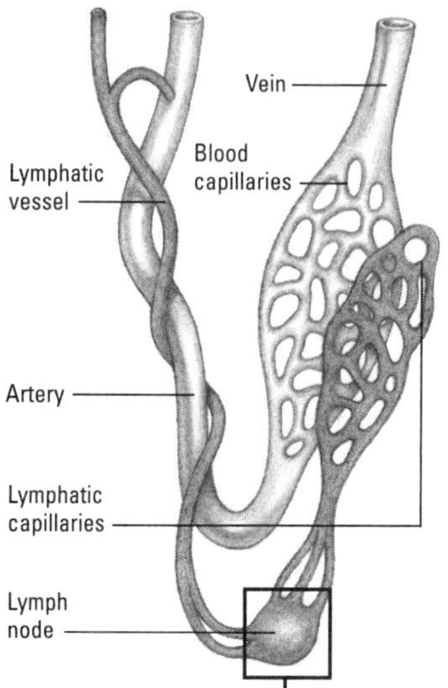

LYMPH NODE

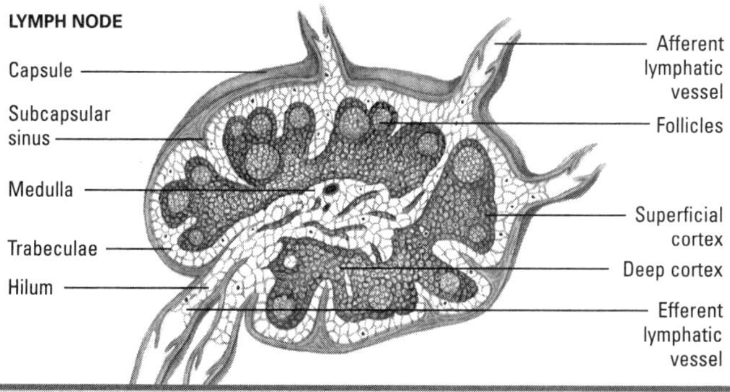

Accessory lymphoid organs and tissues

The tonsils, adenoids, appendix, thymus, and Peyer's patches remove foreign debris in much the same way lymph nodes do. They're located in food and air passages — areas where microbial access is more likely to occur.

Thymus

The *thymus* is a two-lobed mass of lymphoid tissue located above the base of the heart in the mediastinum. It helps to form T lymphocytes in the fetus and infant for several months after birth. After this time, it has no function in the body's immunity. It gradually undergoes atrophy until only a remnant persists in older adults.

Immunity

Immunity refers to the body's capacity to resist invading organisms and toxins and thereby prevent tissue and organ damage. The immune system is designed to recognize, respond to, and eliminate antigens, including bacteria, fungi, viruses, and parasites. It also preserves the body's internal environment by scavenging dead or damaged cells and by patrolling for antigens.

To perform these functions efficiently, the immune system uses three basic strategies:

- protective surface phenomena
- general host defenses
- specific immune responses.

Protective surface phenomena

Strategically placed physical, chemical, and mechanical barriers work to prevent the entry of potentially harmful organisms.

Skin and mucous membranes

Intact and healing skin and mucous membranes provide the first line of defense against microbial invasion, preventing attachment of microorganisms. Skin desquamation (normal cell turnover) and low pH further impede bacterial colonization. Seromucous surfaces, such as the conjunctivae of the eyes and the oral mucous membranes, are protected by antibacterial substances — for instance, the enzyme *lysozyme*, found in tears, saliva, and nasal secretions.

Respiratory defenses

In the respiratory system, nasal hairs and turbulent airflow through the nostrils filter foreign materials. Nasal secretions contain an immunoglobulin that discourages microbe adherence. Also, a mucous layer that's continuously sloughed off and replaced, lines the respiratory tract. Coupled with ciliary action, this mucous layer traps and expels inhaled particles and microbes before they can damage delicate alveolar tissues.

POINT TO REMEMBER
The respiratory system needs special protection because microorganisms can easily enter it from the outside.

GI defenses

In the GI tract, bacteria are mechanically removed by saliva, swallowing, peristalsis, and defecation. What's more, the low pH of gastric secretions is *bactericidal* (bacteria-killing), rendering the stomach virtually free from live bacteria.

Resident bacteria — organisms that normally live in harmony with the body without causing disease — prevent colonization by other microorganisms, protecting the remainder of the GI system through a process known as *colonization resistance.*

Urinary tract defenses

The urinary system is sterile except for the distal end of the urethra and the urinary meatus. Urine flow, low urine pH, immunoglobulin and, in men, the bactericidal effects of prostatic fluid work together to impede bacterial colonization. A series of sphincters also inhibits bacterial migration.

General host defenses

When an antigen does penetrate the skin or mucous membrane, the immune system launches nonspecific cellular responses in an effort to identify and remove the invader. These responses differentiate self from nonself but can't distinguish among specific antigens or respond to them differently.

Inflammatory response

The first of the nonspecific responses against an antigen, the inflammatory response involves vascular and cellular changes that eliminate dead tissue, microorganisms, toxins, and inert foreign matter. Soon after microorganisms invade damaged tissue, basophils release heparin, histamine, and kinins — substances that promote vasodilation and

Focus on function
Understanding the inflammatory response

The flowchart below outlines the sequence of events that occur when the body responds to inflammation.

Microorganisms invade damaged tissue.

↓

Basophils release heparin. Histamine and kinin production occurs.

↓

Vasodilation occurs along with increased capillary permeability.

↓

Blood flow increases to the affected tissues and fluid collects within them.

↓

Neutrophils accumulate at the invasion site and engulf and destroy microorganisms.

↓

Tissue repair occurs.

increase capillary permeability. Blood flow to the affected tissues then increases, and fluid collects in them.

Granulocytes (predominantly neutrophils) promptly flock to the invasion site, where they engulf and destroy the microorganisms, foreign materials, and debris from dying cells. These actions promote tissue repair.

POINT TO REMEMBER
Inflammation causes four characteristic signs and symptoms: heat, redness, swelling, and pain. (See *Understanding the inflammatory response.*)

Phagocytosis
Phagocytosis occurs after inflammation or in chronic infections. In this nonspecific response, neutrophils and macrophages engulf, digest, and dispose of the antigen.

Macrophages and lymphocytes move to the site of insult and infection by two means:

- *diapedesis*, or blood cell migration from the intravascular compartment to tissue sites
- *chemotaxis*, or movement toward a chemical attractor.

Specific immune responses
All foreign substances elicit the same response in general host defenses. In contrast, particular microorganisms or molecules activate specific immune responses and initially can involve specialized sets of immune cells. Such specific responses, classified as either *humoral immunity* or *cell-mediated*

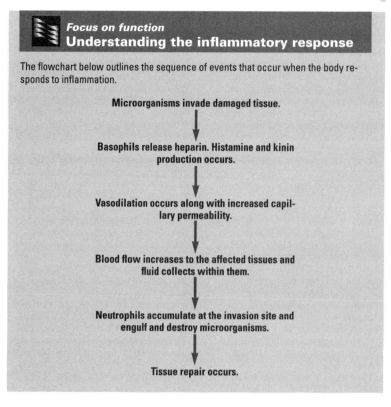

immunity, are produced by lymphocytes (B cells and T cells).

Humoral immunity

In humoral immunity, an invading antigen causes B cells to divide and differentiate into plasma cells. Each plasma cell, in turn, produces and secretes into the bloodstream large amounts of antigen-specific immunoglobulins.

Each of the five types of immunoglobulins — immunoglobulin A (IgA), IgD, IgE, IgG, and IgM — serves a particular function:

- IgA, IgG, and IgM guard against viral and bacterial invasion.
- IgD acts as an antigen receptor of B cells.
- IgE causes an allergic response.

Immunoglobulins have a special molecular structure that creates a Y shape. The crook of the Y is designed to attach to a particular antigen; the stem enables the immunoglobulin to link with other structures in the immune system. (See *Understanding immunoglobulin structure.*)

Depending on the antigen, immunoglobulins may work in one of several ways:

- They may disable certain bacteria by linking with toxins that the bacteria produce; these immunoglobulins are called *antitoxins*.
- They may coat (*opsonize*) bacteria, making them targets for scavenging by phagocytosis. (See *How macrophages accomplish phagocytosis,* page 112.)
- Most commonly, they link to antigens, causing the immune system to produce and circulate enzymes called *complement*.

After the body's initial exposure to an antigen, a time lag occurs during which little or no antibody can be detected. During this time, the B cell recognizes the antigen and the sequence of division, differentiation, and antibody formation begins. This *primary antibody response* occurs 4 to 10 days after first-time antigen exposure. During this response, immunoglobulin levels increase and then quickly dissipate, and IgM antibodies form.

Subsequent exposure to the same antigen initiates a *secondary antibody response.* In this response, memory B cells manufacture antibodies (now mainly IgG), achieving peak levels in 1 to 2 days. These elevated levels persist for months and then fall slowly. Thus, the secondary antibody response is faster, more intense, and more persistent than the primary response. Also, it intensifies with each subsequent exposure to the same antigen.

After the antibody reacts to the antigen, an *antigen-antibody complex* forms. The complex serves several functions. First, a macrophage processes the antigen and presents it to antigen-specific B cells. Then the antibody activates the *complement system*, causing an enzymatic cascade that destroys the antigen.

Complement system

The activated complement system, which bridges humoral and cell-mediated immunity, attracts phagocytic neutrophils and macrophages to the antigen site. Indispensable to the humoral immune response, the complement system consists of about 25 enzymes that "complement" the work of antibodies by destroying bacteria, aiding phagocytosis, or destroying bacteria cells (through puncture of their cell membranes). Complement also helps eliminate antigen-antibody complexes.

Complement proteins travel in the bloodstream in an inactive form. When the first complement substance is triggered (typically by an antibody interlocked with an antigen), it sets in motion a ripple effect. As each component is activated in turn, it acts on the next component in a sequence of carefully controlled steps called the *complement cascade.*

Activation of the complement cascade follows either the *classic pathway,* initiated by antigen-antibody complexes, or the *alternative pathway,* triggered by IgA, some IgG molecules, and certain polysaccharides, lipopolysaccharides, and trypsinlike enzymes.

Both pathways lead to the same result: creation of the *membrane attack*

Understanding immunoglobulin structure

All immunoglobulin molecules consist of two identical light polypeptide chains and two identical heavy polypeptide chains that are connected by disulfide bonds to form a Y shape. The molecules are divided into classes and subclasses based mainly on the type of heavy polypeptide chain.

Five types of heavy chains and two types of light chains exist. These chains are divided into a constant region and a variable region (V), with antigen-binding sites located on the variable region. The enzyme papain separates the immunoglobulin G (IgG) molecule's heavy chain into two parts at the hinge region, creating one Fc (crystallizable) fragment and two Fab (antigen-binding) fragments.

The five different classes of immunoglobulins (IgG, IgA, IgM, IgD, and IgE) differ in size, charge, amino acid composition, and carbohydrate content. IgG, IgD, and IgE have two antigen-binding sites per molecule; IgM has 10 sites per molecule; and dimeric class IgA (usually found in secretions) has four combining sites per molecule. IgG, IgD, and IgE exist only as single, four-chain units; IgM exists as a pentamer with five connected four-chain units; and IgA exists in both single- and multiple-unit forms.

BASIC IMMUNOGLOBULIN STRUCTURE (IgG, IgD, IgE)

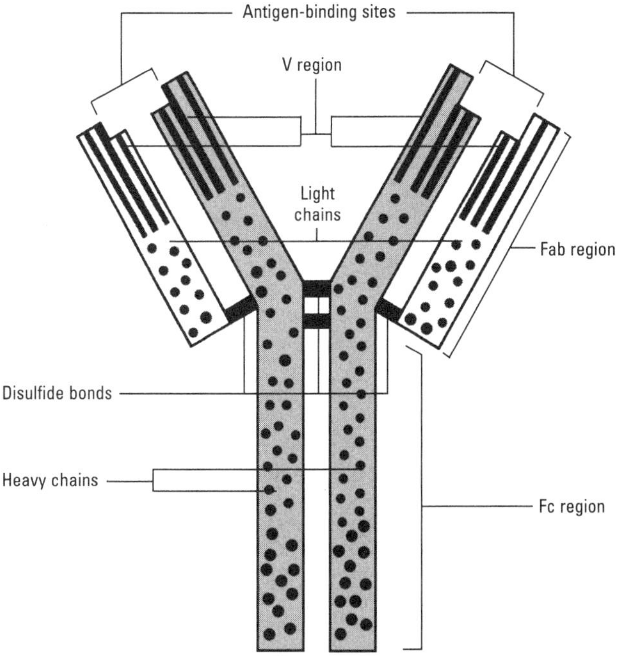

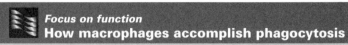

Focus on function

How macrophages accomplish phagocytosis

Microorganisms and other antigens that invade the skin and mucous membranes are removed by phagocytosis, a defense mechanism carried out by macrophages (mononuclear leukocytes) and neutrophils (polymorphonuclear leukocytes). Here's how macrophages accomplish phagocytosis.

Chemotaxis
Chemotactic factors attract macrophages to the antigen site.

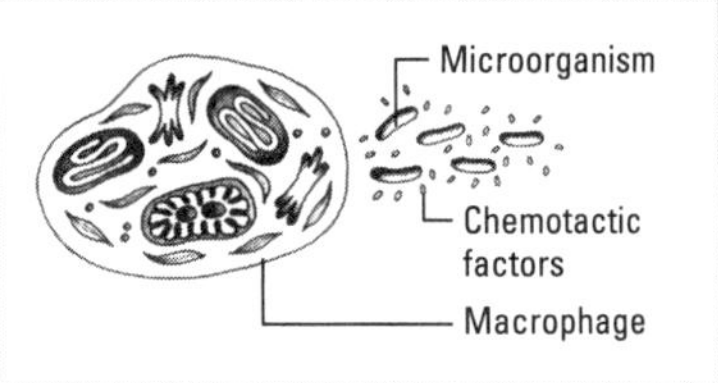

Opsonization
Antibody (immunoglobulin G) or complement fragment coats the microorganism, enhancing macrophage binding to this antigen.

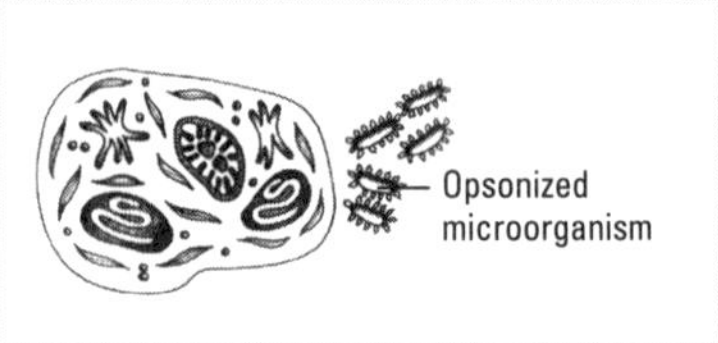

Ingestion
The macrophage extends its membrane around the opsonized microorganism, engulfing it within a vacuole (phagosome).

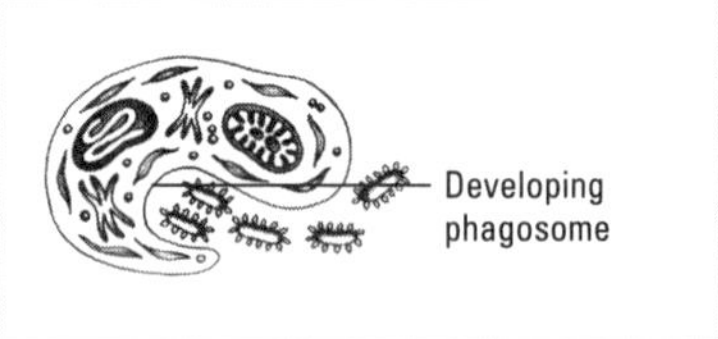

Digestion
As the phagosome shifts away from the cell periphery, it merges with lysosomes, forming a phagolysosome, where antigen destruction occurs

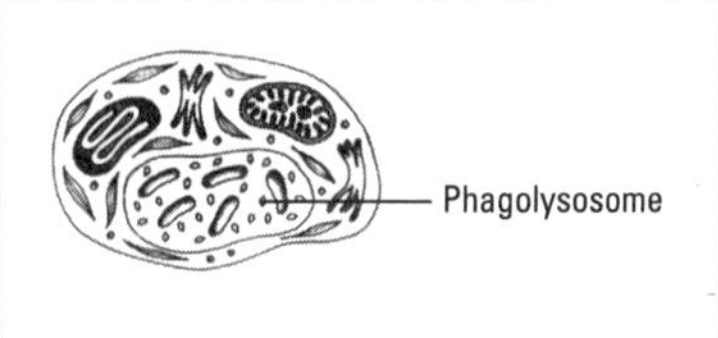

Release
Once digestion is complete, the macrophage expels digestive debris—including lysozymes, prostaglandins, complement components, and interferon—that continue to mediate the immune response.

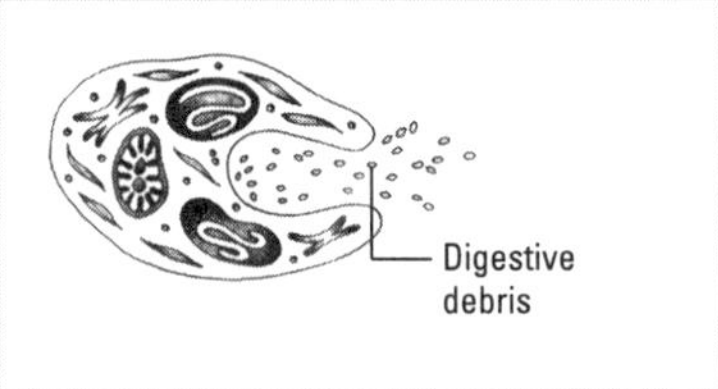

Understanding immune disorders

An immune disorder may take the form of a hypersensitivity disorder, autoimmune disorder, or immunodeficiency.

Hypersensitivity disorders

▸ An exaggerated or inappropriate immune response may lead to various hypersensitivity disorders. Such disorders are classified as Type I through Type IV depending on which immune system activity causes tissue damage, although some overlap exists.

– Type I disorders are anaphylactic (immediate, atopic, immunoglobulin E [IgE]-mediated reaginic) reactions. Examples of Type I disorders include systemic anaphylaxis, hay fever (seasonal allergic rhinitis), reactions to stinging insects, some food and drug reactions, some causes of urticaria, and infantile eczema.
– Type II disorders are cytotoxic (cytolytic, complement-dependent cytotoxicity) reactions. Examples of Type II disorders include Goodpasture's syndrome, autoimmune hemolytic anemia, transfusion reactions, hemolytic disease of the newborn, myasthenia gravis, and some drug reactions.
– Type III disorders are immune complex disease reactions. Examples of Type III disorders may be associated with such infections as hepatitis B and bacterial endocarditis; cancers, in which a serum sickness-like syndrome may occur; and autoimmune disorders such as systemic lupus erythematosus. This hypersensitivity reaction may also follow drug or serum therapy.
– Type IV disorders are delayed (cell-mediated) hypersensitivity reactions. Type IV disorders include tuberculin reactions, contact hypersensitivity, and sarcoidosis.

Autoimmune disorders

Autoimmune disorders are marked by an abnormal tissue response to oneself. Autoimmunity leads to a sequence of tissue reactions and damage that may produce diffuse, systemic signs and symptoms. Among the autoimmune disorders are rheumatoid arthritis, juvenile rheumatoid arthritis, psoriatic arthritis, ankylosing spondylitis, Sjögren's syndrome, and lupus erythematous.

Immunodeficiency

Immunodeficiency disorders are caused by an absent or depressed immune response in various forms. Immunodeficiency disorders include X-linked infantile hypogammaglobulinemia, common variable immunodeficiency, DiGeorge's syndrome, acquired immunodeficiency syndrome, chronic granulomatous disease, ataxiatelangiectasia, severe combined immunodeficiency disease, and complement deficiencies.

complex. Inserted into the membrane of the target cell, this complex creates a channel through which fluids and molecules flow in and out. The target cell then swells and eventually bursts.

By-products of the complement cascade also produce other effects, including:

- inflammatory response (resulting from release of the contents of mast cells and basophils)
- stimulation and attraction of neutrophils, which participate in phagocytosis
- coating of target cells by C3b (an inactivated fragment of the complement protein C3), which makes them attractive to phagocytes.

Too much may be harmful

Studies have shown that a balanced training program of exercise and rest boosts the immune system. However, too much exercise can be harmful, dramatically increasing the risk of upper respiratory infections. The stress of strenuous exercise transiently suppresses immune function. This suppression of immune function can provide opportunities for infection through a variety of infectious diseases, especially viral illnesses such as the common cold. If an athlete continuously overtrains, the immune system weakens, leading to frequent illness and injury.

Cell-mediated immunity

Cell-mediated immunity protects the body against bacterial, viral, and fungal infections and provides resistance against transplanted cells and tumor cells. In this immune response, a macrophage processes the antigen, which is then presented to T cells. Some T cells become sensitized and destroy the antigen; others release *lymphokines*, which activate macrophages that destroy the antigen. Sensitized T cells then travel through the blood and lymphatic systems, providing ongoing surveillance in their quest for specific antigens. (See *Too much may be harmful.*)

Immune disorders

Because of the complexity of immune disorders, the processes involved in host defense and immune response may malfunction. When the body's defenses are exaggerated, misdirected, or either absent or depressed, the result may be a hypersensitivity disorder, autoimmunity, or immunodeficiency, respectively. (See *Understanding immune disorders*, page 113.)

10 Respiratory system

The respiratory system consists of the upper and lower respiratory tracts, the lungs, and the thoracic cage. In addition to maintaining the exchange of oxygen and carbon dioxide in the lungs and tissues, the respiratory system helps to regulate the body's acid-base balance.

Any change in the respiratory system affects every other body system. Conversely, changes in other body systems may compromise the lungs' ability to provide oxygen to body tissues.

Upper respiratory tract

The upper respiratory tract consists primarily of the nose, mouth, nasopharynx, oropharynx, laryngopharynx, and larynx. (See *Structures of the respiratory system,* page 116.) Besides warming and humidifying inhaled air, these structures provide for taste, smell, and the chewing and swallowing of food.

POINT TO REMEMBER

In the upper respiratory tract, involuntary defense mechanisms — sneezing, coughing, gagging, and spasms — help to protect the respiratory system from infection and to prevent foreign body inhalation.

Nostrils and nasal passages

Air enters the body through the nostrils (nares), where small hairs (vibrissae) filter out dust and large foreign particles. Air then passes into the two nasal passages, which are separated by the septum. Cartilage forms the anterior walls of the nasal passages; bony structures (conchae or turbinates) form the posterior walls.

The conchae warm and humidify air before it passes into the nasopharynx. Their mucus layer also traps finer foreign particles, which the cilia carry to the pharynx to be swallowed.

Sinuses and pharynx

The four *paranasal sinuses*, located in the frontal, sphenoid, and maxillary bones, drain through the meatuses near the conchae; the sinuses also provide speech resonance. Air then passes from the nasal cavity into the muscular *nasopharynx* through the *choanae*, a pair of posterior openings in the nasal cavity that constantly remain open.

The *oropharynx*, the posterior wall of the mouth, connects the nasopharynx and the *laryngopharynx*. The laryngopharynx extends to the esophagus and larynx.

Larynx

The *larynx*, which contains the vocal cords, connects the pharynx with the trachea. Muscles and cartilage form the walls of the larynx, including the large, shield-shaped thyroid cartilage situated just under the jawline.

POINT TO REMEMBER

During swallowing, the larynx is protected by the epiglottis, which is made of flexible cartilage that bends to close the larynx to swallowed substances.

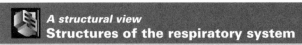

A structural view
Structures of the respiratory system

The respiratory system consists of the organs responsible for external respiration and gas exchange within the lungs.

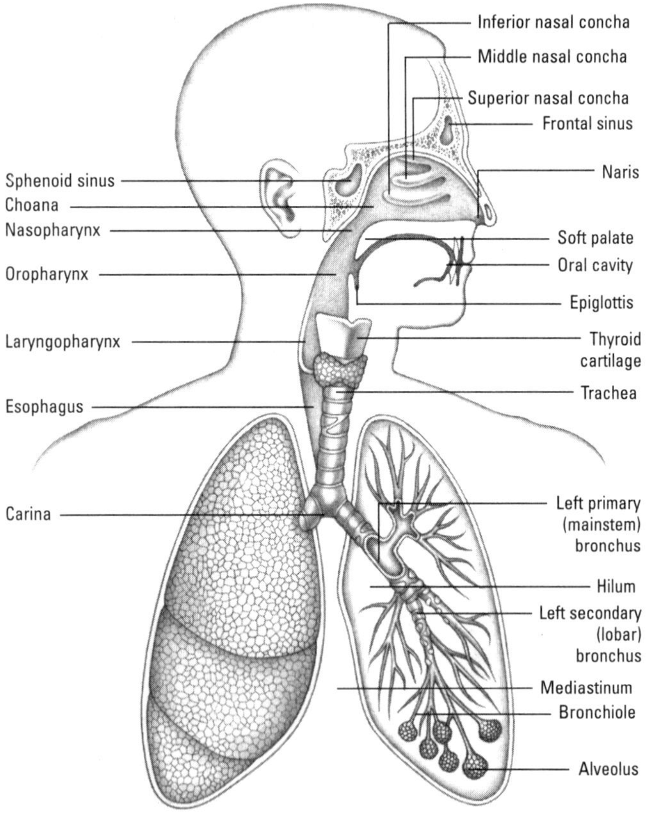

Lower respiratory tract

The lower respiratory tract consists of the trachea, bronchi, and lungs. (See *Structures of the respiratory system.*) Functionally, the lower tract is subdivided into the conducting airways and the *acinus*, which serves as the area of gas exchange. A mucous membrane containing hairlike *cilia* lines the lower tract. The constant movement of mucus by cilia cleans the tract and carries foreign matter upward for swallowing or expectoration.

Conducting airways

The conducting airways are the trachea and the primary, lobar, and segmental bronchi.

Trachea

The tubular *trachea* lies half in the neck and half in the thorax. About 5″ (13 cm) long, the trachea extends from the cricoid cartilage at the top to the *carina* (also called the *tracheal bifurcation*), a ridge-shaped structure at the level of the sixth or seventh thoracic vertebra. C-shaped cartilage rings reinforce and protect the trachea, preventing its collapse.

Bronchi

The *primary bronchi* (mainstem bronchi) begin at the *carina*. The *right mainstem bronchus* — shorter, wider, and more vertical than the left — supplies air to the right lung; the left mainstem bronchus delivers air to the left lung.

The mainstem bronchi divide into the five *lobar bronchi* (secondary bronchi) and, along with blood vessels, nerves, and lymphatics, enter the pleural cavities and the lungs at the *hilum*. Located behind the heart, the hilum is a slit on the lung's medial surface where the lungs are anchored.

Each lobar bronchus enters a lobe in each lung. Within its lobe, each of the lobar bronchi branches into *segmental bronchi* (tertiary bronchi). The segments continue to branch into smaller and smaller bronchi, finally branching into bronchioles.

The larger bronchi consist of cartilage, smooth muscle, and epithelium. As the bronchi become smaller, they lose first cartilage and then smooth muscle until, finally, the smallest bronchioles consist of just a single layer of epithelial cells.

Acinus

Each bronchiole branches into a *lobule*. The lobule includes *terminal bronchioles* and the *acinus* — the chief respiratory unit for gas exchange.

Respiratory bronchioles

Within the acinus, terminal bronchioles branch into yet smaller *respiratory bronchioles*. The respiratory bronchioles feed directly into *alveoli* at sites along their walls.

Alveoli

The respiratory bronchioles eventually become *alveolar ducts*, which terminate in clusters of capillary-swathed alveoli called *alveolar sacs*. Gas exchange takes place throughout the thin-walled respiratory bronchioles and alveoli.

Alveolar walls contain two basic epithelial cell types. Type I cells, the most abundant, are thin, flat, squamous cells across which gas exchange occurs. Type II cells secrete *surfactant*, a substance that coats the alveolus and promotes gas exchange by lowering surface tension.

Respiratory membrane

The alveolar cells, together with a tiny interstitial space, capillary basement membrane, and endothelial cells in the capillary wall, make up the *respiratory membrane* that separates the alveolus and capillary.

The entire respiratory membrane measures less than 1 micron thick. Any increase in its thickness or decrease in surfactant production reduces the rate of gas diffusion across the membrane.

Lungs and accessory structures

The cone-shaped lungs hang suspended in the right and left pleural cavities, straddling the heart. They're freely movable except at the hilum, where they're anchored by root and pulmonary ligaments.

The right lung is shorter, broader, and larger than the left. It has three lobes and handles 55% of gas exchange. The left lung has only two lobes; it shares the left side of the thoracic space with the heart. Each lung's concave base rests on the diaphragm; the apex extends about 1/4″ (1 cm) above the first rib.

Pleura and pleural cavities

The pleura — the membrane that totally encloses the lung — is composed of a visceral layer and a parietal layer. The *visceral pleura* hugs the entire lung surface, including the areas between the lobes. The *parietal pleura* lines the inner surface of the chest wall and upper surface of the diaphragm, then doubles back around the mediastinum and joins the visceral layer at the lung root.

The *pleural cavity* — the tiny area between the visceral and parietal pleural layers — contains a thin film of serous fluid. This fluid has two functions:

- to lubricate the pleural surfaces so that they slide smoothly against each other as the lungs expand and contract
- to create a bond between the layers that causes the lungs to move with the chest wall during breathing.

Thoracic cavity

The *thoracic cavity* is an area within the chest wall surrounded by the diaphragm (below), the scalene muscles and fasciae of the neck (above) and, around the circumference, by the ribs, intercostal muscles, vertebrae, sternum, and ligaments.

Mediastinum

The *mediastinum* — the space between the lungs — contains the following organs and structures:

- heart and pericardium
- thoracic aorta
- pulmonary artery and veins
- vena cavae and azygos veins
- thymus, lymph nodes, and vessels
- trachea, esophagus, and thoracic duct
- vagus, cardiac, and phrenic nerves.

Thoracic cage

Composed of bone and cartilage, the *thoracic cage* supports and protects the lungs and permits them to expand and contract.

Posterior thoracic cage

The vertebral column and 12 pairs of ribs form the posterior portion of the thoracic cage.

POINT TO REMEMBER
Certain landmarks help to identify specific vertebrae. In 90% of patients, the most prominent vertebra on a flexed neck is the seventh cervical vertebra (C7); for the remaining 10%, it's the first thoracic vertebra (T1). Thus, to locate a specific vertebra, count down along the vertebrae from T1.

The ribs, which form the major portion of the thoracic cage, extend from the thoracic vertebrae toward the anterior thorax. Like the vertebrae, they're numbered from top to bottom.

Anterior thoracic cage

The anterior thoracic cage consists of the *manubrium, sternum, xiphoid process*, and ribs. It protects the mediastinal organs that lie between the right and left pleural cavities. Ribs 1 through 7 attach directly to the sternum; ribs 8 through 10 attach to the cartilage of the preceding rib. The other 2 pairs of ribs are "free-floating" — they don't attach to any part of the anterior thoracic cage. Rib 11 ends anterolaterally, and rib 12 ends laterally.

The lower parts of the rib cage *(costal margins)* near the xiphoid process form the borders of the *costal angle* — an angle of about 90 degrees in an average person. (See *Locating lung structures in the thoracic cage.*)

Above the anterior thorax is a depression called the *suprasternal notch.*

POINT TO REMEMBER
Because the suprasternal notch isn't covered by the rib cage like the rest of the thorax, the trachea and aortic pulsations can be palpated here. **(See *Respiratory changes during exercise*, page 121.)**

Atlas of the human body

Inside a cell

The fundamental unit of life, the cell consists of a nucleus, cytoplasm, and organelles. Within the nucleus are the blueprints of heredity — ribonucleic acid and deoxyribonucleic acid.

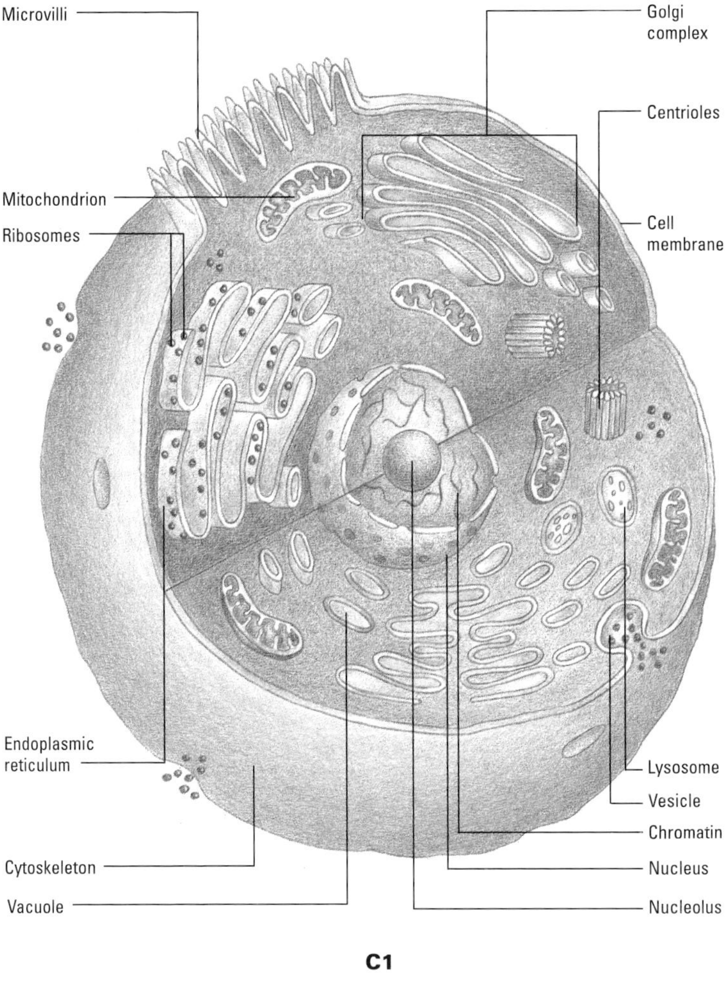

Membrane transport mechanisms

Substances move across the cell membrane either by passive transport mechanisms (diffusion, osmosis, or facilitated diffusion) or active mechanisms (active transport or pinocytosis). Substances can enter or leave the cell by passing through the cell membrane or by moving through pores in the protein molecules embedded in the membrane.

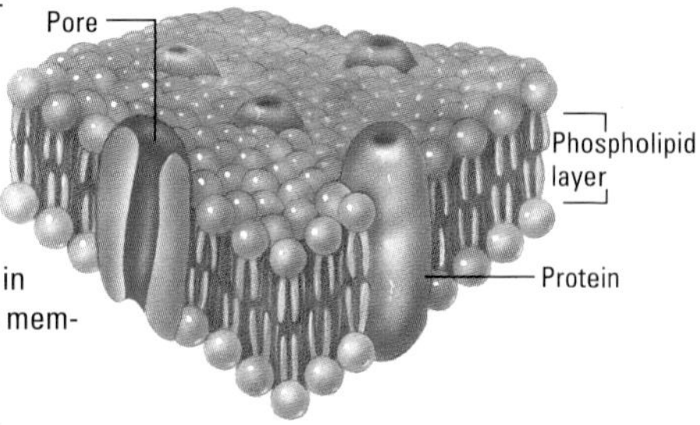

Passive transport mechanisms

In diffusion, substances move from an area of higher concentration to an area of lower concentration. Movement continues until distribution is uniform.

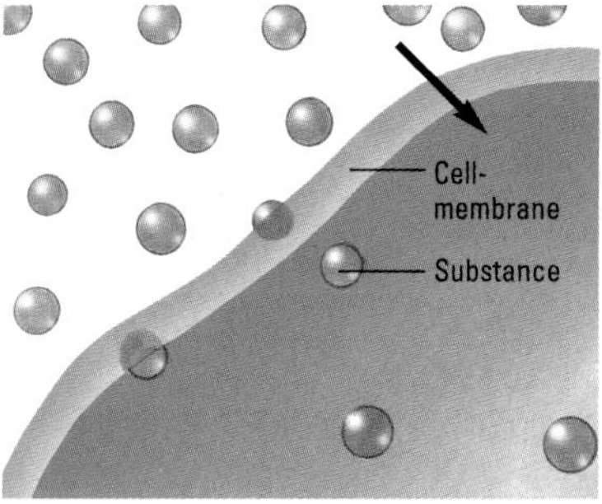

In osmosis, water molecules move from an area of higher water concentration to one of lower concentration.

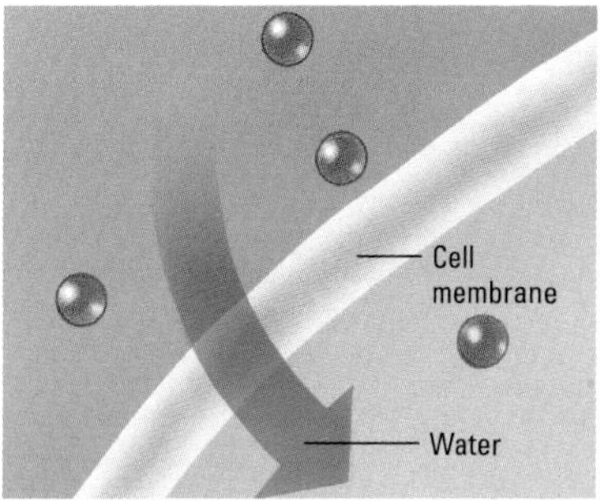

Active transport mechanisms

Active transport moves molecules and ions against a concentration gradient (from lower to higher concentrations). In the sodium-potassium pump, for instance, sodium moves from inside to outside the cell, where sodium concentration is greater; potassium moves from outside to inside the cell, where potassium concentration is greater. In pinocytosis, tiny vacuoles take droplets of fluid containing dissolved substances into the cell. The engulfed fluid is used in the cell.

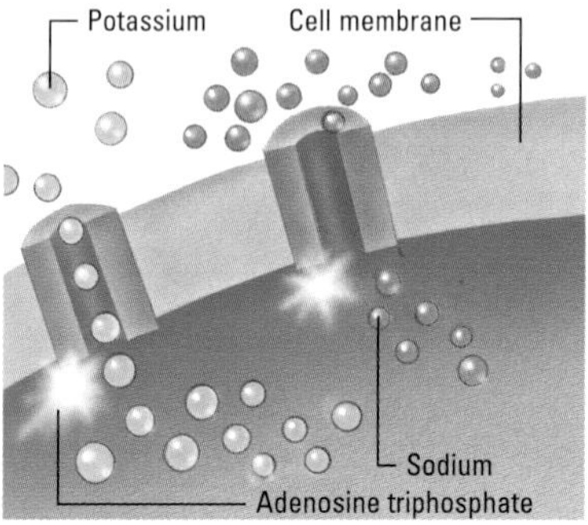

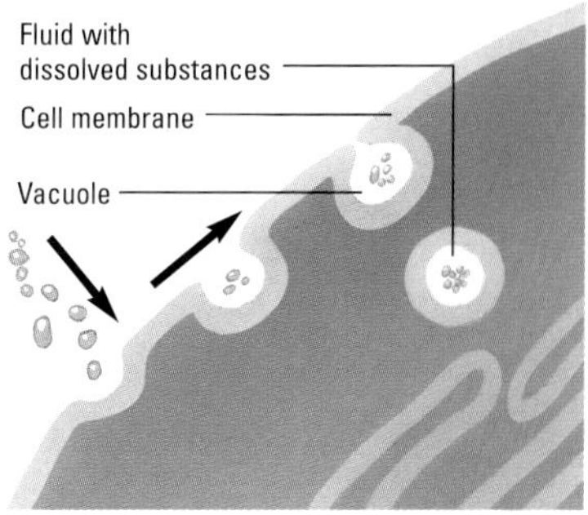

Types of body tissue

The human body contains four basic types of tissue — epithelial, connective, muscle, and nervous. Epithelial tissue may be simple, stratified, or pseudostratified and squamous, columnar, or cuboidal. Types of connective tissue include bone, cartilage, and adipose (fatty) tissue. Muscle tissue may be striated (skeletal), cardiac, or smooth. Nervous tissue consists of neurons and neuroglia.

STRIATED MUSCLE

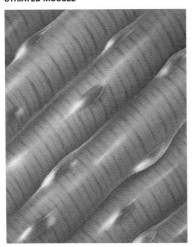

ADIPOSE

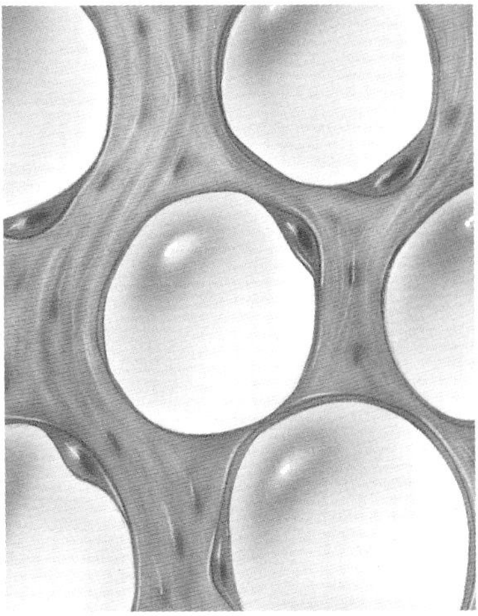

NEUROGLIA

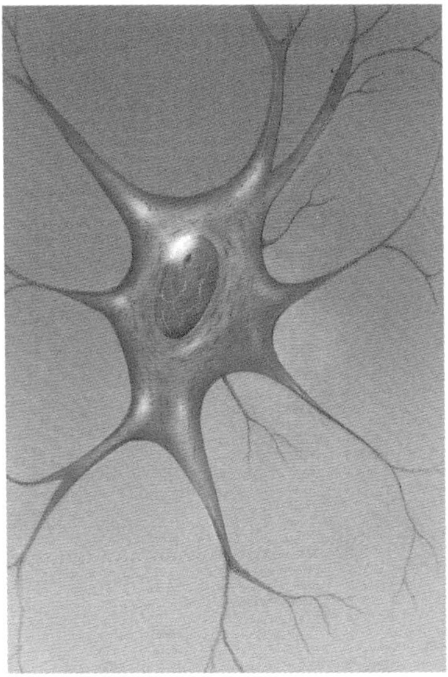

STRATIFIED SQUAMOUS

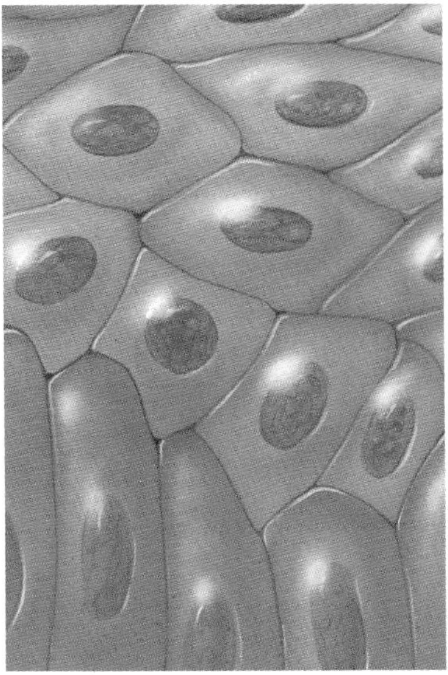

The skin and its structures

SKIN CROSS SECTION

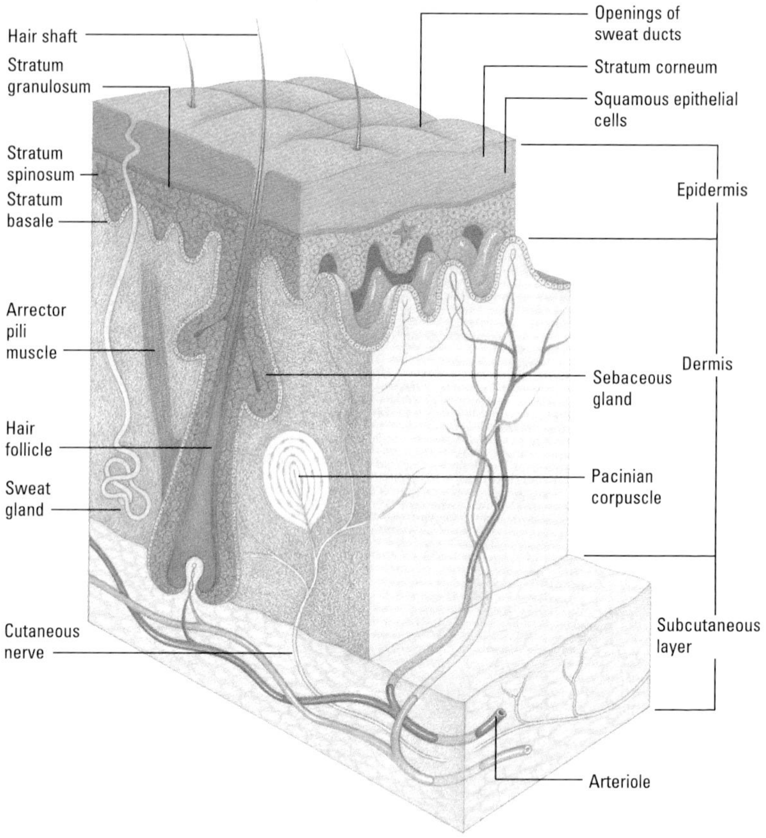

NAIL CROSS SECTION

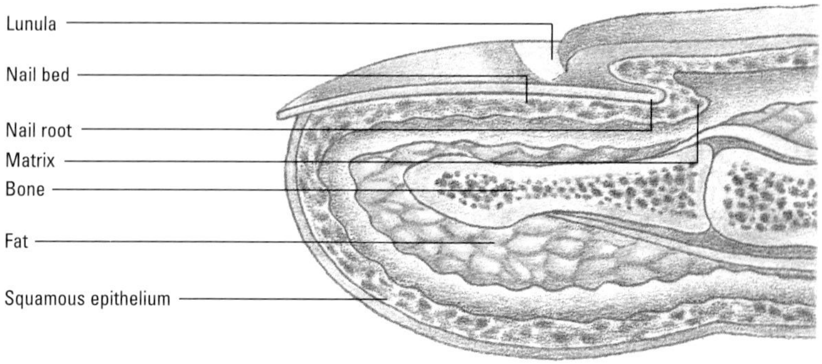

The human skull

LATERAL VIEW

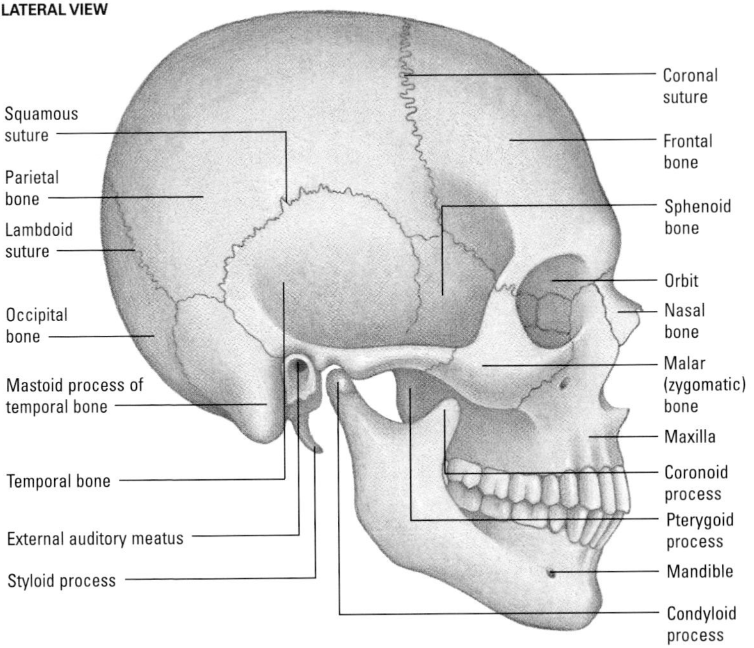
Squamous suture
Parietal bone
Lambdoid suture
Occipital bone
Mastoid process of temporal bone
Temporal bone
External auditory meatus
Styloid process
Coronal suture
Frontal bone
Sphenoid bone
Orbit
Nasal bone
Malar (zygomatic) bone
Maxilla
Coronoid process
Pterygoid process
Mandible
Condyloid process

ANTERIOR VIEW

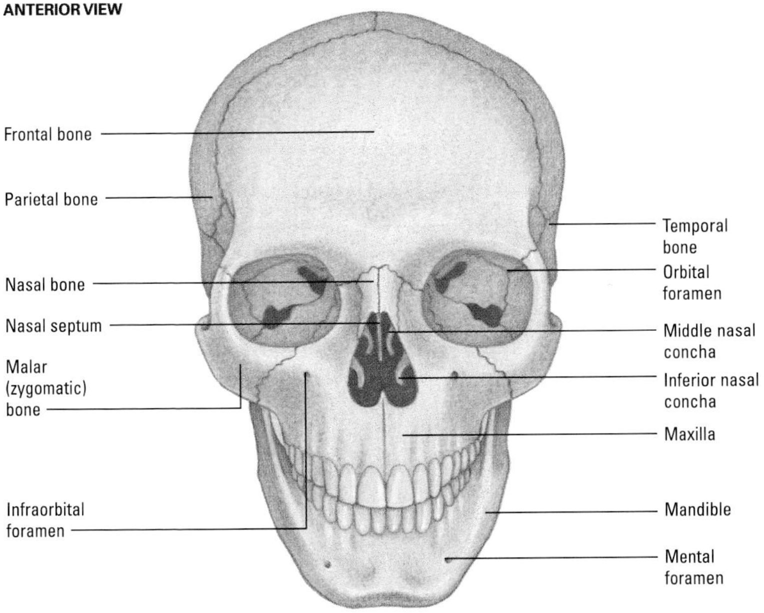
Frontal bone
Parietal bone
Nasal bone
Nasal septum
Malar (zygomatic) bone
Infraorbital foramen
Temporal bone
Orbital foramen
Middle nasal concha
Inferior nasal concha
Maxilla
Mandible
Mental foramen

Vertebral column

LATERAL VIEW

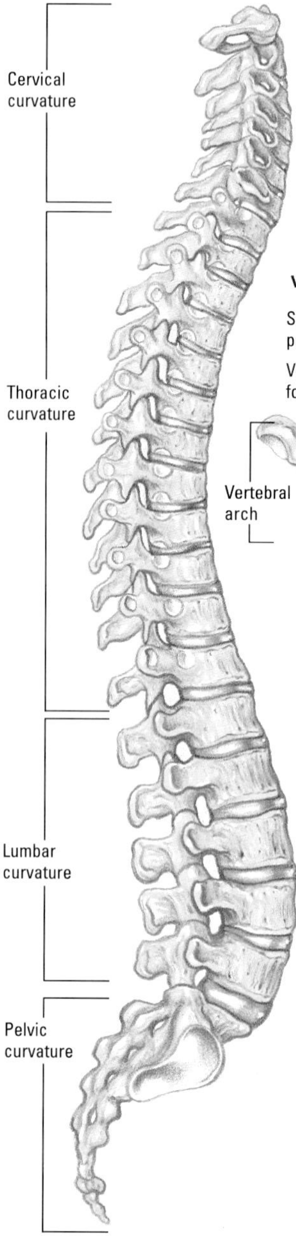

VERTEBRA (SUPERIOR VIEW)

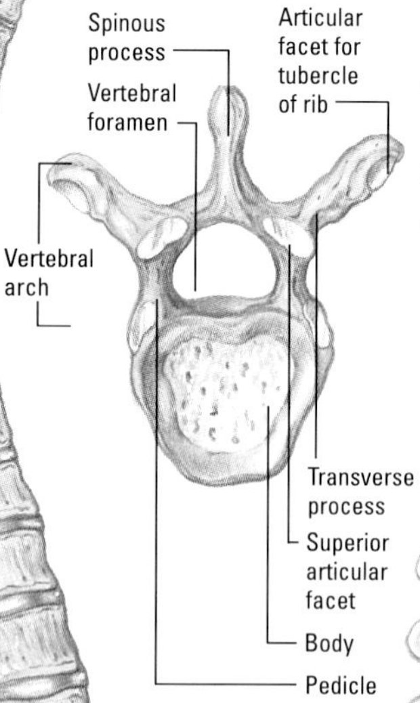

ANTERIOR VIEW

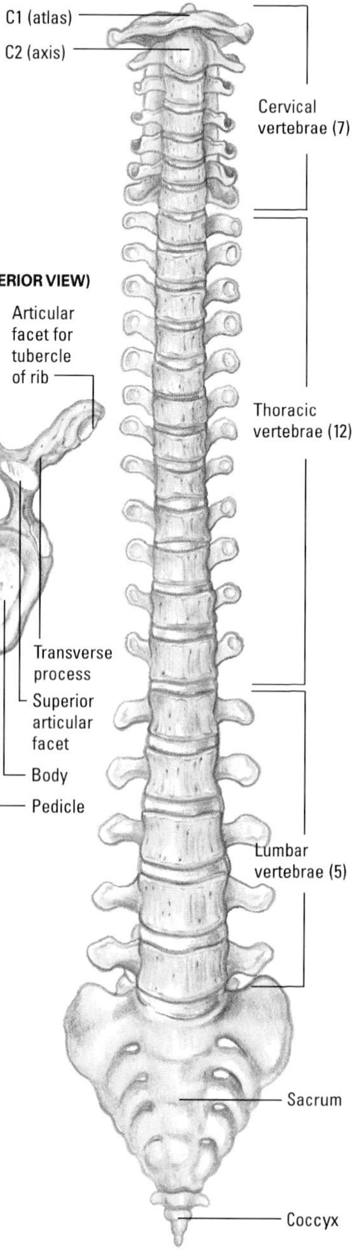

Muscles and tendons

Muscles attach to bone by two tendons of origin and one tendon of insertion.

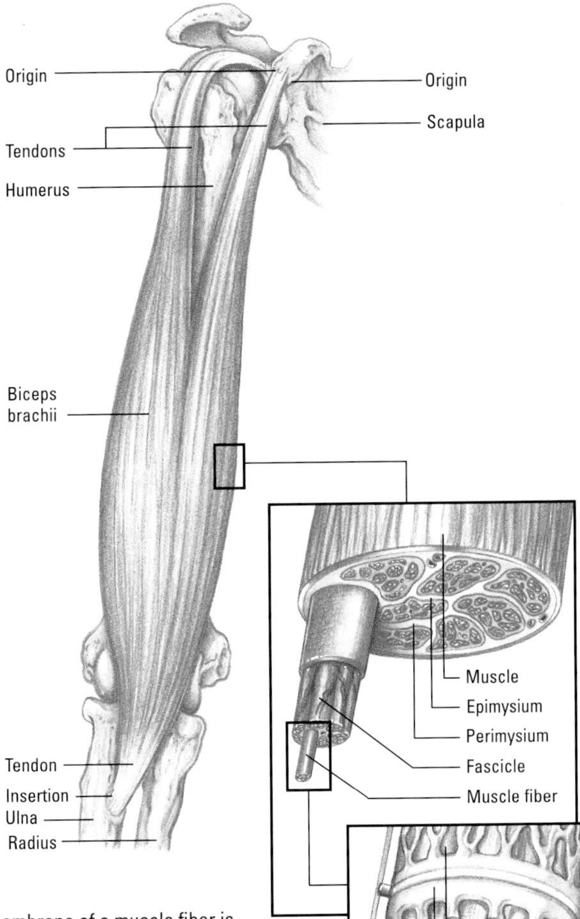

Skeletal muscle

Skeletal muscle is composed of numerous elongated muscle cells, called muscle fibers. Muscle fibers are held together in bundles by fasciae, sheaths of fibrous tissue that extend the entire length of the muscle.

The plasma membrane of a muscle fiber is called the sarcolemma; the cytoplasm, the sarcoplasm. Muscle cells contain a network of tubules and sacs termed the sarcoplasmic reticulum.

Myofibrils, slender threads of protein, extend lengthwise through muscle fibers. Myofibrils contain many finer elements called thick and thin filaments. About 1,500 thick filaments and 3,000 thin filaments form a repeating pattern along the length of the fiber, giving rise to striations. Thick filaments contain myosin, whereas thin filaments contain actin. The interaction between these two proteins leads to muscle contraction.

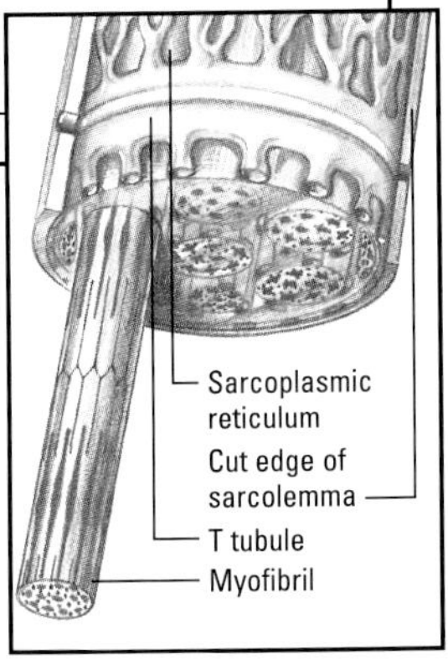

Inside view of a bone

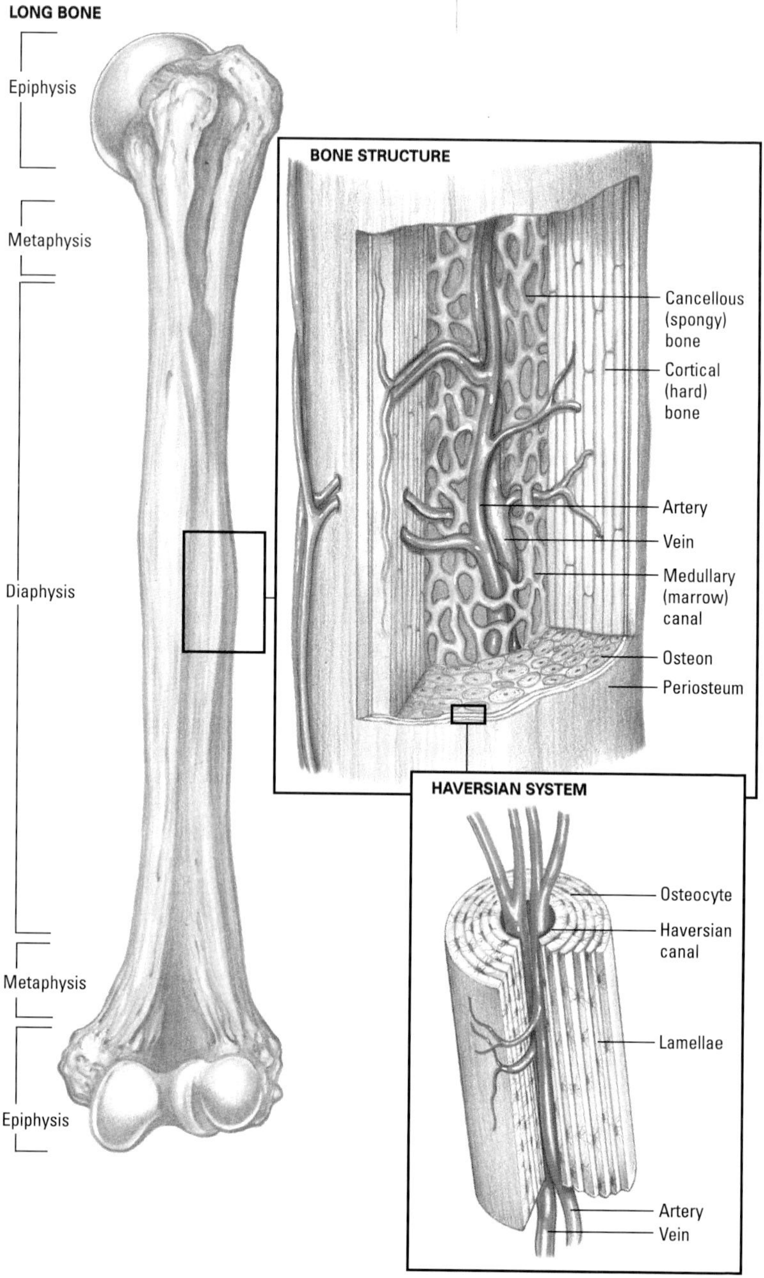
LONG BONE
Epiphysis
Metaphysis
Diaphysis
Metaphysis
Epiphysis
BONE STRUCTURE
Cancellous (spongy) bone
Cortical (hard) bone
Artery
Vein
Medullary (marrow) canal
Osteon
Periosteum
HAVERSIAN SYSTEM
Osteocyte
Haversian canal
Lamellae
Artery
Vein

Major structures of the brain

LATERAL VIEW

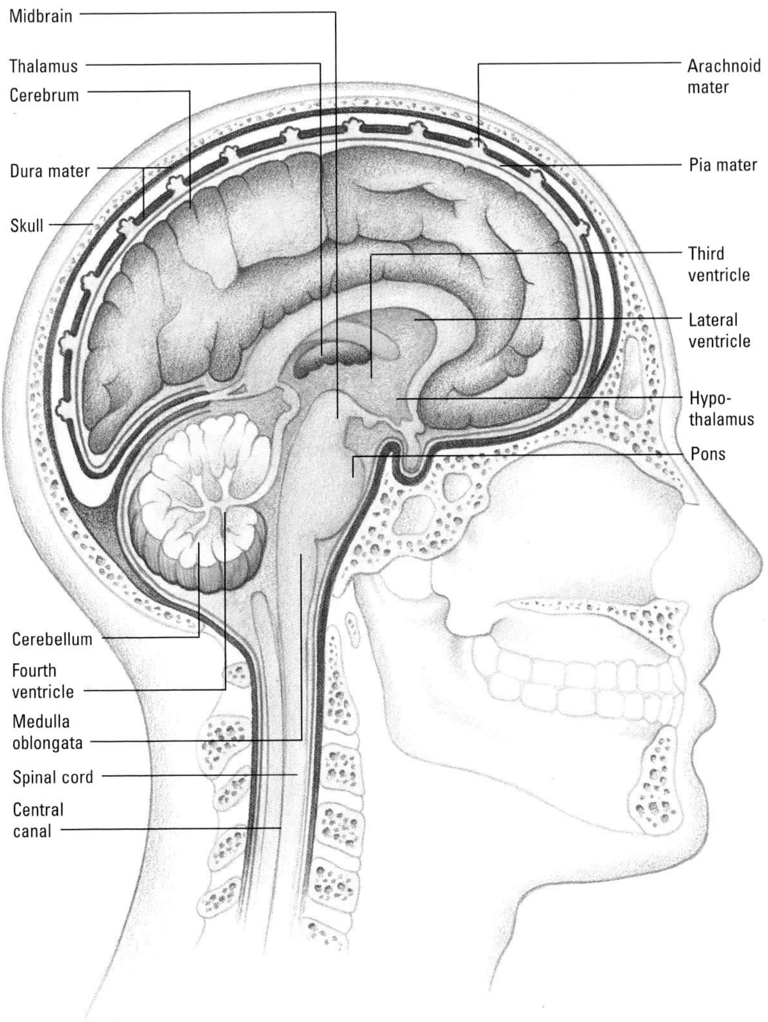

Central nervous system

The nervous system has two major divisions — central and peripheral. The central nervous system includes the brain and spinal cord. The central mass of the cord consists of gray matter (neuronal cell bodies), divided into dorsal and ventral horns.

LATERAL VIEW

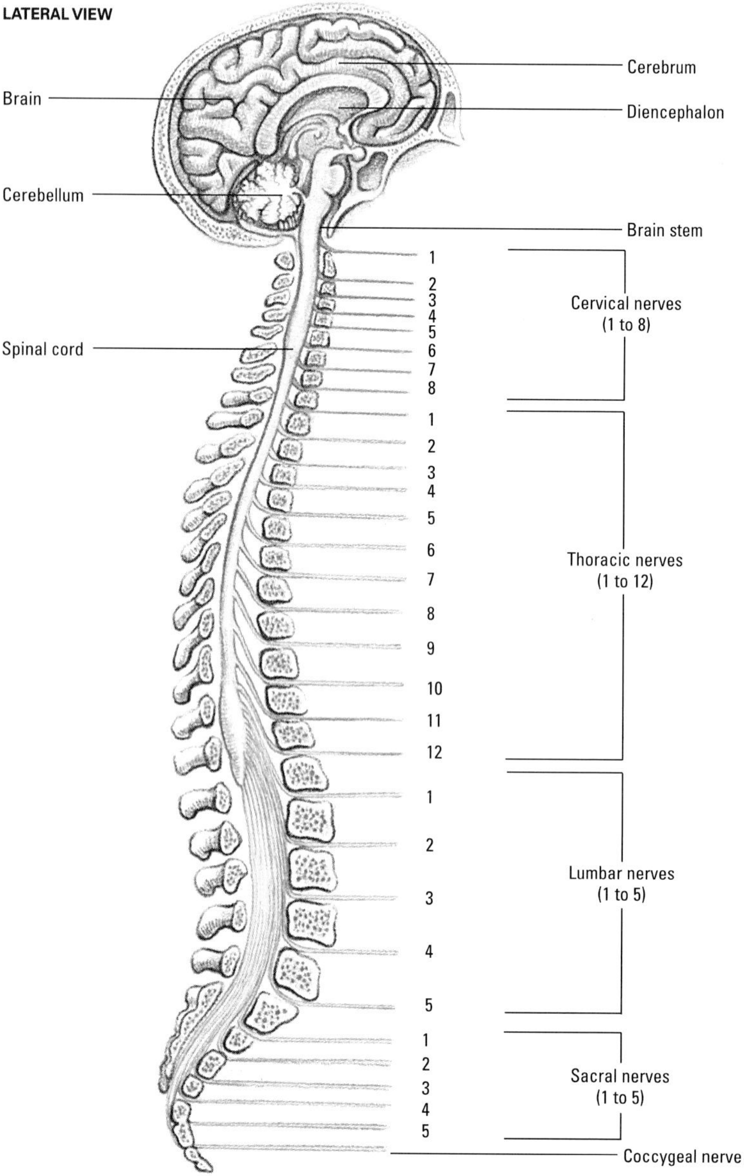

Vision pathways

Images travel along the vision pathways to the brain for interpretation. Each pathway consists of an optic nerve, optic chiasm, lateral geniculate body, optic tract, and visual cortex. In the optic chiasm, fibers from the nasal aspects of both retinas cross to opposite sides, and fibers from the temporal portions remain uncrossed. Both crossed and uncrossed fibers form the optic tracts.

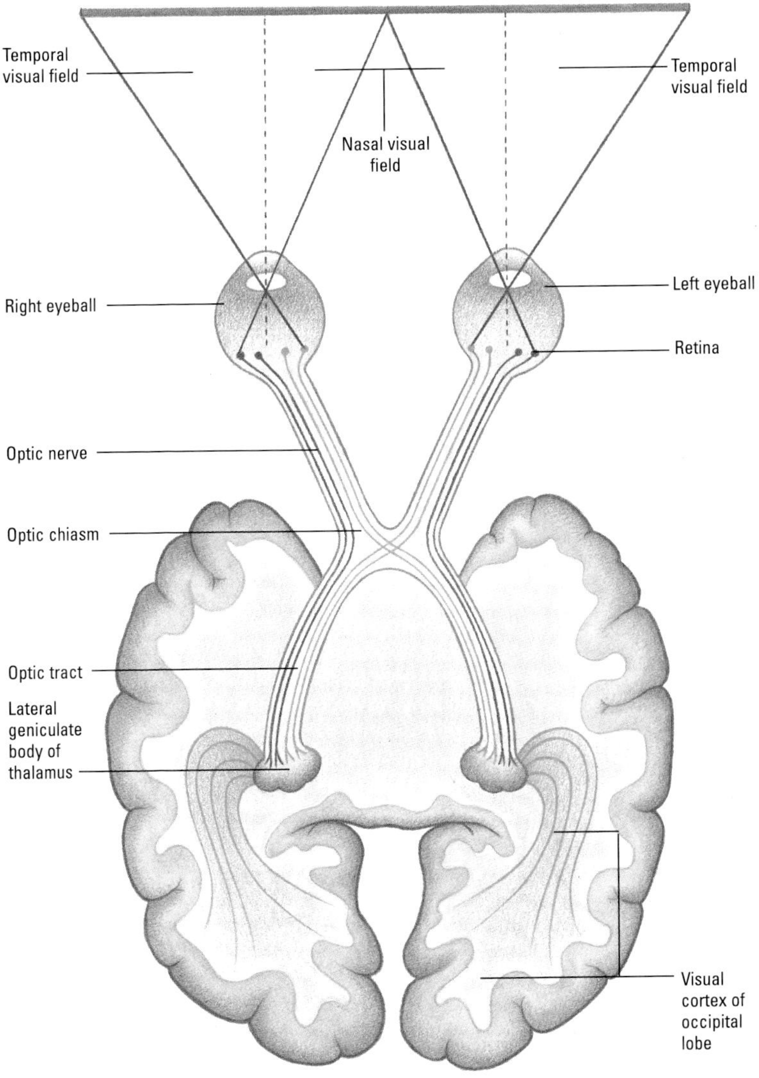

Reflex arc

A reflex arc — the neural relay cycle for quick motor response to a harmful sensory stimulus — requires a sensory (afferent) neuron and a motor (efferent) neuron. The stimulus triggers a sensory impulse, which travels along the dorsal root to the spinal cord. There, two synaptic transmissions occur at the same time. One synapse continues the impulse along a sensory neuron to the brain; the other immediately relays the impulse to an interneuron, which transmits it to a motor neuron. The motor neuron delivers the impulse to a muscle or gland, producing an immediate response.

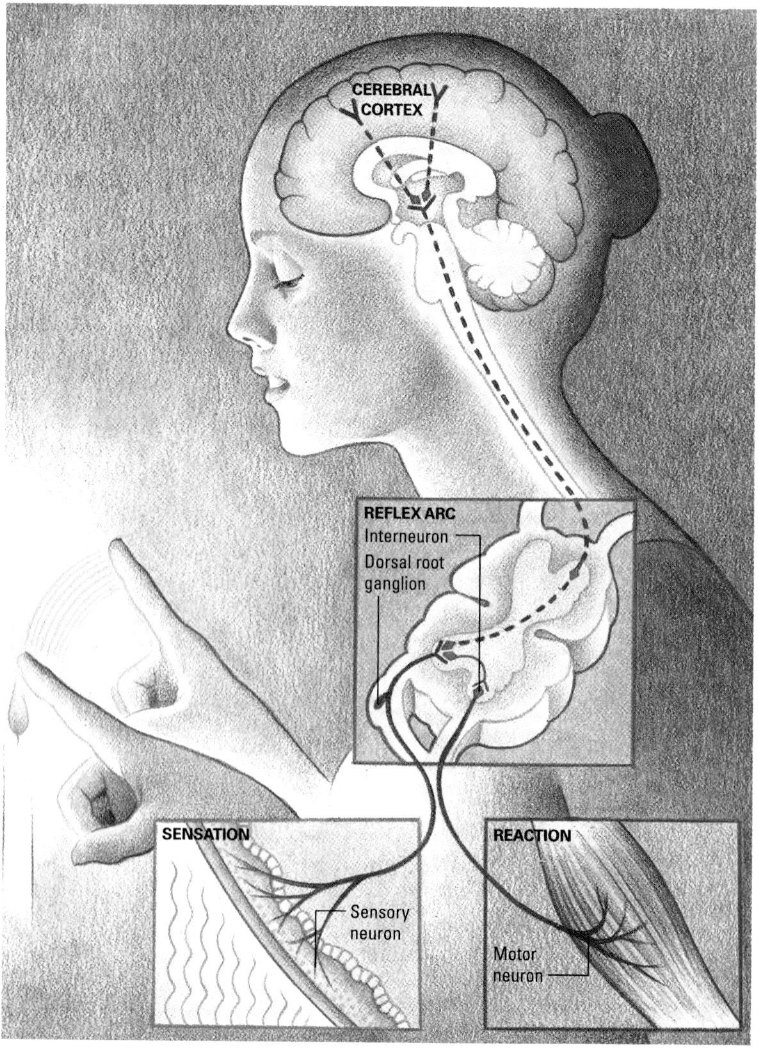

Endocrine gland locations

The hormones of the pituitary gland regulate other endocrine glands and affect many bodily functions. The pituitary gland is directly connected to the brain, making it closely related to the nervous system. Neural stimulation of the posterior pituitary gland triggers secretion of antidiuretic hormone and oxytocin.

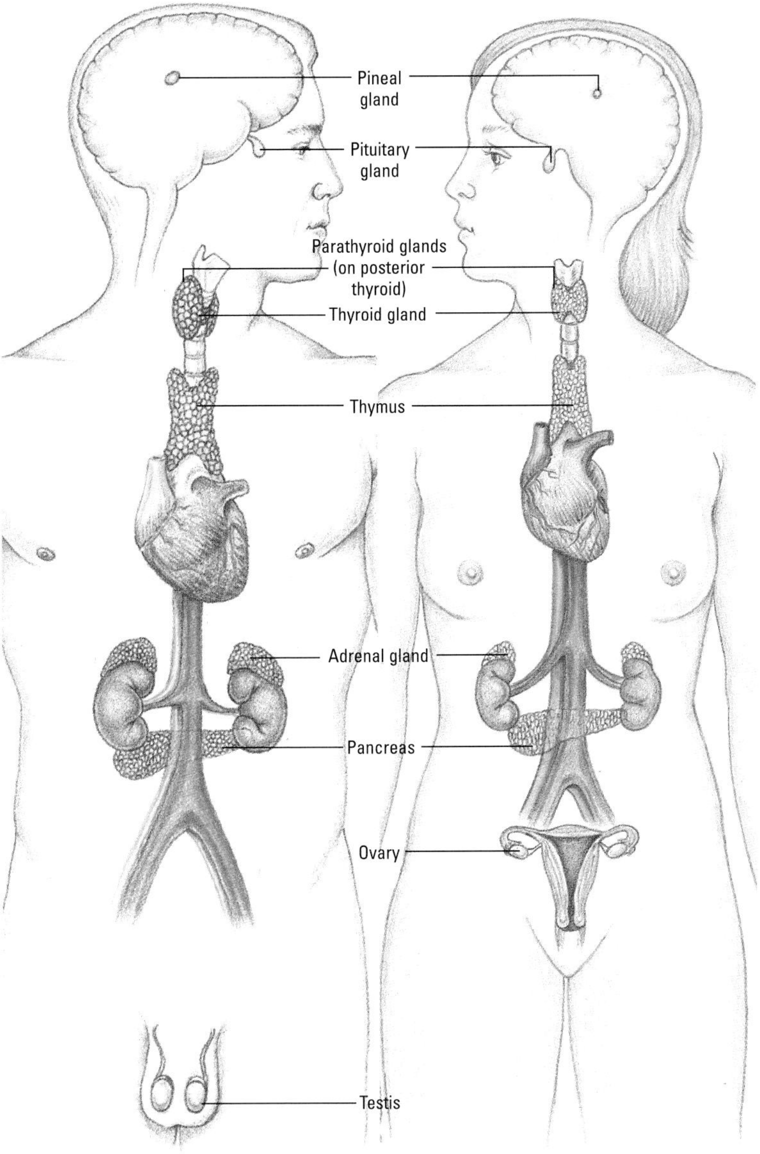

Endocrine glands

The *pituitary gland* is situated at the base of the brain, attached to the hypothalamus. It consists of an anterior lobe and a posterior lobe; the pars intermedia is part of the anterior lobe.

The *thyroid gland,* located in the front of the neck, consists of bilateral lobes joined in the middle by a narrow isthmus.

The *parathyroid glands* are attached to the dorsal surfaces of the lateral lobes of the thyroid gland. Most people have four of these glands. The parathyroid glands are divided, according to their location, into the superior and inferior parathyroids.

The *pancreas,* shaped somewhat like a fish, stretches transversely across the posterior abdominal wall in the epigastric and hypochondriac regions of the body. It is divided into a head, body, and tail. The head is tucked into the curve of the duodenum; the tail is the tapered left extremity of the gland.

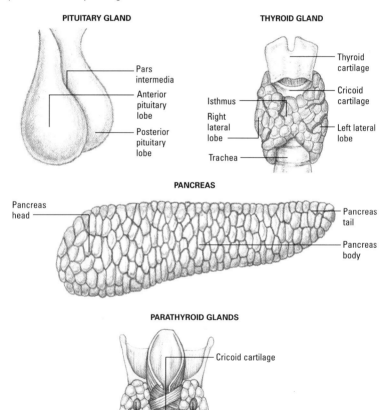

PITUITARY GLAND

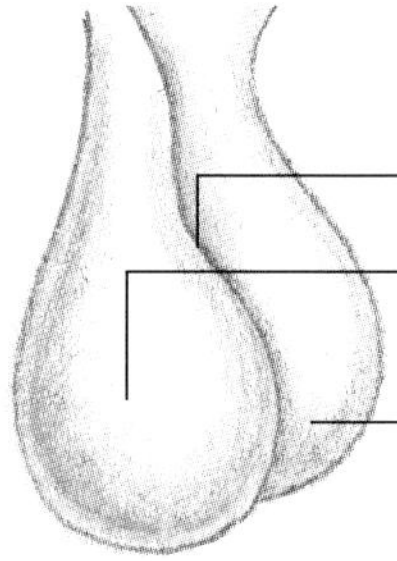

THYROID GLAND

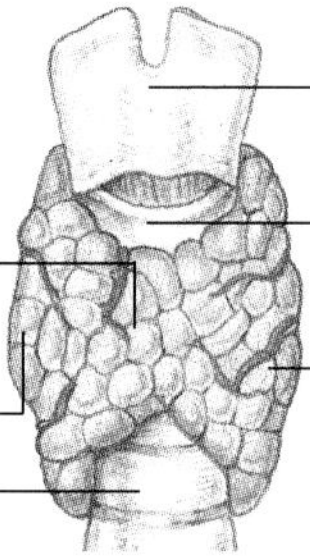

PANCREAS

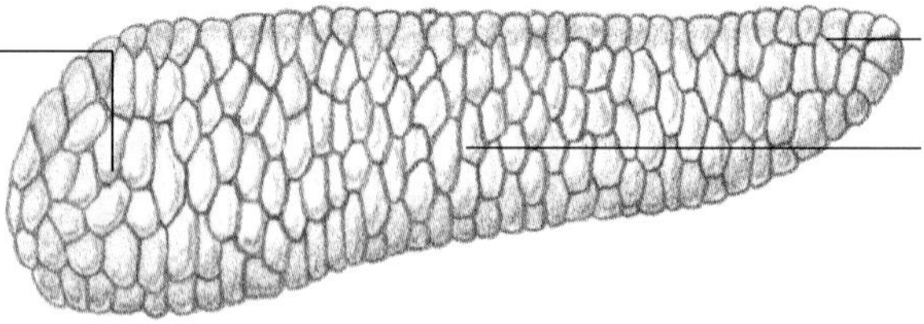

PARATHYROID GLANDS

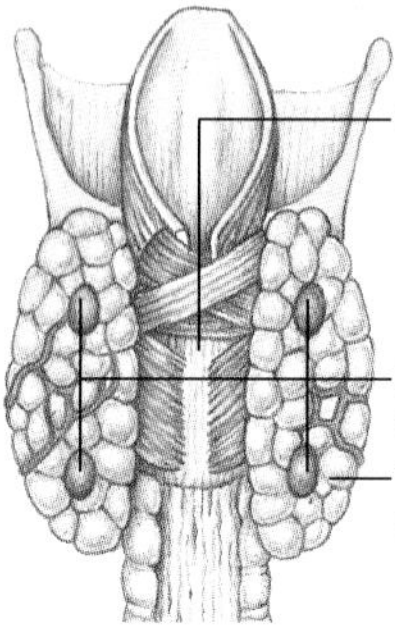

Hormonal feedback mechanisms

Hypothalamic stimulation triggers a complex feedback mechanism that controls the blood levels of many hormones. First, the hypothalamus sends releasing and inhibiting factors or hormones to the anterior pituitary. In response, the anterior pituitary secretes tropic hormones, such as growth hormone (GH), prolactin (PRL), corticotropin, thyroid-stimulating hormone (TSH), follicle-stimulating hormone (FSH), and luteinizing hormone (LH). At the appropriate target gland, these hormones stimulate the target organ to release other hormones that regulate various body functions. When these hormones reach normal levels in body tissue, a feedback mechanism inhibits further hypothalamic and pituitary secretion.

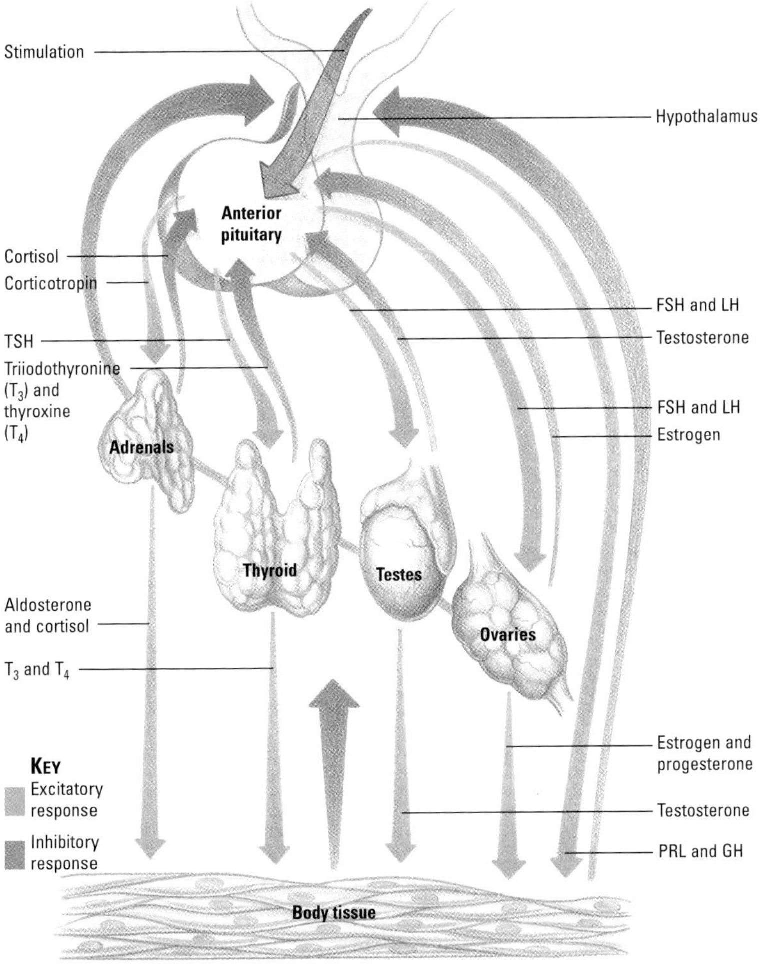

Heart and coronary vessels

ANTERIOR VIEW

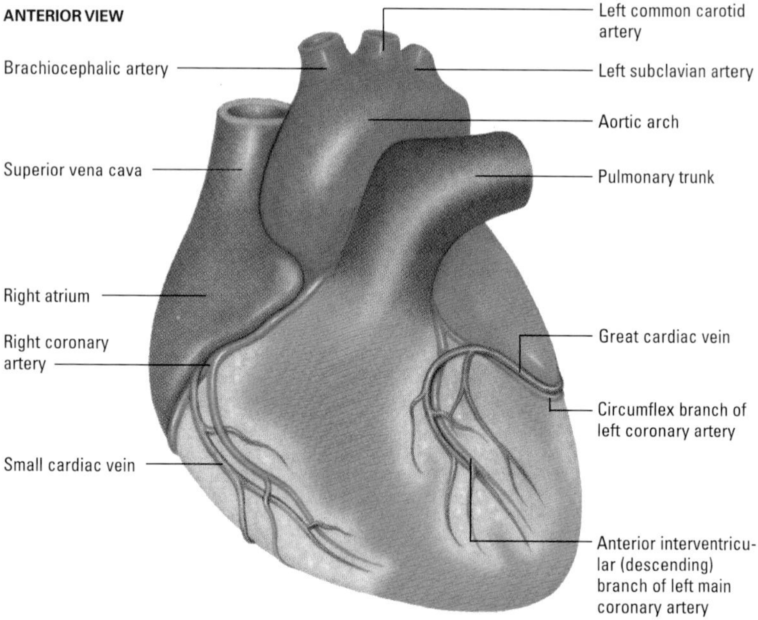

POSTERIOR VIEW

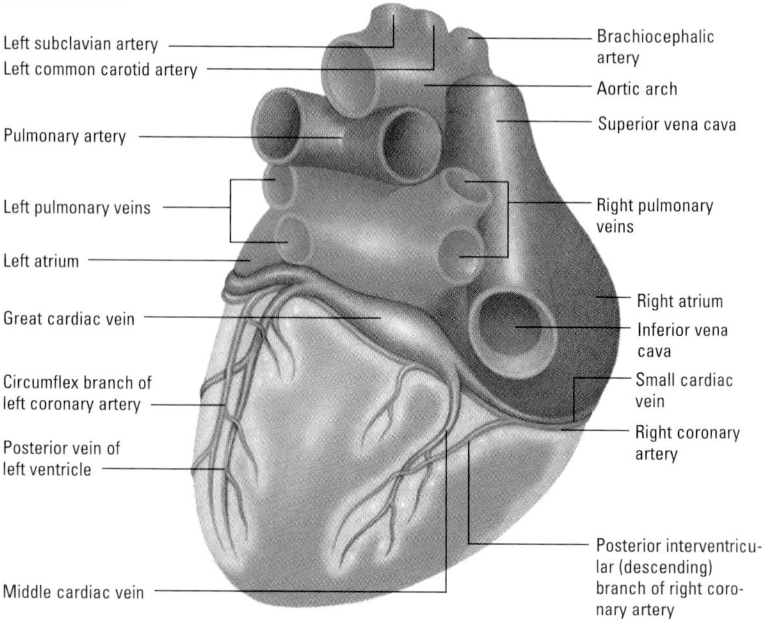

Blood vessel structure

The walls of arteries have three coats: an outer coat (tunica adventitia), a middle coat (tunica media), and an inner coat (tunica intima). Veins have the same three coats but with fewer and thinner elastic fibers. Capillaries have only a tunica intima; they form intricate webs that connect arterioles and venules. The arrows in the illustration below show blood flow.

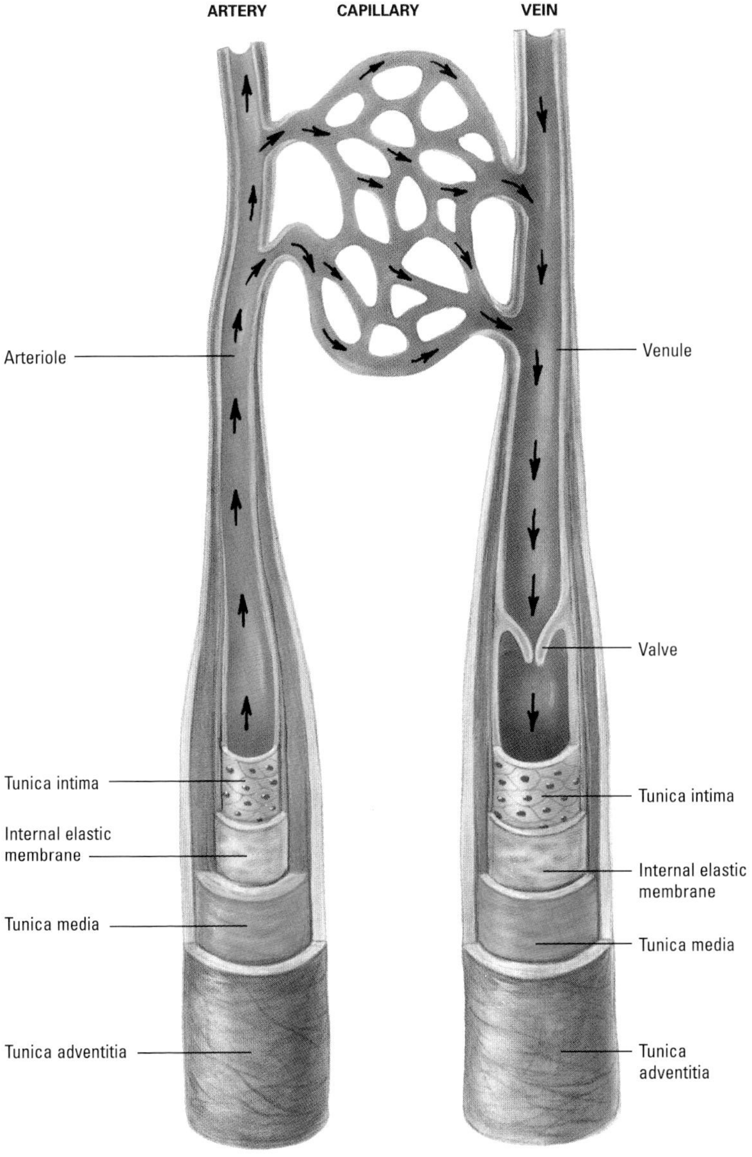

Cardiac conduction system

Specialized fibers in the heart's conduction system generate and conduct rhythmic electrical impulses to stimulate heart contraction. This system includes the sinoatrial (SA) node, atrioventricular (AV) junction, bundle of His and its bundle branches, and ventricular conduction tissue and Purkinje fibers.

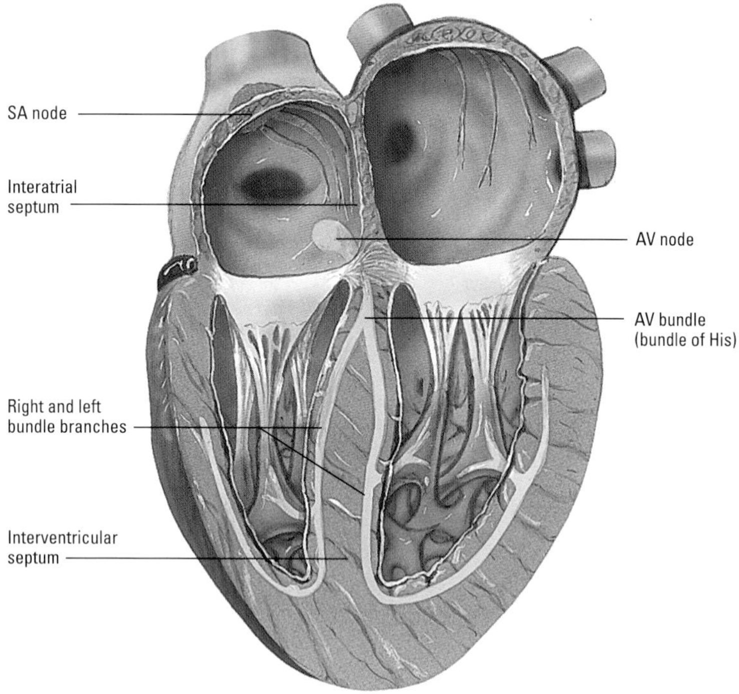

Types of blood cells

Blood cells are categorized as red blood cells (RBCs or erythrocytes), white blood cells (WBCs or leukocytes), and platelets (thrombocytes). WBCs are subdivided into granulocytes (basophils, neutrophils, and eosinophils) and agranulocytes (lymphocytes and monocytes).

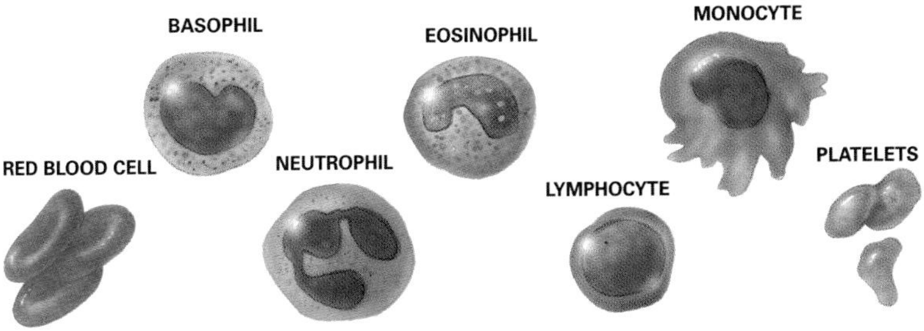
BASOPHIL
EOSINOPHIL
MONOCYTE
RED BLOOD CELL
NEUTROPHIL
LYMPHOCYTE
PLATELETS

ABO blood groups

Blood type refers to the type of antigens present on red blood cell membranes. The four blood types are A, B, AB, and O. Type A has antigen A on its red blood cells (RBCs), type B has antigen B on RBCs, type AB has both antigen A and antigen B on RBCs, and type O has neither antigen.

Plasma never contains antibodies against the antigens present on its RBCs; it does contain antibodies against antigen A or B if these are not present. Thus, type A blood contains anti-B antibodies, type B blood contains anti-A antibodies, type AB blood contains neither anti-A nor anti-B antibodies, and type O blood contains both anti-A and anti-B antibodies.

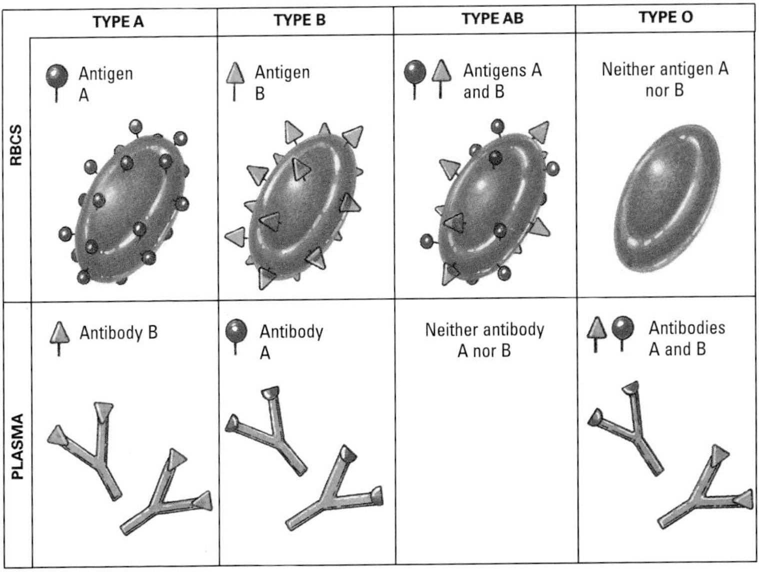
TYPE A
TYPE B
TYPE AB
TYPE O
RBCS
Antigen A
Antigen B
Antigens A and B
Neither antigen A nor B
PLASMA
Antibody B
Antibody A
Neither antibody A nor B
Antibodies A and B

Immune response to bacterial invasion

Invasion of a foreign substance can trigger two types of immune responses — antibody-mediated (humoral) and cell-mediated immunity. Both types involve lymphocytes that share a common origin in stem cells and then undergo differential development to become B cells and T cells.

In *humoral* immunity, antigens stimulate B cells to differentiate into plasma cells and produce circulating antibodies that disable bacteria and viruses before they can enter host cells.

In *cell-mediated* immunity, T cells move directly to attack invaders. Three T-cell subgroups trigger the response to infection. Helper T cells spur B cells to manufacture antibodies. Effector T cells kill antigens and produce lymphokines (proteins that induce inflammatory response and mediate the delayed hypersensitivity reaction). Suppressor T cells regulate T and B types of immune response.

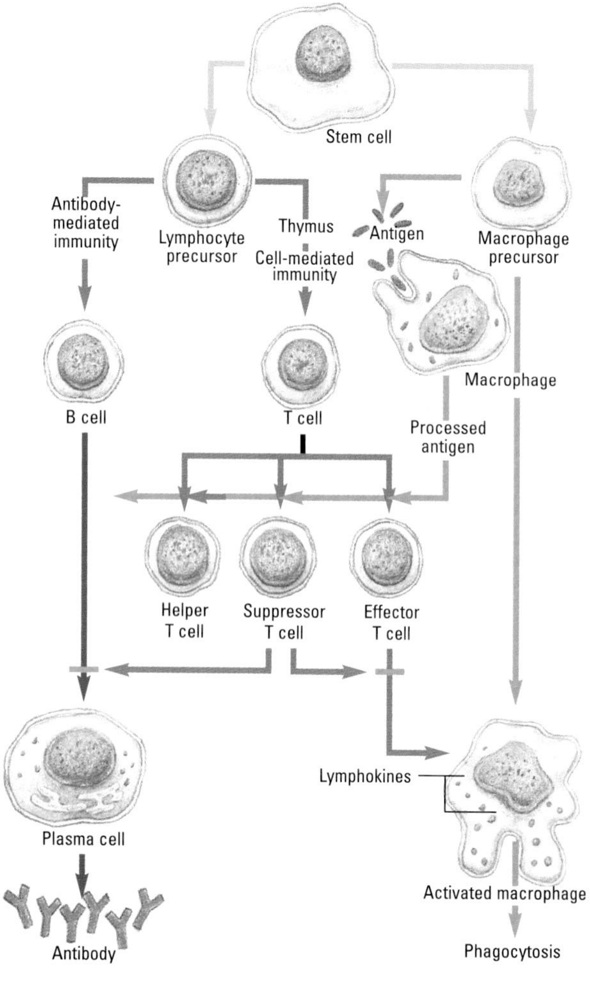

Inflammatory response

The inflammatory response helps the body return to homeostasis after a wound occurs. Its primary function is to bring phagocytic cells (neutrophils and monocytes) to the inflamed area to destroy bacteria and rid the tissue spaces of dead and dying cells so that tissue repair can begin.

Inflammation produces four cardinal signs: redness, swelling, heat, and pain. The first three signs result from local vasodilation, fluid leakage into the extravascular space, and blockage of lymphatic drainage. The fourth results from tissue space distention caused by swelling and pressure and from chemical irritation of nociceptors (pain receptors).

The acute phase of the inflammatory response typically lasts 2 weeks; the subacute phase (a less intense version of the acute phase) lasts 2 weeks.

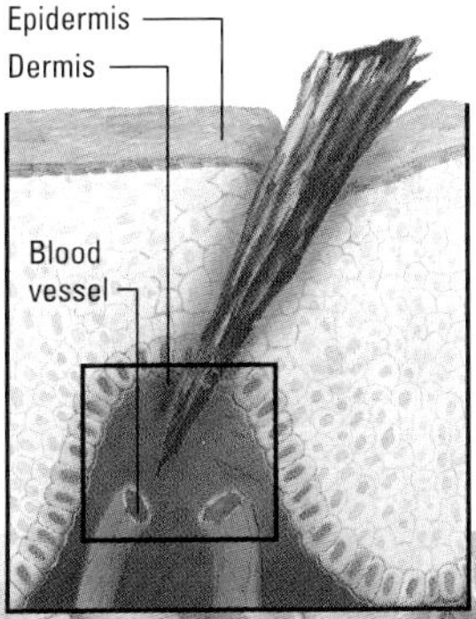

(1) Splinter punctures epidermis
(2) Bacteria introduced
(3) Bacteria implanted in tissue
(4) Injured cells release histamine and kinins, causing capillary dilation
(5) Dilated capillaries make skin hot and red; escaping fluid from blood vessels causes swelling; edema, kinins, and other substances produce pain; phagocytes migrate through vessel walls toward bacteria
(6) Neutrophils and monocytes destroy bacteria by phagocytosis

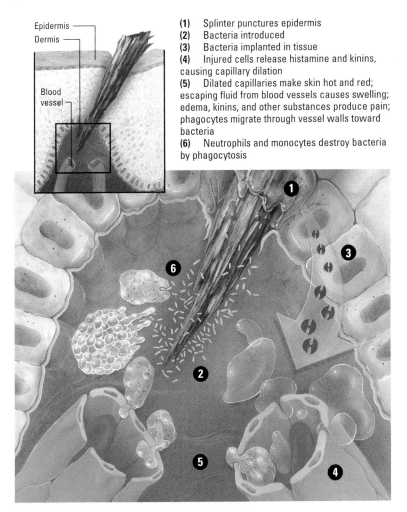

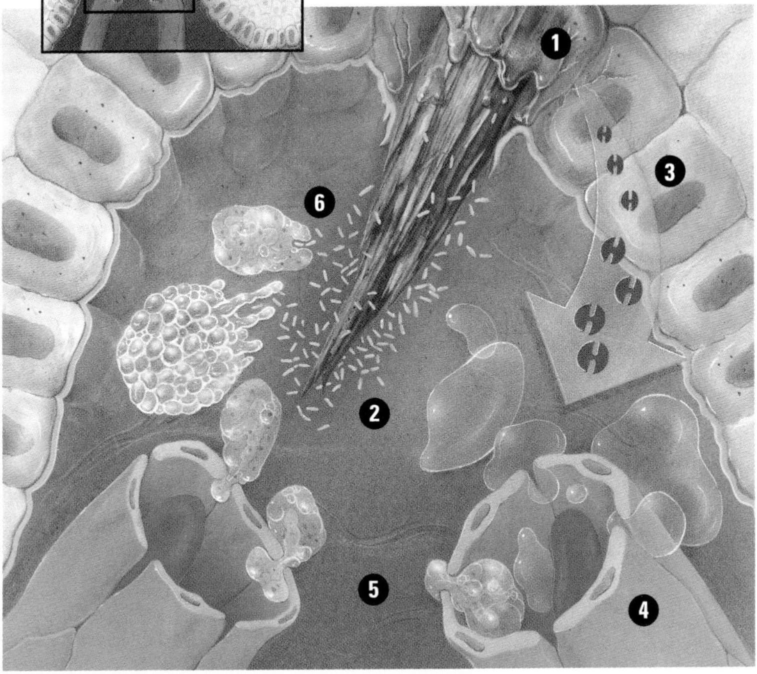

Upper respiratory tract

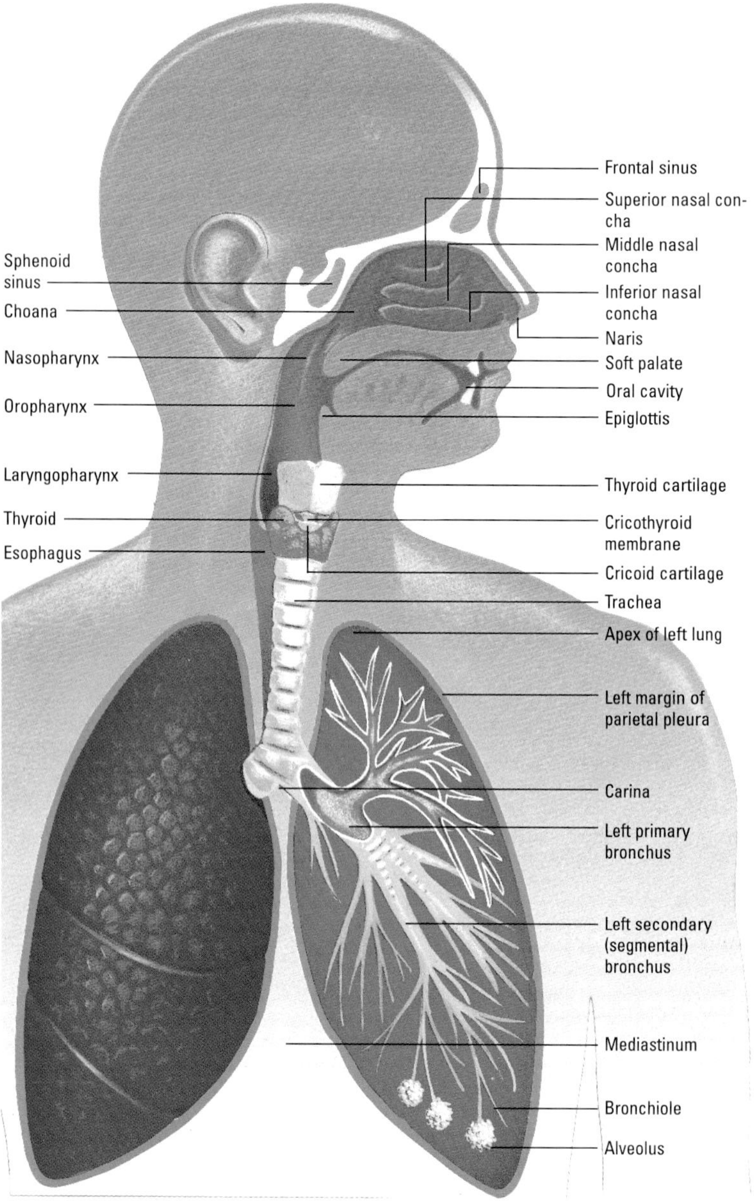
Frontal sinus
Superior nasal concha
Middle nasal concha
Inferior nasal concha
Naris
Soft palate
Oral cavity
Epiglottis
Thyroid cartilage
Cricothyroid membrane
Cricoid cartilage
Trachea
Apex of left lung
Left margin of parietal pleura
Carina
Left primary bronchus
Left secondary (segmental) bronchus
Mediastinum
Bronchiole
Alveolus
Sphenoid sinus
Choana
Nasopharynx
Oropharynx
Laryngopharynx
Thyroid
Esophagus

Lower respiratory tract

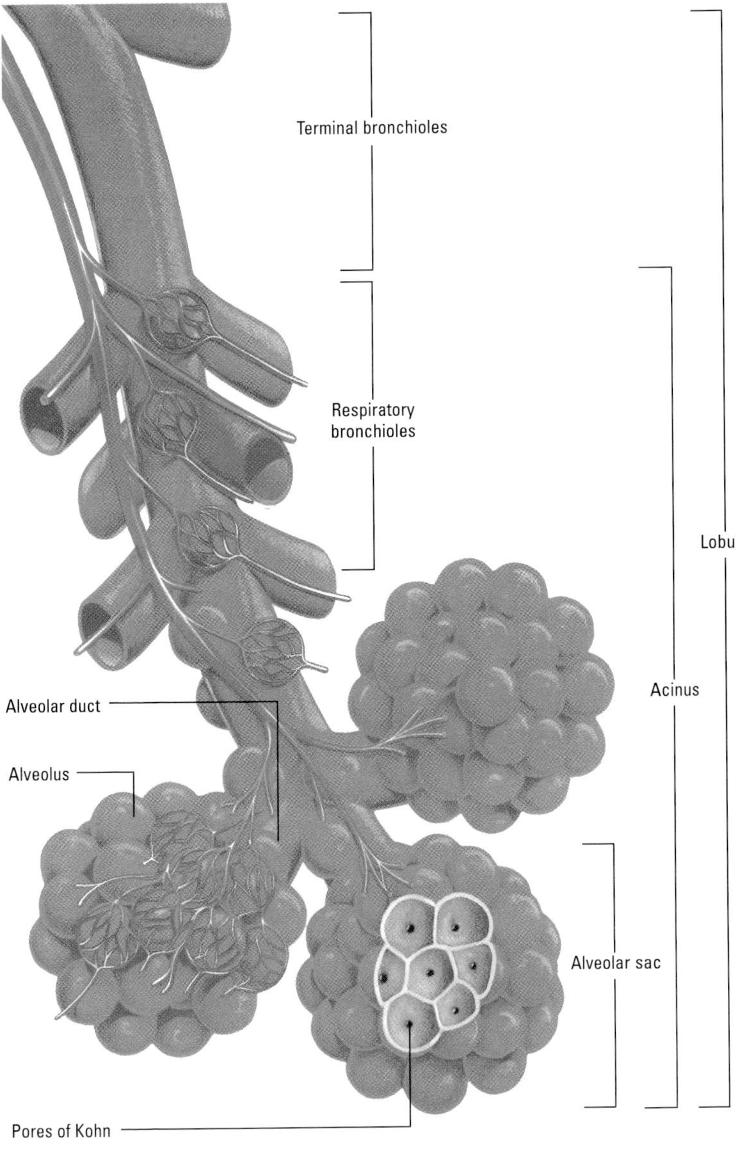

How gas exchange occurs

When the lungs fill with air, oxygen diffuses from the alveoli into the blood and carbon dioxide diffuses in the opposite direction. Gas exchange depends on differences in the partial pressures of the gases.

During inspiration, the partial pressure of water vapor increases, while partial pressures of the other gases decline. Before inspired air enters the alveoli, it mixes with gas that was not exhaled during the previous expiration. Because this gas contains more carbon dioxide and less oxygen than the inspired air, partial pressures change again.

Gas that enters the alveoli undergoes further partial pressure changes but retains a high P_{O_2} and a low P_{CO_2}. This gas meets deoxygenated blood from the right ventricle, which has a low P_{O_2} and a high P_{CO_2}. The pressure differential causes oxygen and carbon dioxide to cross the respiratory membrane toward the lower side of their respective pressure gradients. Oxygen diffuses into blood and carbon dioxide diffuses out, equalizing gas pressures on both sides of the membrane.

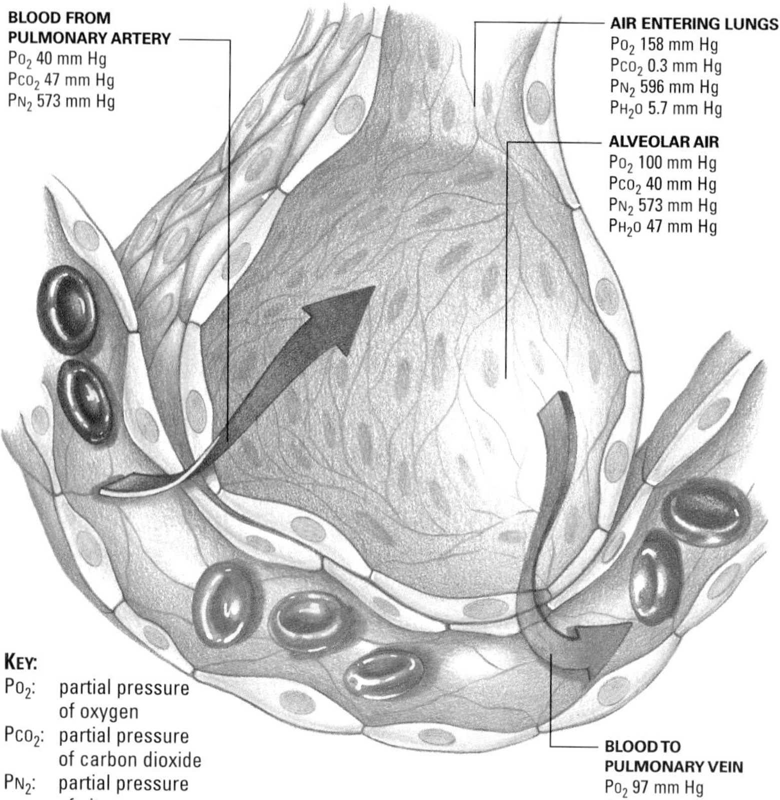

KEY:

P_{O_2}: partial pressure of oxygen

P_{CO_2}: partial pressure of carbon dioxide

P_{N_2}: partial pressure of nitrogen

P_{H_2O}: partial pressure of water vapor

Mechanics of ventilation

Breathing results from differences between atmospheric and intrapulmonary pressures, as described below.

1 Before inspiration, intrapulmonary pressure equals atmospheric pressure, at about 760 mm Hg. Intrapleural pressure equals 756 mm Hg.

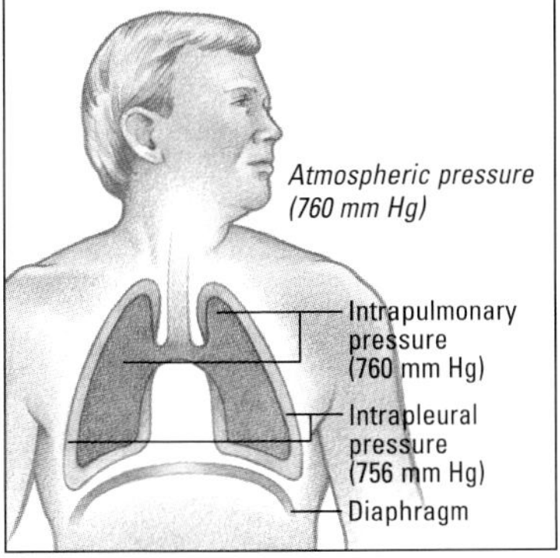

2 During inspiration, the diaphragm and external intercostal muscles contract, enlarging the thorax vertically and horizontally. As the thorax expands, intrapleural pressure decreases and the lungs expand to fill the enlarging thoracic cavity.

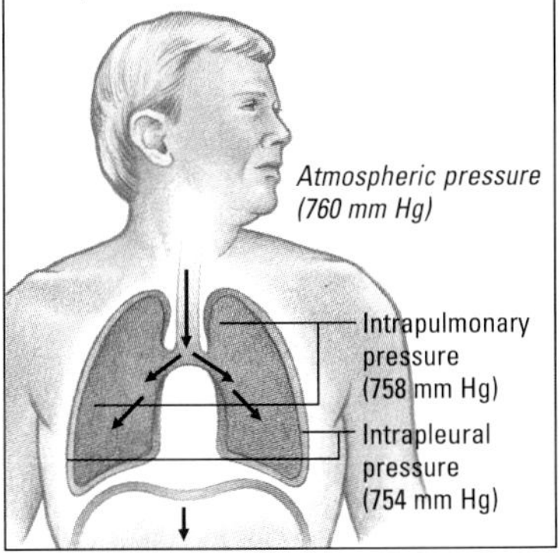

3 The intrapulmonary atmospheric pressure gradient pulls air into the lungs until the two pressures are equal.

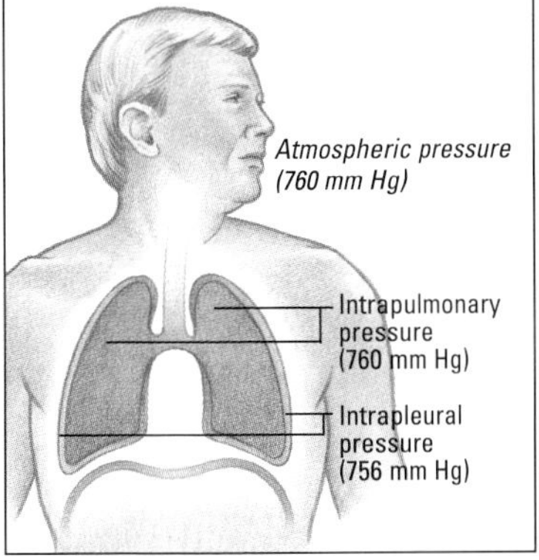

4 During normal expiration, the diaphragm slowly relaxes and the lungs and thorax passively return to resting size and position. During deep or forced expiration, contraction of internal intercostal and abdominal muscles reduces thoracic volume. Lung and thorax compression raises intrapulmonary pressure above atmospheric pressure.

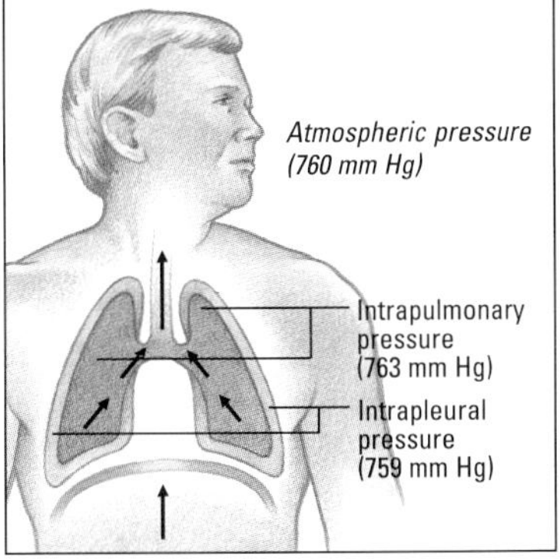

Gastrointestinal system

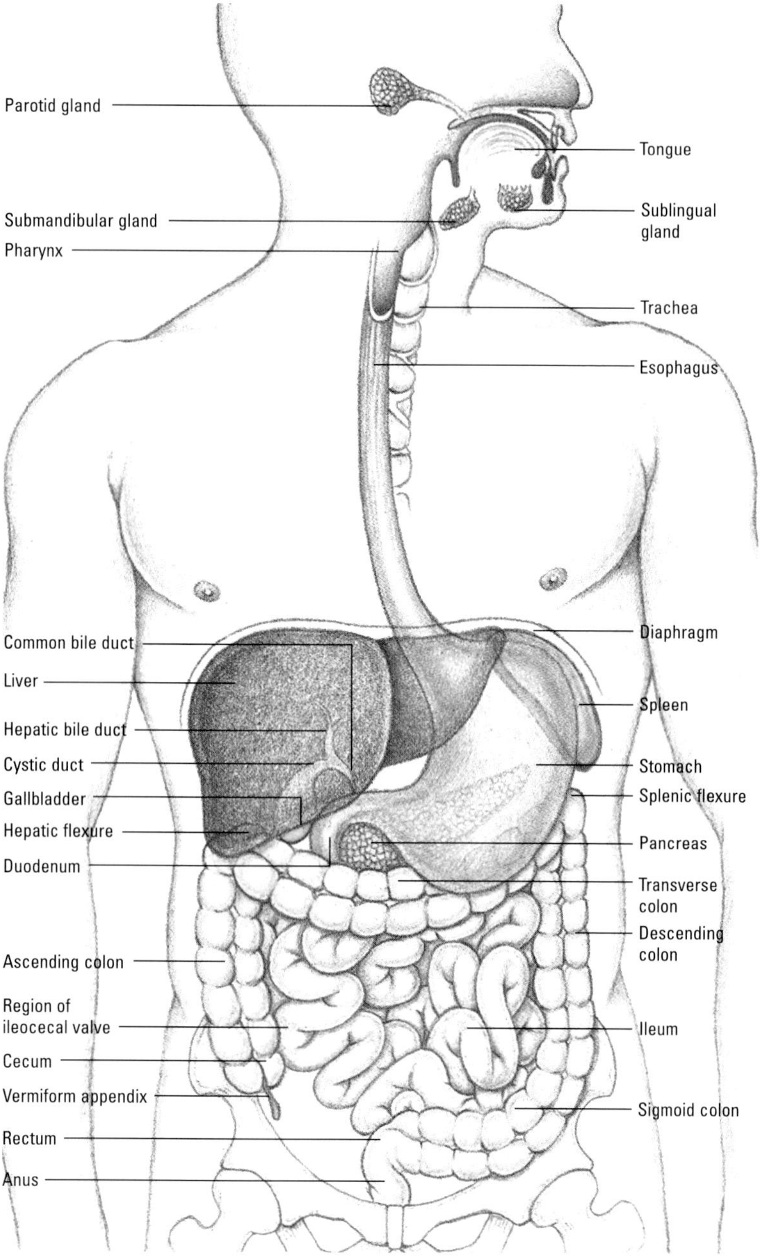
Parotid gland
Tongue
Submandibular gland
Sublingual gland
Pharynx
Trachea
Esophagus
Common bile duct
Diaphragm
Liver
Spleen
Hepatic bile duct
Cystic duct
Stomach
Gallbladder
Splenic flexure
Hepatic flexure
Pancreas
Duodenum
Transverse colon
Descending colon
Ascending colon
Region of ileocecal valve
Ileum
Cecum
Vermiform appendix
Sigmoid colon
Rectum
Anus

Biliary tract

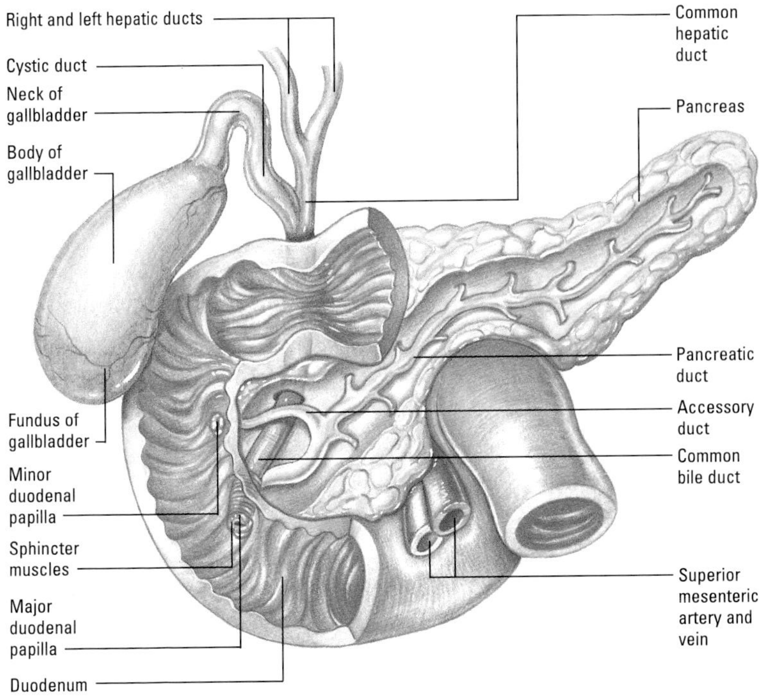
Right and left hepatic ducts
Cystic duct
Neck of gallbladder
Body of gallbladder
Fundus of gallbladder
Minor duodenal papilla
Sphincter muscles
Major duodenal papilla
Duodenum
Common hepatic duct
Pancreas
Pancreatic duct
Accessory duct
Common bile duct
Superior mesenteric artery and vein

Liver lobule

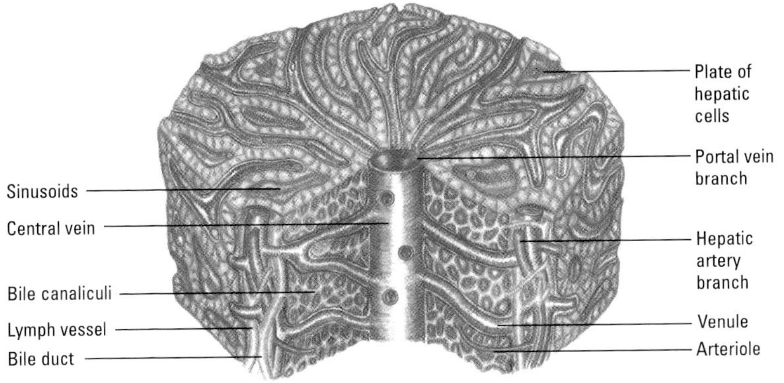
Sinusoids
Central vein
Bile canaliculi
Lymph vessel
Bile duct
Plate of hepatic cells
Portal vein branch
Hepatic artery branch
Venule
Arteriole

Urinary tract

ANTERIOR VIEW

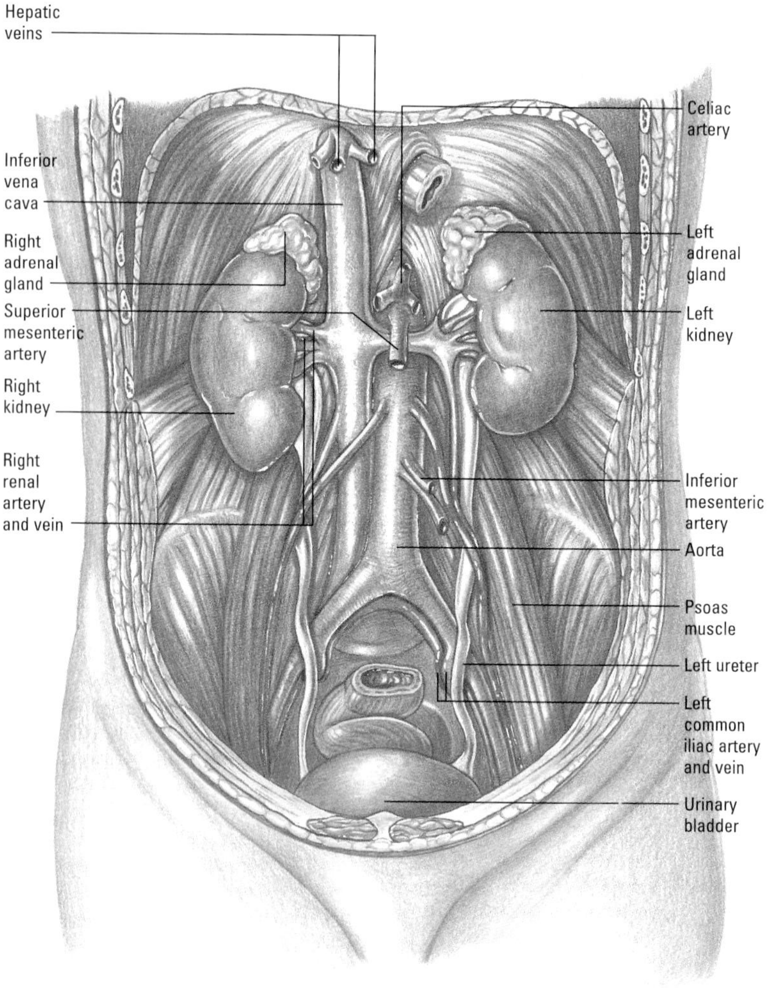
Hepatic veins
Inferior vena cava
Right adrenal gland
Superior mesenteric artery
Right kidney
Right renal artery and vein
Celiac artery
Left adrenal gland
Left kidney
Inferior mesenteric artery
Aorta
Psoas muscle
Left ureter
Left common iliac artery and vein
Urinary bladder

Kidney structures

ANTERIOR VIEW OF KIDNEY

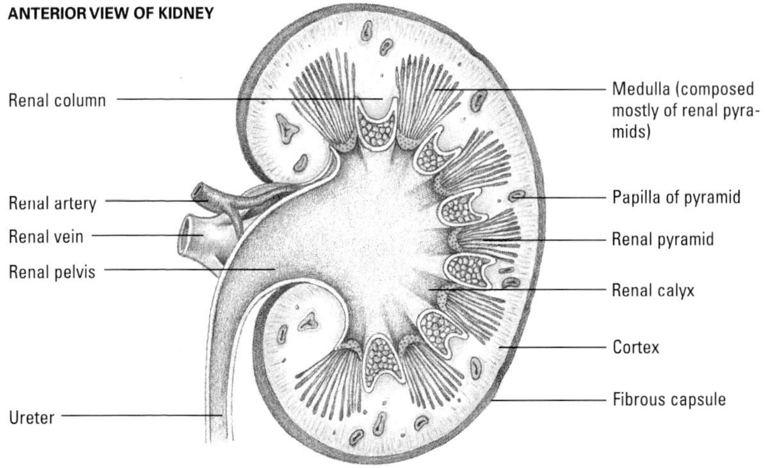

NEPHRON

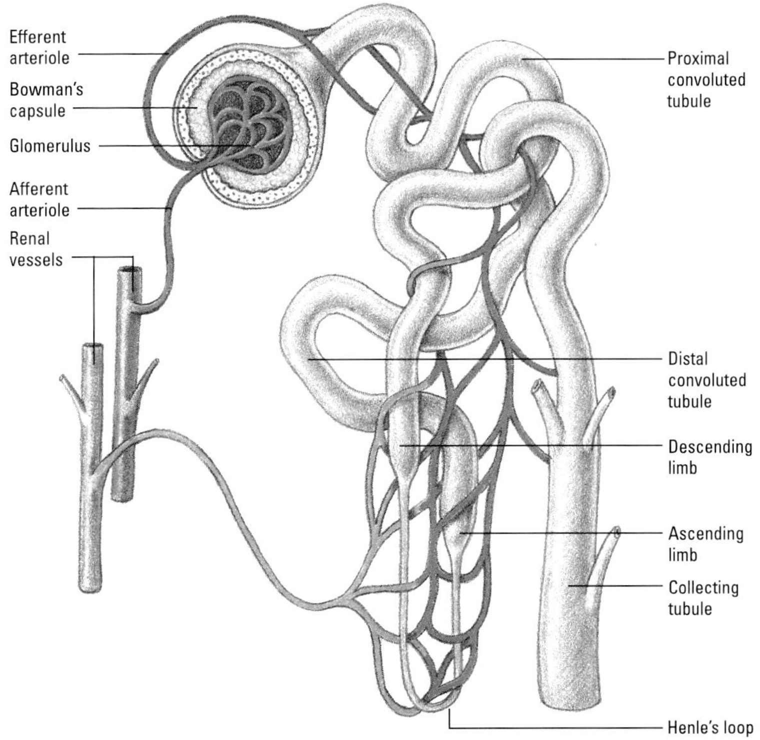

Renin-angiotensin-aldosterone system

The renin-angiotensin-aldosterone system regulates the body's sodium and water levels and blood pressure. Juxtaglomerular cells (1) near the glomeruli in each kidney secrete the enzyme renin into the blood. The renin secretion rate depends on the perfusion rate in the renal afferent arterioles and on the serum sodium level. A low sodium load and low perfusion pressure cause renin secretion to rise; a high sodium load and high pressure cause it to decrease.

Renin circulates throughout the body and converts angiotensinogen, made in the liver (2), into angiotensin I. In the lungs (3), angiotensin I is converted by hydrolysis to angiotensin II. Angiotensin II acts on the adrenal cortex (4) to stimulate production of the hormone aldosterone. Aldosterone acts on the juxtaglomerular cells to increase sodium and water retention and to stimulate or depress further renin secretion, completing the feedback system that automatically readjusts homeostasis.

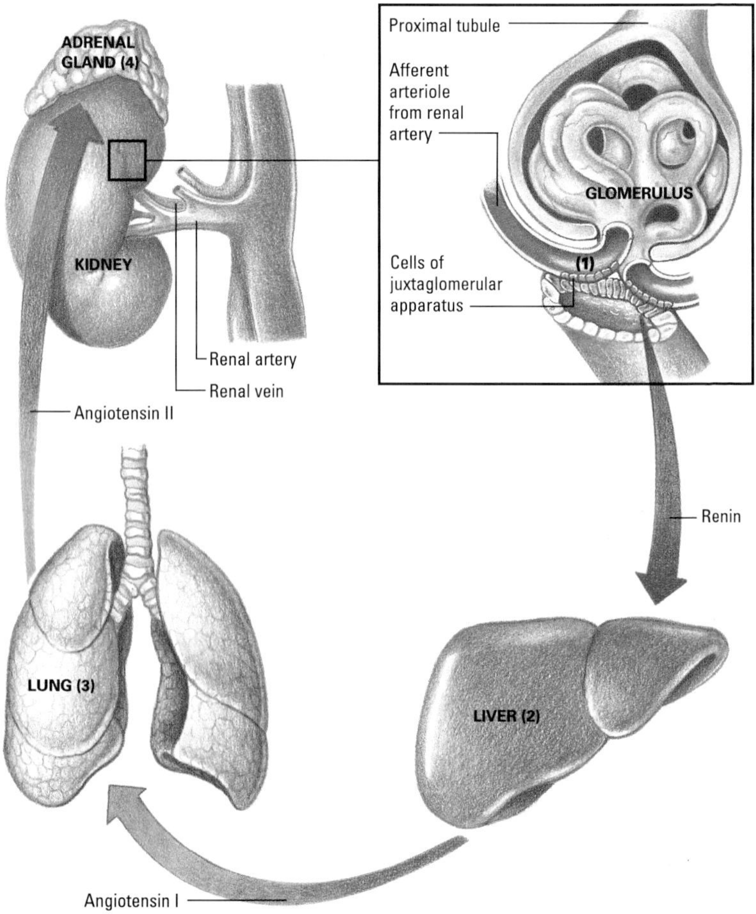

Male reproductive system

The male reproductive system consists of the penis, scrotum, testes, duct system, and accessory structures (prostate gland, seminal vesicles, bulbourethral glands, and urethral glands).

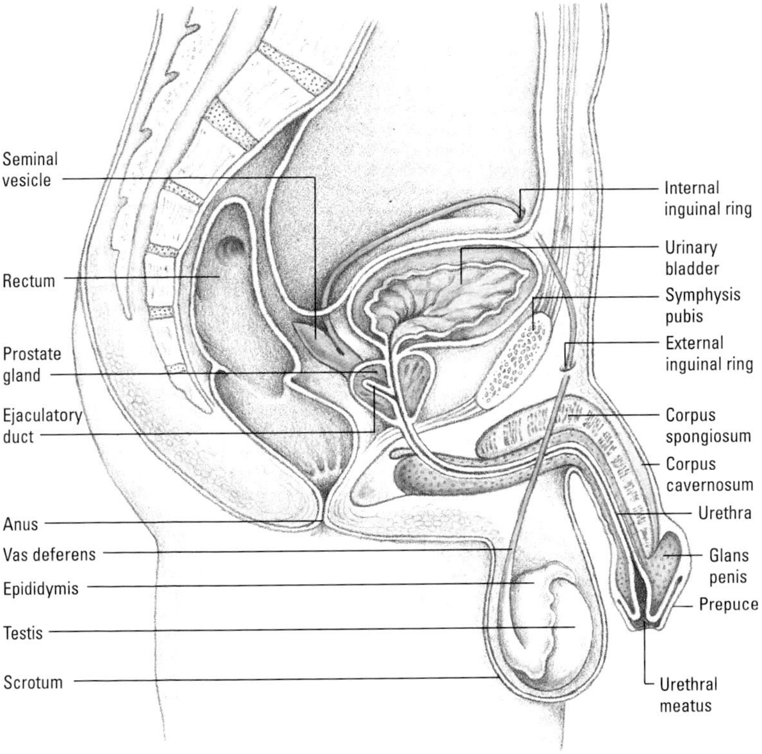

SPERMATOZOON (MALE REPRODUCTIVE CELL)

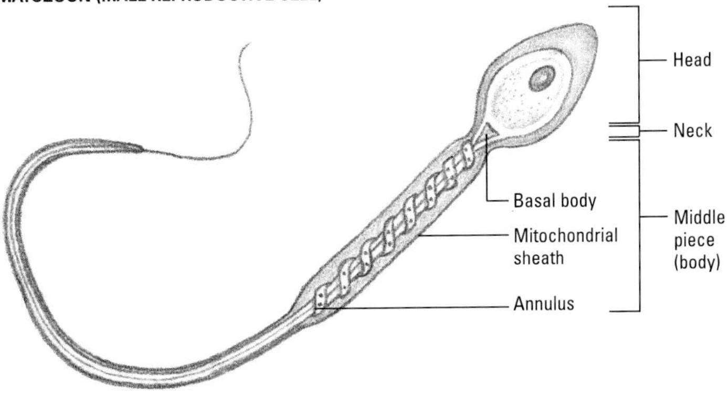

Female reproductive system

The female reproductive system includes the vagina, uterus, fallopian tubes, and ovaries, which are shown below. It also includes external genitalia — mons pubis, labia majora, labia minora, urethral meatus, ducts from Skene's and Bartholin's glands, and vaginal orifice — that aren't shown here.

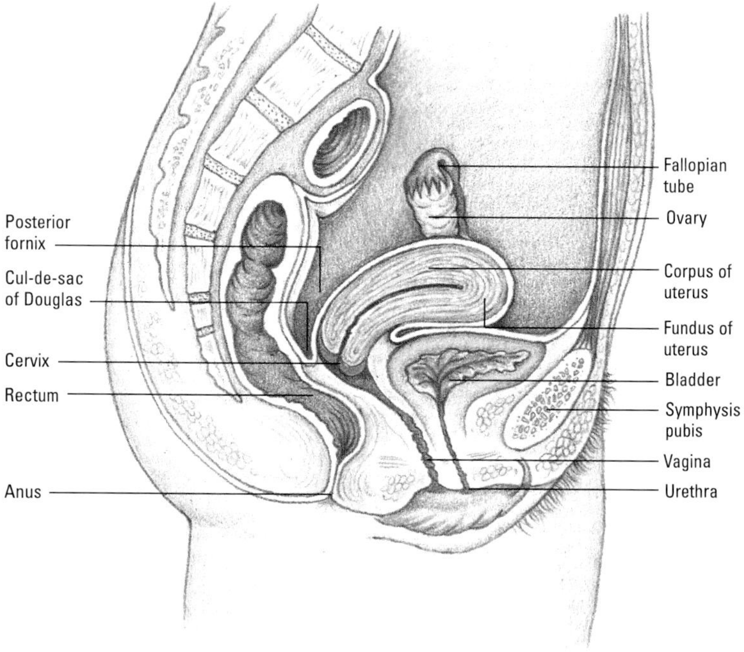

OVUM (FEMALE REPRODUCTIVE CELL)

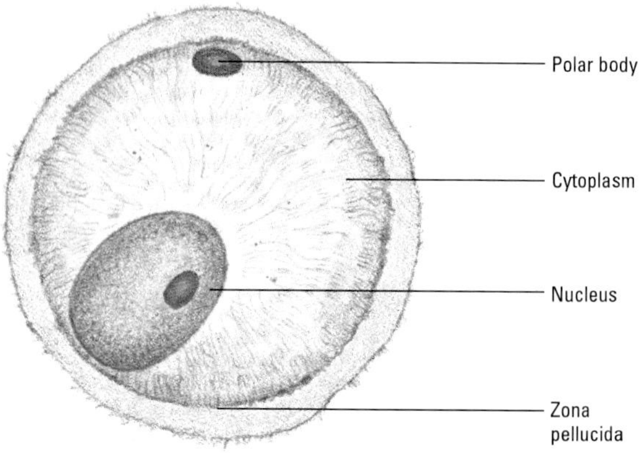

A structural view

Locating lung structures in the thoracic cage

The ribs, vertebrae, and other structures of the thoracic cage—along with the imaginary lines shown in these illustrations—act as landmarks that you can use to identify underlying structures.

From an anterior view

- The base or bottom of each lung rests at the level of the sixth rib at the midclavicular line and the eighth rib at the midaxillary line.
- The apex (pointed upper part) of each lung extends about ¾" to 1 ½" (2 to 4 cm) above the inner aspects of the clavicles.
- The upper lobe of the right lung ends level with the fourth rib at the midclavicular line and with the fifth rib at the midaxillary line.
- The middle lobe of the right lung extends triangularly from the fourth to the sixth rib at the midclavicular line and to the fifth rib at the midaxillary line.
- Because the left lung doesn't have a middle lobe, the upper lobe of the left lung ends level with the fourth rib at the midclavicular line and with the fifth rib at the midaxillary line.

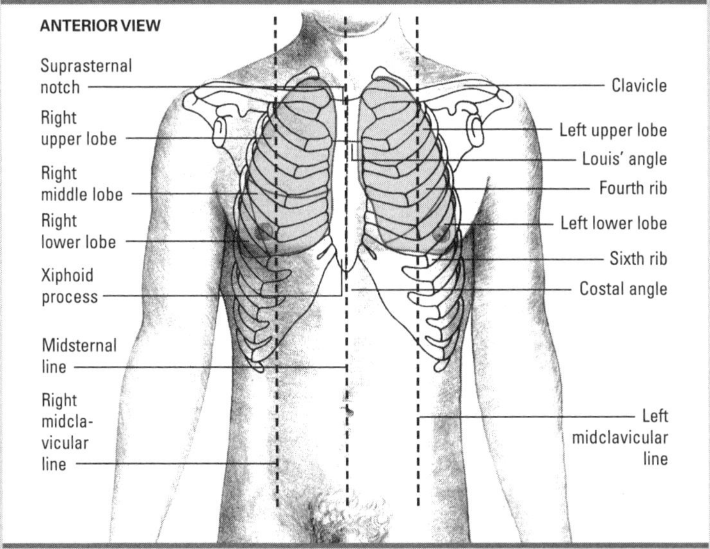

(continued)

Locating lung structures in the thoracic cage *(continued)*

From a posterior view

- The lungs extend from the cervical area to the level of the tenth thoracic vertebra (T10). On deep inspiration, the lungs may descend to T12.
- An imaginary line stretching from the T3 level along the inferior border of the scapulae to the fifth rib at the midaxillary line separates the upper lobes of both lungs.
- The upper lobes exist above T3; the lower lobes exist below T3 and extend to the level of T10.
- The diaphragm originates around the ninth or tenth rib.

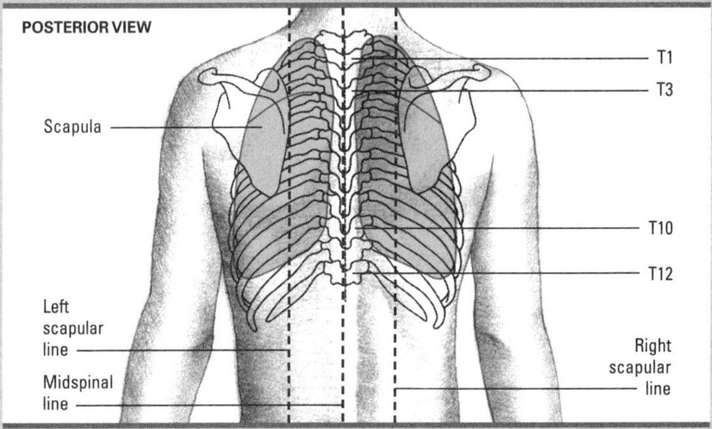

From a lateral view

- The right and left lateral rib cages cover the lobes of the right and left lungs, respectively.
- Beneath these structures, the lungs extend from just above the clavicles to the level of the eighth rib.
- The left lateral thorax allows access to two lobes; the right lateral thorax, to three lobes.

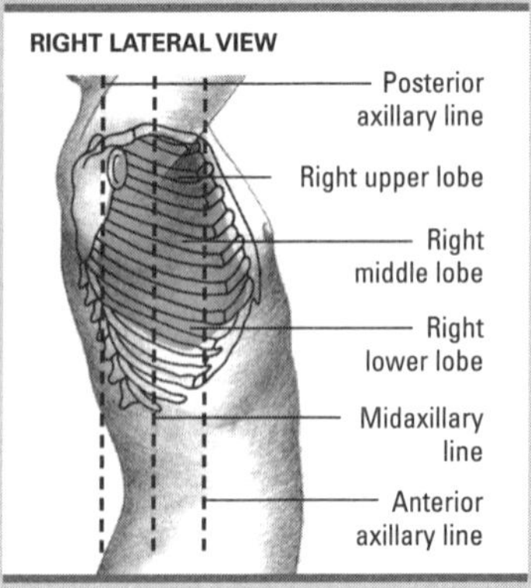

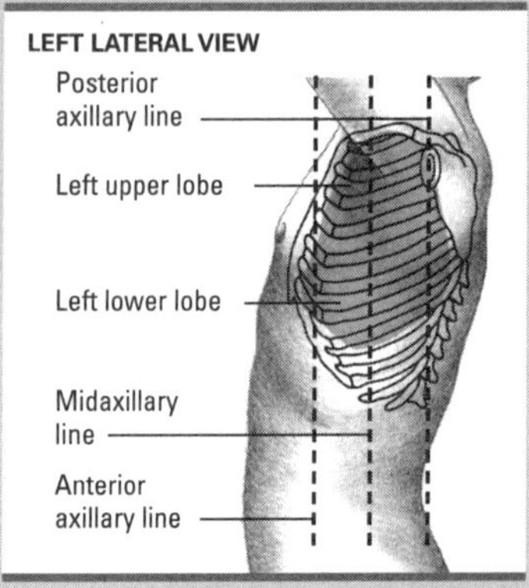

Respiratory changes during exercise

Healthy lungs can easily expand to meet the added demands for oxygen during exercise. During the deep inspirations that occur during exercise, accessory muscles work to increase thoracic volume. These muscles, including the scalenes, sternocleidomastoids, and pectoralis minor, raise the ribs more than during normal inspiration to accommodate increased oxygen demands.

Inspiration and expiration

Breathing involves two actions: *inspiration,* an active process, and *expiration,* a relatively passive one. Both actions rely on respiratory muscle function and the effects of pressure differences in the lungs.

Normal respiration

During normal respiration, the external intercostal muscles aid the *diaphragm,* the major muscle of respiration. The diaphragm descends to lengthen the chest cavity, while the external intercostal muscles (located between and along the lower borders of the ribs) contract to expand the anteroposterior diameter. This coordinated action causes inspiration. Rising of the diaphragm and relaxation of the intercostal muscles causes expiration. (See *Mechanics of respiration,* page 122.)

Forced inspiration and active expiration

During exercise, when the body needs increased oxygenation, or in certain disease states that require forced inspiration and active expiration, the *accessory muscles* of respiration also participate. These muscles include:

- internal intercostal muscles on the inner surface of the ribs
- pectoral muscles in the upper chest
- sternocleidomastoid muscles on the sides of the neck
- scalene muscles in the neck
- posterior trapezius muscle in the upper back
- abdominal rectus muscles.

During forced inspiration, the pectoral muscles raise the chest to increase the anteroposterior diameter; the sternocleidomastoid muscles raise the sternum; the scalene muscles elevate, fix, and expand the upper chest; and the posterior trapezius muscles raise the thoracic cage.

During active expiration, the internal intercostals contract to shorten the chest's transverse diameter and the abdominal rectus muscles pull down the lower chest, thus depressing the lower ribs.

Gas exchange

Oxygen-depleted blood enters the lungs from the pulmonary artery of the heart's right ventricle and then flows through the main pulmonary arteries into the smaller vessels of the pleural cavities and the main bronchi, through the arterioles and, eventually, to the capillary networks in the alveoli. (See *Tracing the pulmonary circulation,* page 123.)

In the alveoli, gas exchange — oxygen and carbon dioxide diffusion — takes place. After passing through the pulmonary capillaries, oxygenated blood flows through the end branches of the pulmonary veins, or *venules.* From there, the blood flows through progressively larger vessels, eventually reaching the left atrium of the heart through the pulmonary veins. From the heart's left side, oxygenated blood is distributed throughout the body.

External and internal respiration

Effective respiration consists of gas exchange in the lungs, called *external respiration,* and gas exchange in the tissues, called *internal respiration.*

A structural view

Mechanics of respiration

The muscles of respiration help the chest cavity expand and contract. Pressure differences between atmospheric air and the lungs help produce air movement. These drawings illustrate the muscles that work together to allow inspiration and expiration.

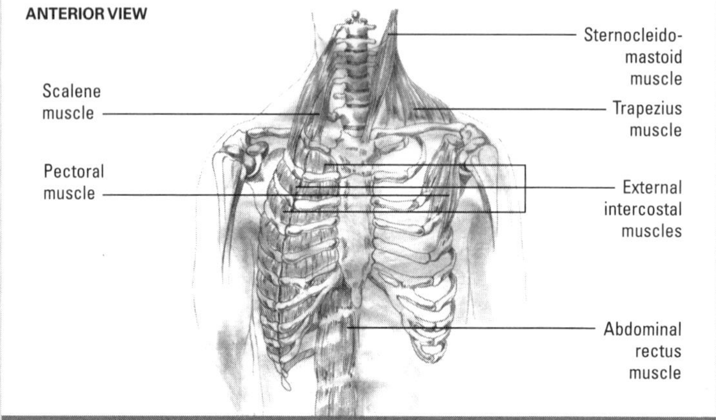

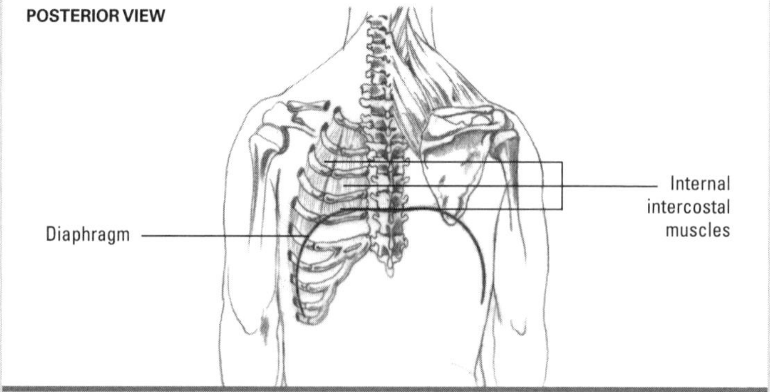

External respiration occurs through three processes:

- *ventilation* — gas distribution into and out of the pulmonary airways
- *pulmonary perfusion* — blood flow from the right side of the heart, through the pulmonary circulation, and into the left side of the heart
- *diffusion* — gas movement through a semipermeable membrane from an area of greater concentration to one of lesser concentration (internal respiration occurs only through diffusion).

POINT TO REMEMBER

All three processes — ventilation, pulmonary perfusion,

Focus on function
Tracing the pulmonary circulation

The right and left pulmonary arteries carry deoxygenated blood from the right side of the heart to the lungs. These arteries divide into distal branches, called arterioles, which eventually terminate as a concentrated capillary network in the alveoli and alveolar sac, where gas exchange occurs.

Venules—the end branches of the pulmonary veins—collect oxygenated blood from the capillaries and transport it to larger vessels, which in turn lead to the pulmonary veins. The pulmonary veins enter the left side of the heart and distribute oxygenated blood throughout the body.

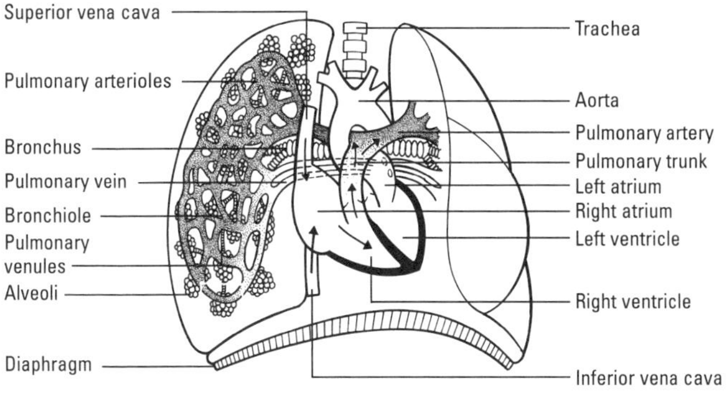

and diffusion — are vital to maintaining adequate oxygenation and acid-base balance.

Ventilation
Adequate ventilation depends on the nervous, musculoskeletal, and pulmonary systems to accomplish the necessary changes in lung pressure. If any of these systems fails to function properly, breathing effort increases and breathing effectiveness decreases.

Nervous system influence
Although ventilation is largely involuntary, a person can control its rate and depth by performing breathing exercises to reduce stress. Involuntary breathing results from stimulation of the respiratory center in the medulla and the pons of the brain. The medulla controls the rate and depth of respiration; the pons moderates the rhythm of the switch from inspiration to expiration.

Musculoskeletal influence
The adult thorax is flexible; its shape can be changed by contracting the chest muscles. The medulla controls ventilation primarily by stimulating contraction of the diaphragm and external intercostals, the major muscles of breathing. The diaphragm flattens and descends to expand the length of the chest cavity, while the external intercostals contract to expand the anteroposterior diameter. These actions produce the intrapulmonary pressure changes that cause inspiration.

Pulmonary influence

During inspiration, air flows through the right and left mainstem bronchi into increasingly smaller bronchi and then into bronchioles, alveolar ducts, and alveolar sacs. Finally, it reaches the alveolar membrane. This normal airflow distribution can be affected by many factors, including:

- airflow pattern (see *Comparing airflow patterns*)
- volume and location of the functional reserve capacity (air retained in the alveoli that prevents their collapse during respiration)
- degree of intrapulmonary resistance
- presence of lung disease.

If airflow is disrupted, airflow distribution follows the path of least resistance. For example, an obstruction in one of the lungs or forced inspiration causes uneven distribution of air.

Other musculoskeletal and intrapulmonary factors can affect airflow and, in turn, may affect breathing. For instance, forced breathing, as in emphysema, activates accessory muscles of respiration, which require additional oxygen to work. This results in less efficient ventilation with an increased workload.

Other airflow alterations can also increase oxygen and energy demand and cause respiratory muscle fatigue. These conditions include interference with expansion of the lungs or thorax (changes in compliance) and interference with airflow in the tracheobronchial tree (changes in resistance).

Pulmonary perfusion

Perfusion aids external respiration. Normal pulmonary blood flow allows alveolar gas exchange, but many factors may interfere with gas transport to the alveoli. Here are some examples:

- Cardiac output less than the average of 5 L/minute decreases gas exchange by reducing blood flow.
- Elevations in pulmonary and systemic resistance reduce blood flow.
- Abnormal or insufficient hemoglobin picks up less oxygen for exchange.

Ventilation-perfusion ($\dot{V}/\dot{Q}$) match

Gravity can affect oxygen and carbon dioxide transport in a positive way by influencing pulmonary circulation. Gravity causes more unoxygenated blood to travel to the lower and middle lung lobes than to the upper lobes.

This explains why ventilation and perfusion differ in the various parts of the lungs. Areas where perfusion and ventilation are similar have what's referred to as a *$\dot{V}/\dot{Q}$ match*; in such areas, gas exchange is most efficient.

$\dot{V}/\dot{Q}$ mismatch

Other areas of the lung may have unequal ventilation and perfusion, known as a *$\dot{V}/\dot{Q}$ mismatch.* (See *What happens in ventilation-perfusion mismatch,* page 126.)

Optimal conditions for diffusion

In diffusion, oxygen and carbon dioxide molecules move between the alveoli and capillaries. *Partial pressure* — the pressure exerted by one gas in a mixture of gases — dictates the direction of movement, which is always from an area of greater concentration to one of lesser concentration. In the process, oxygen moves across the alveolar and capillary membranes, dissolves in the plasma, and then passes through the red blood cell (RBC) membrane. Carbon dioxide moves in the opposite direction.

For diffusion to succeed, the epithelial membranes lining the alveoli and capillaries must be intact. Both the alveolar epithelium and the capillary endothelium are composed of a single layer of cells. Between these layers are tiny interstitial spaces filled with elastin and collagen.

Normally, oxygen and carbon dioxide move easily through all of these layers. Oxygen moves from the alveoli into the bloodstream, where it's taken up by hemoglobin in the RBCs. Once there, it displaces carbon dioxide (the by-product of metabolism), which diffuses from RBCs into the blood and then to the alveoli.

Focus on function
Comparing airflow patterns

The pattern of airflow through the respiratory passages affects airway resistance.

Laminar flow
Laminar flow, a linear pattern that occurs at low flow rates, offers minimal resistance. This flow type occurs mainly in the small peripheral airways of the bronchial tree.

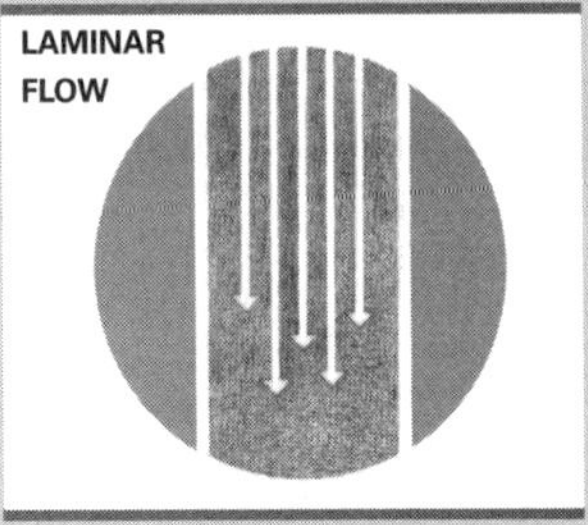

Turbulent flow
The eddying pattern of *turbulent flow* creates friction and increases resistance. Turbulent flow is normal in the trachea and large central bronchi. However, if the smaller airways become constricted or clogged with secretions, turbulent flow may occur there also.

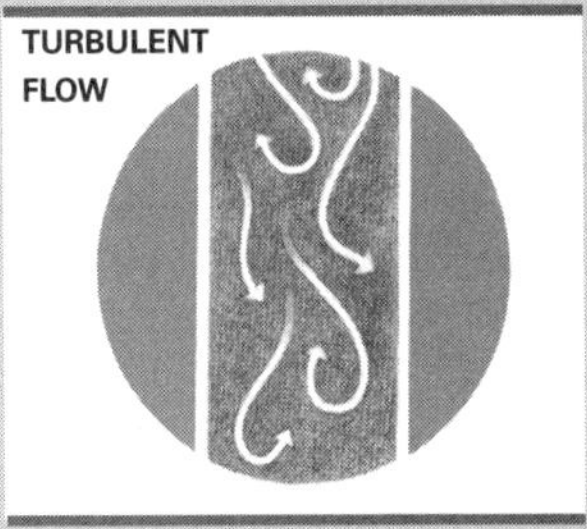

Transitional flow
A mixed pattern known as *transitional flow* is common at lower flow rates in the larger airways, especially where the airways narrow from obstruction, meet, or branch.

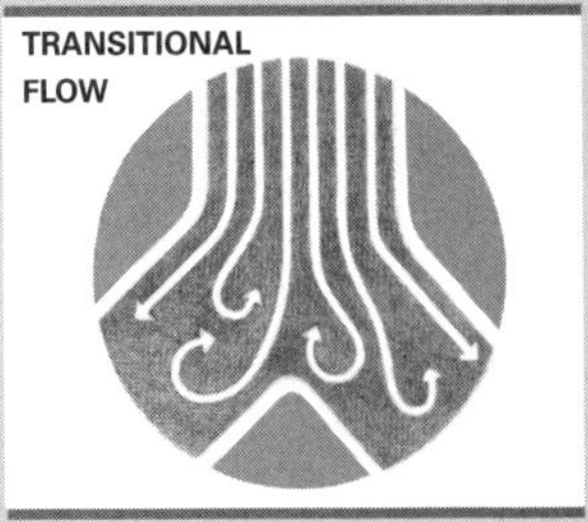

Most transported oxygen binds with hemoglobin to form *oxyhemoglobin*, while a small portion dissolves in the plasma. (The portion that dissolves in plasma can be measured as the partial pressure of arterial oxygen, or Pa_{O_2}).

After oxygen binds to hemoglobin, RBCs travel to the tissues. Internal respiration occurs when, through cellular diffusion, RBCs release oxygen and absorb carbon dioxide. The RBCs then transport the carbon dioxide back to the lungs for removal during expiration.

Role of the lungs in acid-base balance

The lungs help sustain acid-base balance in the body by maintaining exter-

What happens in ventilation-perfusion mismatch

Ideally, the amount of air in the alveoli (a reflection of ventilation) matches the amount of blood in the capillaries (a reflection of perfusion). This allows gas exchange to proceed smoothly.

Actually, this ventilation-perfusion ($\dot{V}/\dot{Q}$) ratio is unequal: The alveoli receive air at a rate of approximately 4 L/minute, while the capillaries supply blood at a rate of about 5 L/minute. This creates a $\dot{V}/\dot{Q}$ mismatch of 4:5 or 0.8.

Keep in mind, however, that this ratio is an average and varies in different areas of lung tissue. Only those areas with a low $\dot{V}/\dot{Q}$ ratio are at risk for impaired gas exchange.

Effects of $\dot{V}/\dot{Q}$ mismatch

$\dot{V}/\dot{Q}$ mismatch accounts for most of the defective gas exchange in respiratory disorders. When ineffective gas exchange results from a physiologic abnormality, the effect may be reduced ventilation to a unit (shunt), reduced perfusion to a unit (dead-space ventilation), or both (silent unit). Variations of the three $\dot{V}/\dot{Q}$ abnormalities exist, depending on the overall lung $\dot{V}/\dot{Q}$ ratio.

Respiratory disorders are commonly categorized physiologically as shunt producing if the $\dot{V}/\dot{Q}$ ratio falls below 0.8, or as dead-space producing if the $\dot{V}/\dot{Q}$ exceeds 0.8.

NORMAL

In the normal lung, ventilation closely matches perfusion.

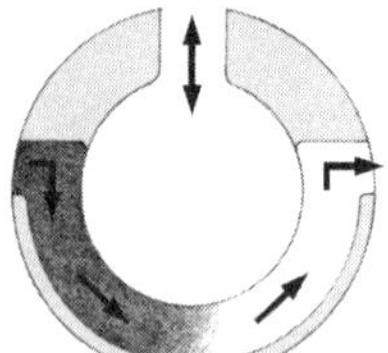

SHUNT

Perfusion without ventilation usually results from airway obstruction, particularly that caused by acute diseases, such as atelectasis or pneumonia.

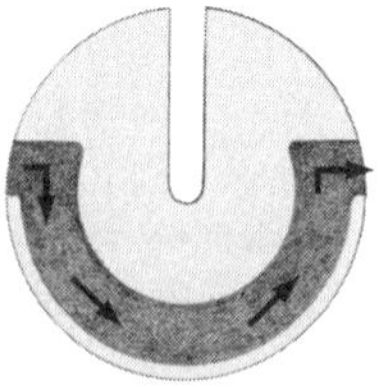

DEAD-SPACE VENTILATION

Normal ventilation without perfusion usually results from a perfusion defect such as pulmonary embolism.

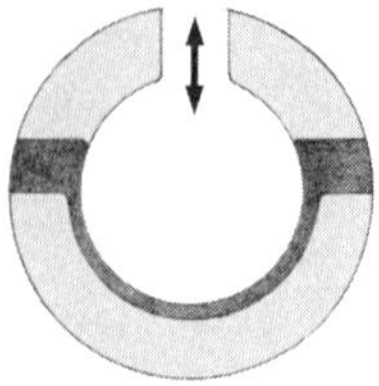

SILENT UNIT

Absence of ventilation and perfusion usually stems from multiple causes, such as pulmonary embolism with resultant adult respiratory distress syndrome or emphysema.

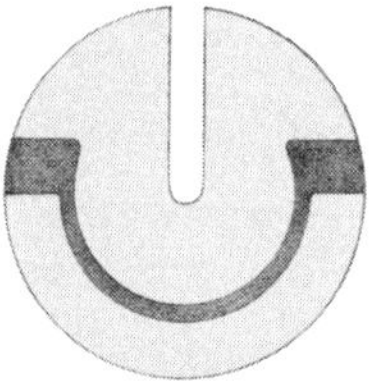

nal and internal respiration. Oxygen taken up in the lungs is transported to the tissues by the circulatory system, which exchanges it for carbon dioxide produced by metabolism in body cells. Because carbon dioxide is more soluble than oxygen, it dissolves in the blood, where most of it forms bicarbonate (base) and smaller amounts form carbonic acid (acid).

Respiratory responses

The lungs control bicarbonate levels by converting bicarbonate to carbon dioxide and water for excretion. In response to signals from the medulla, the lungs can change the rate and depth of breathing. This change allows for adjustments in the amount of carbon dioxide lost to help maintain acid-base balance.

For example, in metabolic alkalosis (a condition resulting from excess bicarbonate retention), the rate and depth of ventilation decrease so that carbon dioxide can be retained; this increases carbonic acid levels. In metabolic acidosis (a condition resulting from excess acid retention or excess bicarbonate loss), the lungs increase the rate and depth of ventilation to eliminate excess carbon dioxide, thus reducing carbonic acid levels.

Hypoventilation and hyperventilation

When the lungs don't function properly, they can produce an acid-base imbalance. For example, they can cause respiratory acidosis through *hypoventilation* (reduced rate and depth of ventilation), which leads to carbon dioxide retention. (For more information on acid-base balance, see chapter 14, Fluid, electrolyte, and acid-base balance.)

11 Gastrointestinal system

The GI system has two major components: the alimentary canal (also called the GI tract) and the accessory GI organs. Together, the alimentary canal and accessory organs serve two major functions:

- digestion — the breaking down of food and fluid into simple chemicals that can be absorbed into the bloodstream and transported throughout the body
- elimination of waste products from the body through excretion of feces.

Alimentary canal

The *alimentary canal* consists essentially of a hollow muscular tube that begins in the mouth and extends to the anus. It includes the pharynx, esophagus, stomach, small intestine, and large intestine. (See *Structures of the GI system.*)

Mouth

Also called the *buccal cavity* or oral cavity, the mouth is bounded by the lips (labia), cheeks, *palate* (the roof of the mouth), and tongue. It also contains the teeth. Ducts connect the mouth with the three major pairs of *salivary glands* (parotid, submandibular, and sublingual glands), which secrete saliva to moisten food during chewing. The mouth initiates the mechanical breakdown of food.

Pharynx

A cavity extending from the base of the skull to the esophagus, the *pharynx* aids swallowing by grasping food and propelling it toward the esophagus.

Esophagus

A muscular tube measuring about 10" (25 cm), the *esophagus* extends from the pharynx through the mediastinum to the stomach.

POINT TO REMEMBER
Swallowing triggers the passage of food from the pharynx to the esophagus.

Peristalsis — the rhythmic contraction and relaxations of smooth muscle — propels liquids and solids through the esophagus into the stomach. The *cricopharyngeal sphincter* — a sphincter at the upper border of the esophagus — must relax for food to enter the esophagus.

Stomach

The *stomach* is a collapsible, pouchlike structure in the left upper part of the abdominal cavity, just below the diaphragm. Measuring about 10" long, it lies in the left side of the superior part of the abdominal cavity, its upper border attaching to the lower end of the esophagus. The lateral surface of the stomach is called the *greater curvature;* the medial surface, the *lesser curvature.*

POINT TO REMEMBER
The size of the stomach varies with the degree of distention. With marked distention, such as from eating a very large meal, stomach size impedes the diaphragm as it falls on inspiration. This causes the shortness of breath that sometimes accompanies overeating.

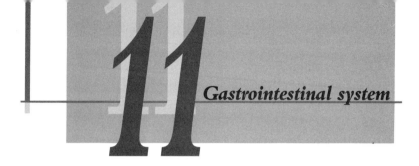

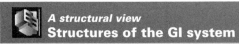

A structural view
Structures of the GI system

The GI system includes the alimentary canal (pharynx, esophagus, stomach, and small and large intestines) and the accessory organs (liver, biliary duct system, and pancreas).

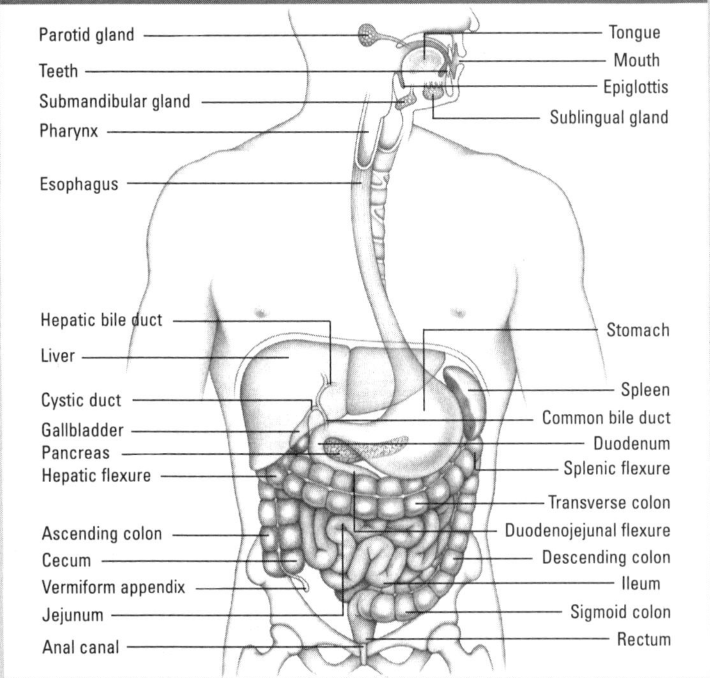

Regions

The stomach has four main regions:

- The *cardia* lies near the junction of the stomach and esophagus.
- The *fundus* is the enlarged portion above and to the left of the esophageal opening into the stomach.
- The *body* is the middle portion of the stomach.
- The *pylorus* is the lower portion, lying near the junction of the stomach and duodenum.

Functions

The stomach serves as a temporary storage area for food, with a capacity of 2 to 4 qt (2 to 4 L). The stomach also begins digestion. Structural folds called *rugae*, located in the inside wall of the stomach, help with the mechanical breakdown of food and help mix the food with gastric secretions.

After the food mixes with gastric secretions, the stomach breaks it down into *chyme*, a semifluid substance, and then moves the gastric contents into the small intestine.

Small intestine

The longest organ of the GI tract, the small intestine is a tube measuring about 20′ (6 m) long. It has three major divisions:

- The *duodenum* is the most superior division. It measures roughly 10″ (25 cm) long.
- The *jejunum,* the middle portion, is about 8′ (2.5 m) long.
- The *ileum,* the most inferior portion, is approximately 12′ (3.5 m) long.

Intestinal wall features

Structural features of the wall of the small intestine significantly increase its absorptive surface area. These features include:

- *plicae circulares*—circular folds of the intestinal mucosa, or mucous membrane lining
- *villi*—fingerlike projections on the mucosa
- *microvilli*—tiny cytoplasmic projections on the surface of epithelial cells.

Other structures

The small intestine also contains *intestinal crypts*, simple glands lodged in the grooves separating villi; *Peyer's patches*, collections of lymphatic tissue within the submucosa; and *Brunner's glands,* which secrete mucus.

Functions

The small intestine completes food digestion. Food molecules are absorbed through the wall of the small intestine into the circulatory system, from which they're delivered to body cells.

The small intestine also secretes hormones that help control the secretion of bile, pancreatic juice, and intestinal juice.

Large intestine

The large intestine extends from the *ileocecal valve* (the valve between the ileum of the small intestine and the first segment of the large intestine) to the anus. Measuring roughly 5′ (1.5 m) long, the large intestine has five segments:

- The *cecum,* a saclike structure, makes up the first few inches of the large intestine, beginning just below the ileocecal valve.
- The *ascending colon* rises on the right posterior abdominal wall and then turns sharply under the liver at the hepatic flexure.
- The *transverse colon* is situated above the small intestine, passing horizontally across the abdomen and below the liver, stomach, and spleen. At the left colic flexure, it turns downward.
- The *descending colon* starts near the spleen and extends down the left side of the abdomen into the pelvic cavity.
- The *sigmoid colon* descends through the pelvic cavity, where it becomes the rectum.
- The *rectum,* the last few inches of the large intestine, terminates at the anus.

Functions

The large intestine absorbs water, secretes mucus, and eliminates digestive wastes.

GI tract wall structures

The wall of the GI tract consists of several layers: mucosa, submucosa, tunica muscularis, and visceral peritoneum.

Mucosa

The innermost layer, the mucosa (also called *tunica mucosa*) consists of epithelial and surface cells and loose connective tissue. In the small intestine, epithelial cells on the mucosal surface form millions of *villi* that vastly increase the absorptive surface area. These cells also secrete gastric and protective juices and absorb nutrients.

Surface cells overlie connective tissue (*lamina propria*), supported by a thin layer of smooth muscle (*muscularis mucosae*).

Submucosa

The submucosa (also called *tunica submucosa*) encircles the mucosa. It's composed of loose connective tissue, blood and lymphatic vessels, and a nerve network (*submucosal plexus*, or *Meissner's plexus*).

Tunica muscularis

Around the submucosa lies the *tunica muscularis*, composed of skeletal muscle in the mouth, pharynx, and upper esophagus and of longitudinal and circular smooth muscle fibers elsewhere in the tract. During peristalsis, longitudinal fibers shorten the lumen length and circular fibers reduce the lumen diameter. At points along the tract, circular fibers thicken to form sphincters.

In the large intestine, circular and longitudinal fibers of the tunica muscularis move and mix intestinal contents; longitudinal fibers give the large intestine its shape. These fibers gather into three narrow bands *(taeniae coli)* down the middle of the colon and pucker the intestine into characteristic pouches *(haustra)*.

Between the two muscle layers lies another nerve network — the *myenteric plexus*, also known as *Auerbach's plexus*.

The stomach wall contains a third muscle layer made up of oblique fibers.

Visceral peritoneum

The *visceral peritoneum* is the GI tract's outer covering. In the esophagus and rectum, it's also called the *tunica adventitia*; elsewhere in the GI tract, it's called the *tunica serosa*.

The visceral peritoneum covers most of the abdominal organs and lies next to an identical layer, the *parietal peritoneum*, that lines the abdominal cavity. The visceral peritoneum becomes a double-layered fold around the blood vessels, nerves, and lymphatics supplying the small intestine, and attaches the jejunum and ileum to the posterior abdominal wall to prevent twisting. A similar fold attaches the transverse colon to the posterior abdominal wall. (See *Features of the GI tract wall,* page 132.)

GI tract innervation

Distension of the submucosal plexus or myenteric plexus stimulates transmission of nerve signals to the smooth muscle, which initiates peristalsis and mixing contractions. Parasympathetic stimulation of the vagus nerve (for most of the intestines) and the sacral spinal nerves (for the descending colon and rectum) increases gut and sphincter tone as well as the frequency, strength, and velocity of smooth muscle contractions. Vagal stimulation also increases motor and secretory activities. Sympathetic stimulation, by way of the spinal nerves from levels T6 to L2, reduces peristalsis and inhibits GI activity.

Accessory organs of digestion

Accessory organs — the liver, biliary duct system, and pancreas — contribute hormones, enzymes, and bile vital to digestion. They deliver their secretions to the duodenum through the *hepatopancreatic ampulla*, also called the *ampulla of Vater* or *Oddi's sphincter*.

Liver

The body's largest gland, the 3-lb (1.4-kg) liver is enclosed in a fibrous capsule in the right upper quadrant of the abdomen. The liver is highly vascular.

The *lesser omentum*, a fold of peritoneum, covers most of the liver and anchors the liver to the lesser curvature of the stomach. The hepatic artery and hepatic portal vein as well as the common bile duct and hepatic veins pass through the lesser omentum.

Lobes and lobules

The liver consists of four lobes — a left lobe, right lobe, caudate lobe (behind the right lobe), and quadrate lobe (behind the left lobe).

The liver's functional unit, the *lobule,* consists of a plate of hepatic cells, or *hepatocytes*, that encircle a central vein and radiate outward. Separating the hepatocyte plates from each other are *sinusoids*, the liver's capillary system. Reticuloendothelial macrophages *(Kupffer's cells)* lining the sinusoids remove bacteria and toxins that have entered the blood through the intestinal capillaries.

A structural view

Features of the GI tract wall

Several layers—the tunica mucosa, tunica submucosa, and tunica adventitia—form the wall of the GI tract. This illustration depicts the cellular anatomy of the wall, including special features (such as the villi), the peritoneum, the muscles, and a nerve network.

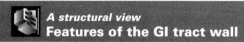

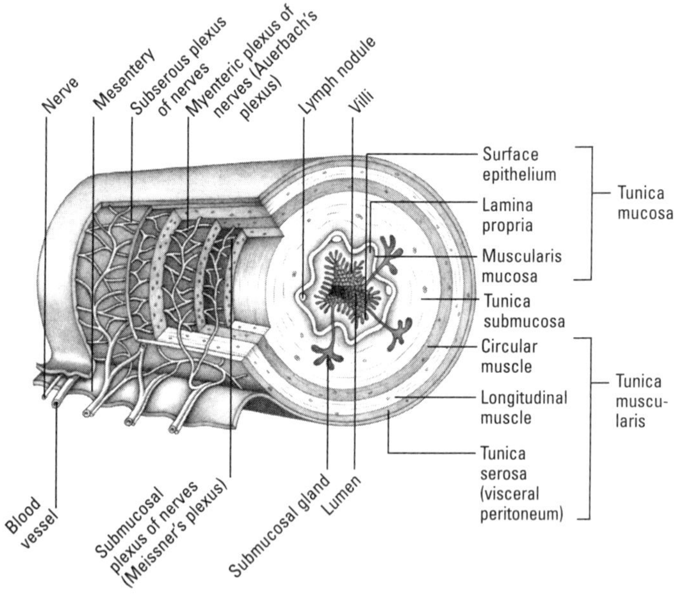

The sinusoids carry oxygenated blood from the hepatic artery and nutrient-rich blood from the portal vein. Unoxygenated blood leaves through the central vein and flows through hepatic veins to the inferior vena cava.

Ducts

Bile, recycled from bile salts in the blood, leaves through bile ducts *(canaliculi)* that merge into the right and left hepatic ducts to form the *common hepatic duct*. This duct joins the *cystic duct* from the gallbladder to form the *common bile duct* leading to the duodenum.

Functions

The liver performs complex and important functions related to digestion and nutrition:

- It plays an important role in carbohydrate metabolism.
- It detoxifies various endogenous and exogenous toxins in plasma.

- It synthesizes plasma proteins, nonessential amino acids, and vitamin A.
- It stores essential nutrients, such as vitamins K, D, and B_{12} and iron.
- It removes ammonia from body fluids, converting it to urea for excretion in urine.
- It secretes bile.

Function of bile

A greenish liquid, *bile* is composed of water, cholesterol, bile salts, electrolytes, and phospholipids. Important in fat emulsification (breakdown), bile promotes intestinal absorption of fatty acids, cholesterol, and other lipids. When bile salts are absent from the intestinal tract, lipids are excreted and fat-soluble vitamins are absorbed poorly.

POINT TO REMEMBER
Bile helps prevent jaundice by aiding excretion of conjugated bilirubin (an end product of hemoglobin degradation) from the liver.

The liver recycles about 80% of bile salts into bile, combining them with *bile pigments* (biliverdin and bilirubin, the breakdown products of red blood cells) and cholesterol. The liver produces this alkaline bile in continuous secretion.

Bile production may increase from stimulation of the vagus nerve, release of the hormone secretin, increased blood flow in the liver, and the presence of fat in the intestine.

Blood glucose regulation

The liver metabolizes digestive end products by regulating blood glucose levels. As glucose is absorbed through the intestine (anabolic state), the liver stores glucose as glycogen. When glucose isn't being absorbed or when blood glucose levels fall (catabolic state), the liver mobilizes glucose to restore blood levels necessary for brain function.

Gallbladder

A pear-shaped organ measuring roughly 3″ to 4″ (7.5 to 10 cm) long, the gallbladder is joined to the ventral surface of the liver by the cystic duct. It's covered with visceral peritoneum.

Functions

The gallbladder stores and concentrates bile produced by the liver. Secretion of the hormone *cholecystokinin* stimulates gallbladder contraction and relaxation of Oddi's sphincter. These actions in turn lead to bile release into the common bile duct for delivery to the duodenum. When the sphincter closes, bile is shunted to the gallbladder for storage. (See *GI hormones: Production and function,* page 134.)

Pancreas

A somewhat flat organ about 6″ to 9″ (15 to 23 cm) long, the pancreas lies behind the stomach. Its head and neck extend into the curve of the duodenum and its tail lies against the spleen.

Functions

The pancreas performs both exocrine and endocrine functions. Its exocrine function involves scattered cells that secrete more than 1,000 ml of digestive enzymes every day. Lobules and lobes of the clusters *(acini)* of enzyme-producing cells release their secretions into ducts that merge into the pancreatic duct.

Running the length of the pancreas, the *pancreatic duct* joins the bile duct from the gallbladder before entering the duodenum. Vagal stimulation and release of the hormones secretin and cholecystokinin control the rate and amount of pancreatic secretion.

The endocrine function of the pancreas involves the *islets of Langerhans,* located between the acinar cells. Over 1 million of these islets house two cell types: beta and alpha. *Beta cells* secrete *insulin* to promote carbohydrate metabolism; *alpha cells* secrete *glucagon,* a hormone that stimulates glycogenolysis in the liver. Both hormones flow directly into the blood, their release stimulated by blood glucose levels.

GI hormones: Production and function

When stimulated, GI structures secrete four hormones. Each hormone plays a different part in digestion.

Hormone and production site	Stimulating factor or agent	Function
Gastrin		
Produced in pyloric antrum and duodenal mucosa	▸ Pyloric antrum distension ▸ Vagal stimulation ▸ Protein digestion products ▸ Alcohol	Stimulates gastric secretion and motility
Gastric inhibitory peptides		
Produced in duodenal and jejunal mucosa	▸ Gastric acid ▸ Fats ▸ Fat digestion products	Inhibits gastric secretion and motility
Secretin		
Produced in duodenal and jejunal mucosa	▸ Gastric acid ▸ Fat digestion products ▸ Protein digestion products	Stimulates secretion of bile and alkaline pancreatic fluid
Cholecystokinin		
Produced in duodenal and jejunal mucosa	▸ Fat digestion products ▸ Protein digestion products	Stimulates gallbladder contraction and secretion of enzyme-rich pancreatic fluid

Digestion and elimination

Digestion starts in the oral cavity, where chewing (mastication), salivation (the beginning of starch digestion), and swallowing (deglutition) all take place.

When a person swallows a food bolus, *hypopharyngeal sphincter* — the sphincter in the upper esophagus — relaxes, allowing food to enter the esophagus. (See *What happens in swallowing.*) In the esophagus, the glossopharyngeal nerve activates peristalsis, which moves the food down toward the stomach.

As food passes through the esophagus, glands in the esophageal mucosal layer secrete mucus, which lubricates the bolus and protects the mucosal membrane from damage caused by poorly chewed foods.

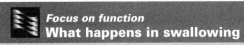

Focus on function
What happens in swallowing

Before peristalsis can begin, the neural pattern to initiate swallowing, illustrated here, must occur:

- Food pushed to the back of the mouth stimulates swallowing receptor areas that surround the pharyngeal opening.
- These receptor areas transmit impulses to the brain by way of the sensory portions of the trigeminal (V) and glossopharyngeal (IX) nerves.
- Then the brain's swallowing center relays motor impulses to the esophagus by way of the trigeminal (V), glossopharyngeal (IX), vagus (X), and hypoglossal (XII) nerves, causing swallowing to occur.

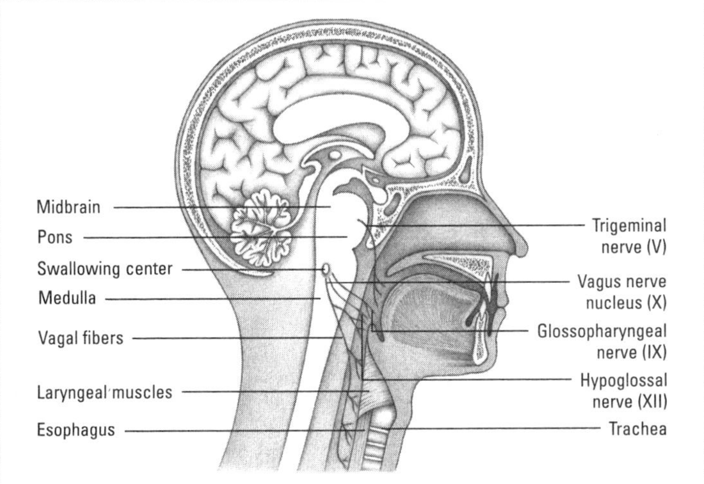

What happens in the stomach

The stomach's three major motor functions are storing food, mixing food with gastric juices, and slowly parcelling food into the small intestine for further digestion and absorption.

Cephalic phase of digestion

By the time the food bolus is traveling toward the stomach, the *cephalic phase* of digestion has already begun. In this phase, the stomach secretes digestive juices (hydrochloric acid and pepsin).

POINT TO REMEMBER
Digestive juices are secreted in response to stimuli aroused by smelling, tasting, chewing, or thinking about food.

Gastric phase of digestion

When food enters the stomach through the cardiac sphincter, the stomach wall stretches, initiating the *gastric phase* of digestion. In this phase, distention of the stomach wall stimulates the stomach to release *gastrin*. Gastrin, in turn, stimulates the stomach's motor functions and secretion of gastric juice by the gastric glands. Highly acidic (pH of 0.9 to 1.5), these digestive secretions consist mainly of pepsin, hydrochloric acid, intrinsic factor, and proteolytic enzymes. (See *Sites and mechanisms of gastric secretion.*)

Intestinal phase of digestion

Normally, except for alcohol, little food absorption occurs in the stomach. Peristaltic contractions churn the food into tiny particles and mix it with gastric juices, forming chyme.

Next, stronger peristaltic waves move the chyme into the *antrum*, where it backs up against the *pyloric sphincter* before being released into the duodenum and triggering the *intestinal phase* of digestion.

The rate of stomach emptying depends on a complex interplay of factors, including gastrin release, neural signals generated when the stomach wall distends, and the *enterogastric reflex*. In this reaction, the duodenum releases secretin and gastric-inhibiting peptide, and the jejunum secretes cholecystokinin — all of which act to decrease gastric motility.

What happens in the small intestine

The small intestine performs most of the work of digestion and absorption. (See *Small intestine: How form affects absorption*, page 138.) Here, intestinal contractions and various digestive secretions break down carbohydrates, proteins, and fats — actions that enable the intestinal mucosa to absorb these nutrients into the bloodstream (along with water and electrolytes) and subsequently for use by the body.

What happens in the large intestine

By the time chyme passes through the small intestine and enters the ascending colon of the large intestine, it has been reduced to mostly indigestible substances.

The food bolus begins its journey through the large intestine where the ileum and cecum join with the *ileocecal pouch*. Then the bolus moves up the ascending colon, past the right abdominal cavity to the liver's lower border. It crosses horizontally below the liver and stomach by way of the transverse colon and descends the left abdominal cavity to the *iliac fossa* through the descending colon.

From there, the bolus travels through the sigmoid colon to the lower midline of the abdominal cavity, then to the rectum, and finally to the anal canal. The anus opens to the exterior through two sphincters. The *internal sphincter* contains thick, circular smooth muscle under autonomic control; the *external sphincter* contains skeletal muscle under voluntary control.

Role in absorption

Although the large intestine produces no hormones or digestive enzymes, it continues the absorptive process. Through blood and lymph vessels in the submucosa, the proximal half of the large intestine absorbs all but about 100 ml of the remaining water in the colon. It also absorbs large amounts of both sodium and chloride.

Bacterial actions

The large intestine harbors the bacteria *Escherichia coli, Enterobacter aerogenes, Clostridium perfringens*, and *Lactobacillus bifidus*, which help synthesize vitamin K and break down cellulose into usable carbohydrate. Bacterial action also produces flatus, which helps propel feces toward the rectum.

In addition, the mucosa of the large intestine produces alkaline secretions from tubular glands composed of goblet cells. This alkaline mucus lubricates the intestinal walls as food pushes through, protecting the mucosa from acidic bacterial action.

Mass movements

In the lower colon, long and relatively sluggish contractions cause propulsive waves, or *mass movements*. Normally occurring several times per day, these movements propel intestinal contents

Sites and mechanisms of gastric secretion

The body of the stomach lies between the cardiac sphincter, also called the lower esophageal sphincter (LES), and the pyloric sphincter. Between these sphincters lie the fundus, body, antrum, and pylorus. These areas have a rich variety of mucosal cells that help the stomach carry out its tasks (see enlargement).

Cardiac gland and gastric gland secretions

Three types of glands secrete 2 to 3 L of gastric juice daily through the stomach's gastric pits. Cardiac glands near the LES and pyloric glands in the pylorus secrete a thin mucus. Gastric glands in the stomach's body and fundus secrete hydrochloric acid (HCl), pepsinogen, intrinsic factor, and mucus.

Specialized cells line the gastric glands, gastric pits, and surface epithelium. Mucous cells in the necks of the gastric glands produce a thin mucus; those in the surface epithelium, a protective alkaline mucus. Both substances lubricate food and protect the stomach from self-digestion by corrosive enzymes and acids.

Gastrin and pepsinogen

Argentaffin cells in gastric glands produce the hormone gastrin. Chief cells, primarily in the fundus, produce pepsinogen—the inactive precursor of the proteolytic enzyme pepsin, which breaks proteins into polypeptides.

Hydrochloric acid and intrinsic factor

Large parietal cells scattered throughout the fundus secrete HCl and intrinsic factor. HCl degrades pepsinogen by enzymatic action into pepsin and maintains the acid environment favorable for pepsin activity. It also helps disintegrate nucleoproteins and collagens, hydrolyzes sucrose, and inhibits excess growth of bacteria. Intrinsic factor promotes vitamin B_{12} absorption in the small intestine.

STOMACH STRUCTURES

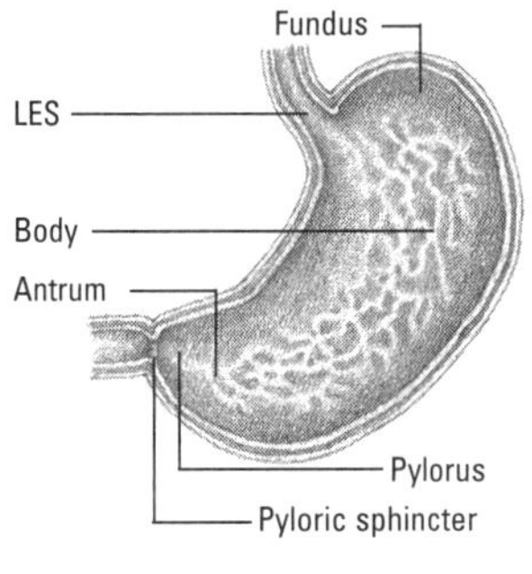

GASTRIC MUCOSA

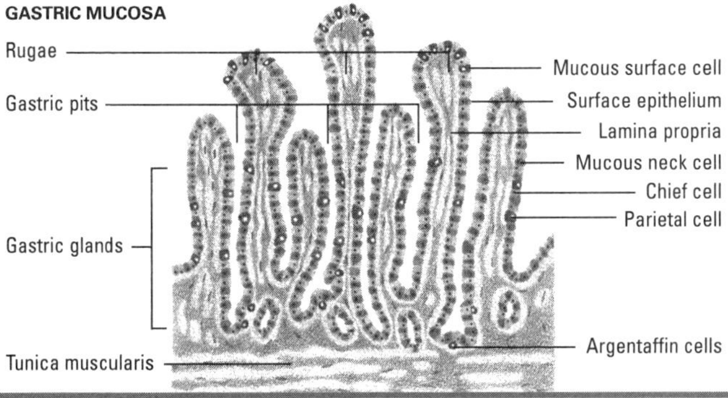

Small intestine: How form affects absorption

Nearly all digestion and absorption takes place in the 20′ (6 m) of small intestine.

Specialized mucosa

Multiple projections of the intestinal mucosa increase the surface area for absorption several hundredfold, as shown in the enlarged views below.

Circular projections *(Kerckring's folds)* are covered by villi, each containing a lymphatic vessel *(lacteal)*, a venule, capillaries, an arteriole, nerve fibers, and smooth muscle.

Each villus is densely fringed with about 2,000 microvilli resembling a fine brush. The villi are lined with columnar epithelial cells, which dip into the lamina propria between the villi to form intestinal glands *(crypts of Lieberkühn).*

Types of epithelial cells

The type of epithelial cell dictates its function. Mucus-secreting *goblet cells* are found on and between the villi on the crypt mucosa. In the proximal duodenum, specialized Brunner's glands also secrete large amounts of mucus to lubricate and protect the duodenum from potentially corrosive acidic chyme and gastric juices.

Paneth's cells are thought to regulate intestinal flora. Duodenal *argentaffin cells* produce the hormones secretin and cholecystokinin. *Undifferentiated cells* deep within the intestinal glands replace the epithelium. *Absorptive cells* consist of large numbers of tightly packed microvilli over a plasma membrane containing transport mechanisms for absorption and producing enzymes for the final step in digestion.

Intestinal glands

The intestinal glands primarily secrete a watery fluid that bathes the villi with chyme particles. Fluid production results from local irritation of nerve cells and possibly from hormonal stimulation by secretin and cholecystokinin. The microvillous brush border secretes various hormones and digestive enzymes that catalyze final nutrient breakdown.

SMALL INTESTINE

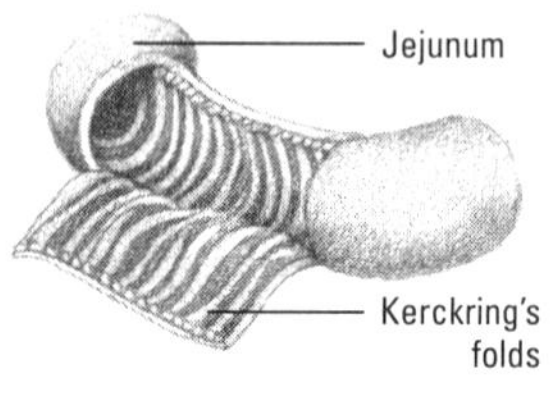

DETAIL OF VILLI

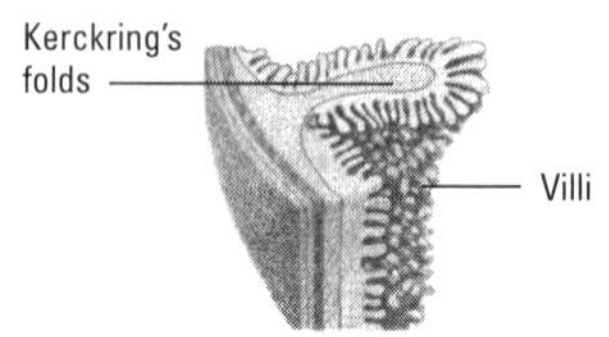

DETAIL OF INTESTINAL MUCOSA

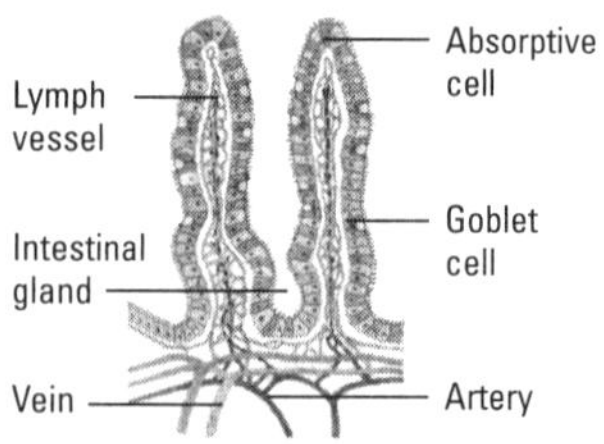

TRANSVERSE SECTION OF VILLUS

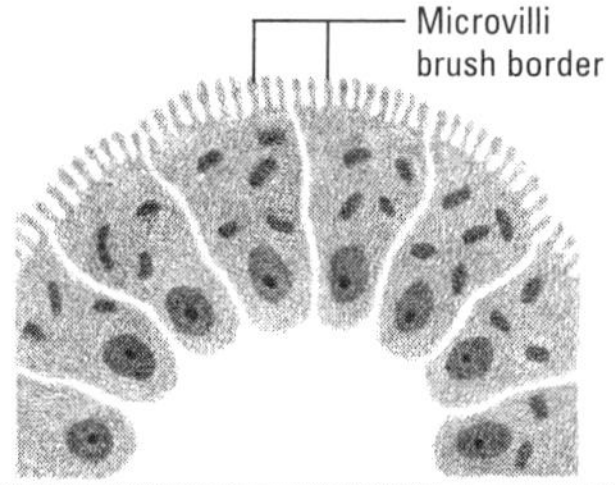

into the rectum and produce the urge to defecate.

Defecation normally results from the *defecation reflex,* a sensory and parasympathetic nerve-mediated response, along with the voluntary relaxation of the external anal sphincter.

12 Nutrition and metabolism

To maintain life, human beings must obtain nutrients from food and beverages. *Nutrition* refers to the processes involved in taking in, assimilating, and utilizing nutrients.

The crucial nutrients in food must be broken down into components. Within cells, the products of digestion undergo further chemical reactions. *Metabolism* refers to the sum of these chemical reactions. Through metabolism, food substances are transformed into energy or materials that the body can use or store.

Metabolism involves two processes:

- *anabolism*—synthesis of simple substances into complex ones
- *catabolism*—breakdown of complex substances into simpler ones or into energy.

Nutrition

The body needs a continuous supply of water and various nutrients to provide energy for its activities and to obtain building materials for growth and repair. Virtually all nutrients come from digested food. The three major types of nutrients required by the body are carbohydrates, proteins, and lipids.

POINT TO REMEMBER

The energy in nutrients is measured in kilocalories (kcal), or calories, per gram of nutrient. Adults need approximately 2,000 kcal daily.

Vitamins—essential for normal metabolism—contribute to the enzyme reactions that promote the metabolism of carbohydrates, proteins, and lipids. *Minerals* participate in such essential functions as enzyme metabolism and membrane transfer of essential elements.

Carbohydrates

Carbohydrates are organic compounds composed of carbon, hydrogen, and oxygen; they yield 4 kcal/g when used for energy. Carbohydrates are classified as monosaccharides, disaccharides, and polysaccharides.

Monosaccharides

Simple sugars that can't be split into smaller units by hydrolysis, *monosaccharides* are subdivided into polyhydroxy aldehydes or ketones based on whether the molecule consists of an aldehyde group or a ketone group. An *aldehyde* contains the characteristic group CHO; the term *polyhydroxy* refers to linking of the carbon atoms to a hydroxyl (OH) group. A *ketone*, on the other hand, contains the carbonyl group CO and carbon groups attached to the carbonyl carbon. The ringlike, or cyclic, structure of monosaccharides results from the chemical attraction between the aldehyde or ketone at one end of the chain and the OH group at the other end.

Monosaccharides are also classified by the number of carbon atoms they contain. A *pentose*, for instance, contains five carbon atoms; pentoses include *ribose* in ribonucleic acid (RNA) and *deoxyribose* in deoxyribonucleic acid (DNA).

A *hexose*, in contrast, contains six carbon atoms in its molecule. Hexoses include glucose, fructose, and galactose. (See *Comparing monosaccharides*.)

Disaccharides

Disaccharides are synthesized from monosaccharides; a disaccharide molecule consists of two monosaccharides minus a water molecule. The joining of a glucose molecule with a fructose molecule yields the disaccharide sucrose; the joining of a glucose molecule with a galactose molecule results in the disaccharide lactose.

Polysaccharides

Like disaccharides, *polysaccharides* are synthesized from monosaccharides. A polysaccharide consists of a long chain (polymer) of more than 10 monosaccharides linked by glycoside bonds. The polysaccharide starch is a polymer of glucose.

Comparing monosaccharides

Based on the number of carbon atoms they contain, monosaccharides fall into the following categories:

- dioses, which contain two carbon atoms
- trioses, which contain three carbon atoms
- tetroses, which contain four carbon atoms
- pentoses, which contain five carbon atoms
- hexoses, which contain six carbon atoms
- heptoses, which contain seven carbon atoms.

Proteins

Proteins are complex nitrogenous organic compounds containing amino acid chains; some also contain sulfur. Proteins are used mainly for growth and repair of body tissues; when used for energy, they yield 4 kcal/g. Some proteins combine with lipids to form lipoproteins or with carbohydrates to form glycoproteins.

Amino acids

The building blocks of proteins, *amino acids* each contain a carbon atom to which a carboxyl (COOH) group and an amino group are attached. Amino acids show structural differences in their side chains; the nature of the side chain identifies the amino acid.

Peptide bonds

Amino acids unite by condensation of the COOH group on one amino acid with the amino group of the adjacent amino acid. This reaction releases a water molecule and creates a linkage called a *peptide bond*.

A chain of 2 to 10 amino acids forms a *peptide*; a chain of 10 or more amino acids forms a *polypeptide*; a chain of more than 50 amino acids forms a protein. The sequence and types of amino acids in the chain determine the nature of the protein. Each protein is synthesized on a ribosome as a straight chain. Chemical attractions between the amino acids in various parts of the chain cause the chain to coil or twist into a specific shape. A protein's shape, in turn, determines its function.

Lipids

Lipids are organic compounds that don't dissolve in water but do dissolve in alcohol and other organic solvents. A concentrated form of fuel, lipids yield approximately 9 kcal/g when used for energy. The major lipids include fats (the most common lipids), phospholipids, and steroids.

Fats

A *fat*, or *triglyceride*, contains three molecules of fatty acid combined with one molecule of glycerol. A *fatty acid* is a long-chain compound with an even number of carbon atoms and a terminal COOH group.

Glycerol, for example, is a three-carbon compound (alcohol) with an OH group attached to each carbon atom. The COOH group on each fatty acid molecule joins to one OH group on the glycerol molecule; this results in the

Common fatty acids

Fatty acids (a simple lipid type) can be saturated, monounsaturated, or polyunsaturated.

Saturated fatty acids
- Arachidic acid
- Behenic acid
- Butyric acid
- Capric acid
- Caproic acid
- Caprylic acid
- Lauric acid
- Myristic acid
- Palmitic acid
- Stearic acid

Monounsaturated fatty acids
- Erucic acid
- Oleic acid
- Palmitoleic acid

Polyunsaturated fatty acids
- Arachidonic acid
- Linoleic acid
- Linolenic acid

release of a water molecule. Linking of the COOH and OH groups produces an ester linkage.

Fats can be classified by the number of double bonds between carbon atoms in their fatty acid molecules. In a *saturated fat,* all available bonds of the hydrocarbon chains are filled (saturated) with hydrogen atoms; thus, a saturated fat contains no double bonds between carbon atoms. A *monounsaturated fat* has one double bond between carbon atoms. A *polyunsaturated fat* has multiple double bonds between carbon atoms. (See *Common fatty acids.*)

Phospholipids

Phospholipids are complex lipids similar to fats, but with a phosphorus- and nitrogen-containing compound replacing one of the fatty acid molecules. Phospholipids are major structural components of cell membranes.

Steroids

Steroids are complex molecules in which the carbon atoms form four cyclic structures attached to various side chains. They contain no glycerol or fatty acid molecules. Examples of steroids include cholesterol, bile salts, and sex hormones.

Vitamins and minerals

Vitamins are organic compounds needed in small quantities for normal metabolism, growth, and development. Vitamins are classified as water-soluble or fat-soluble. Water-soluble vitamins include the B complex and C vitamins; fat-soluble vitamins include vitamins A, D, E, and K. (See *Guide to vitamins and minerals.*)

POINT TO REMEMBER
The body must obtain adequate vitamins from the diet because it can't manufacture many vitamins itself.

Minerals are inorganic substances that play important roles in enzyme metabolism, membrane transfer of essential compounds, regulation of acid-base balance and osmotic pressure, muscle contractility, nerve impulse transmission, and growth. Minerals are found in bones, hemoglobin, thyroxine, and vitamin B_{12}.

Minerals may be classified as *major minerals* (more than 0.005% of body weight) or *trace minerals* (less than 0.005% of body weight). Major minerals include calcium, chloride, magnesium, phosphorus, potassium, sodium, and sulfur. Trace minerals include chromium, cobalt, copper, fluorine, iodine, iron, manganese, molybdenum, selenium, and zinc.

Nutrient digestion and absorption

Nutrients must be digested in the GI tract by enzymes that split large units into smaller ones. In this process, called *hydrolysis,* a compound unites with water and then splits into simpler

(Text continues on page 150.)

Guide to vitamins and minerals

Good health requires intake of adequate amounts of vitamins and minerals to meet the body's metabolic needs. A vitamin or mineral excess or deficiency, although rare, can lead to various disorders.

The chart below reviews main food sources, major functions, and deficiency and toxicity findings for vitamins and minerals.

Water-soluble vitamins

Major functions	Deficiency and toxicity findings
Vitamin C (ascorbic acid) *Main food sources: Fresh fruits and vegetables*	
Collagen production, digestion, fine bone and tooth formation, iodine conservation, healing (burns and wounds), red blood cell (RBC) formation, infection resistance, vitamin protection, epinephrine and anti-inflammatory steroid synthesis	**Deficiency:** Scurvy, bleeding gums, capillary wall rupture (easy bruising), dyspnea, low infection resistance, nosebleeds, tooth decay, anorexia, fatigue, irritability, muscle and joint pain, skin lesions **Toxicity (rare):** GI signs and symptoms, impaired leukocyte bactericidal activity, excessive iron absorption, uricosuria with resultant renal calculi, pancreatic damage resulting in decreased insulin production
Vitamin B_1 (thiamine) *Main food sources: Meats, fish, poultry, pork, molasses, brewer's yeast, brown rice, nuts, wheat germ, whole and enriched grains*	
Appetite stimulation, blood building, carbohydrate metabolism, circulation, digestion, growth, learning ability, muscle tone maintenance, pain inhibition, energy metabolism, acetylcholine synthesis	**Deficiency:** Beriberi, weakness, appetite loss, constipation, digestive problems, dyspnea, fatigue, irritability, memory loss, myocardial pain, nervousness, hand and foot numbness, pain and noise sensitivity **Toxicity:** Edema, sweating, tremors, tachycardia, vascular hypotension
Vitamin B_2 (riboflavin) *Main food sources: Meats, fish, poultry, milk, molasses, brewer's yeast, eggs, fruit, green leafy vegetables, nuts, whole grains*	
Antibody and RBC formation; energy metabolism; cell respiration; epithelial, eye, and mucosal tissue maintenance	**Deficiency:** Cataracts, cheilosis, digestive problems, dizziness, eye fatigue, itching and burning eyes, light sensitivity, oily skin, retarded growth, tongue redness and soreness **Toxicity:** No known effects

(continued)

Guide to vitamins and minerals *(continued)*

Water-soluble vitamins *(continued)*

Major functions	Deficiency and toxicity findings
Vitamin B_6 (pyridoxine)	
Main food sources: Meats, poultry, bananas, molasses, brewer's yeast, desiccated liver, fish, green leafy vegetables, peanuts, raisins, walnuts, wheat germ, whole grains	
Antibody formation, digestion, deoxyribonulecic acid (DNA) and ribonucleic acid (RNA) synthesis, fat and protein utilization, amino acid metabolism, hemoglobin production, magnesium and linoleic acid function, sodium and potassium balance, myelin sheath development	**Deficiency:** Seborrheic dermatitis, acne, arthritis, glossitis, cheilosis, convulsions (in infants), depression, dizziness, hair loss, irritability, learning disabilities, weakness **Toxicity (rare):** Occurs only with 3 g/kg dose
Folic acid (folacin; pteroylglutamic acid)	
Main food sources: Citrus fruits, eggs, green leafy vegetables, milk products, organ meats, seafood, whole grains	
Appetite stimulation, cell growth and reproduction, circulation, DNA production, hydrochloric acid production, liver function, nucleic acid formation, protein metabolism, RBC formation	**Deficiency:** Macrocytic or megaloblastic anemia, fatigue, weakness, fainting, pallor, digestive problems, graying hair, growth problems, insomnia, tongue inflammation, memory impairment **Toxicity:** No known effects
Niacin (nicotinic acid, nicotinamide, niacinamide)	
Main food sources: Eggs, lean meats, milk products, organ meats, peanuts, poultry, seafood, whole grains	
Circulation, cholesterol level reduction, growth, hydrochloric acid production, metabolism (carbohydrate, protein, fat), sex hormone production, electron transport, pigment metabolism	**Deficiency:** Pellagra, diarrhea, depression, appetite loss, canker sores, fatigue, halitosis, headaches, indigestion, insomnia, memory impairment, muscle weakness, nervous disorders, skin eruptions **Toxicity:** Flushing or vascular dilation (only with large nicotinic acid doses)

Guide to vitamins and minerals *(continued)*

Water-soluble vitamins *(continued)*	
Major functions	**Deficiency and toxicity findings**
Vitamin B_{12} (cyanocobalamin) *Main food sources: Beef, eggs, fish, milk products, organ meats, pork*	
Appetite stimulation, RBC formation, cellular and nutrient metabolism, cell longevity, iron absorption, tissue growth, nerve cell maintenance	**Deficiency (most common in vegetarians):** Fatigue, memory impairment, mental depression and confusion, nervousness, reduced reflex responses, walking and speech problems, glossitis, headache, pernicious anemia **Toxicity:** No known effects
Biotin *Main food sources: Egg yolks, legumes, organ meats, whole grains, yeast, milk, seafood*	
Cell growth; fatty acid production; metabolism (carbohydrate, fat, protein); vitamin B utilization; skin, hair, nerve, and bone marrow maintenance	**Deficiency:** Depression, dry skin, anemia, glossitis, gray skin tone, insomnia, muscle pain, poor appetite **Toxicity:** Essentially nontoxic
Pantothenic acid (formerly called vitamin B_3) *Main food sources: Eggs, legumes, mushrooms, organ meats, salmon, wheat germ, whole grains, fresh vegetables, yeast*	
Antibody formation; conversion of carbohydrates, fats, and protein; cortisone production; growth stimulation; stress tolerance; vitamin utilization	**Deficiency:** Diarrhea, eczema, hair loss, intestinal disorders, kidney problems, muscle cramps, nervousness, premature aging, respiratory infections, fatigue, numbness **Toxicity:** Essentially nontoxic
Fat-soluble vitamins	
Vitamin A (called retinol when preformed) *Main food sources: Fish, green and yellow fruits and vegetables, milk products*	
Body tissue repair and maintenance, infection resistance, bone growth, nervous system development, cell membrane metabolism and structure, RNA synthesis, visual purple production (for night vision)	**Deficiency:** Allergies; appetite loss; blemishes; dry hair; fatigue; frequent infections; itching and burning eyes; smell loss; night blindness; rough, dry skin; sinus problems; softened tooth enamel **Toxicity:** Skin dryness and desquamation, hair loss, bone pain and fragility, enlarged liver and spleen

(continued)

Guide to vitamins and minerals *(continued)*

Fat-soluble vitamins *(continued)*	
Major functions	**Deficiency and toxicity findings**
Vitamin D (calciferol; subtypes include D_2 [ergocalciferol] and D_3 [cholecalciferol]) *Main food sources: Bone meal, egg yolks, organ meats, butter, cod liver oil, fatty fish*	
Calcium and phosphorus metabolism (bone formation), myocardial function, nervous system maintenance, normal blood clotting	**Deficiency:** Burning sensation (in mouth and throat), diarrhea, insomnia, myopia, nervousness, softened bones and teeth, rickets (in infants and children), osteomalacia (in adults) **Toxicity:** Polyuria, nocturia, weight loss, nausea, diarrhea (With severe toxicity, soft tissue calcification.)
Vitamin E (tocopherol) *Main food sources: Butter, dark green vegetables, eggs, fruits, nuts, organ meats, vegetable oils, wheat germ*	
Aging retardation, anticlotting factor, capillary wall strengthening, diuresis, fertility, lung protection (antipollution), male potency, muscle and nerve cell membrane maintenance, myocardial perfusion, serum cholesterol reduction, synthesis of heme (hemoglobin component)	**Deficiency:** Dry or dull hair, enlarged prostate gland, GI problems, hair loss, impotence, miscarriage, muscle wasting, sterility **Toxicity:** Bleeding, intestinal problems, disturbed vitamin A and K utilization
Vitamin K (menadione; subtypes include K_2 [menaquinone] and K_3) *Main food sources: Green leafy vegetables, safflower oil, yogurt, liver, molasses*	
Liver synthesis of prothrombin and other blood clotting factors	**Deficiency:** Diarrhea, increased hemorrhaging tendency, miscarriage, nosebleeds **Toxicity (most common in infants):** Vomiting, increased albumin and porphyrin excretion
Macronutrients	
Calcium *Main food sources: Bonemeal, cheese, milk, molasses, yogurt, whole grains, nuts, legumes, leafy vegetables*	
Blood clotting, bone and tooth formation, cardiac rhythm, cell membrane permeability, muscle growth and contraction, nerve impulse transmission	**Deficiency:** Arm and leg numbness, brittle fingernails, heart palpitations, insomnia, muscle cramps, nervousness, tooth decay, tetany, rickets, osteoporosis, osteomalacia **Toxicity:** No known effects

Guide to vitamins and minerals *(continued)*

Macronutrients *(continued)*	
Major functions	**Deficiency and toxicity findings**
Chloride *Main food sources: Fruits, vegetables, table salt*	
Maintenance of fluid, electrolyte, acid-base, and osmotic pressure balance; hydrochloric acid formation; enzyme regulation; carbon dioxide transfer (from blood to lungs)	**Deficiency (rare):** Hypochloremic alkalosis **Toxicity:** No known effects
Magnesium *Main food sources: Green leafy vegetables, nuts, seafood, cocoa, whole grains*	
Acid-base balance, metabolism, protein synthesis, muscle relaxation, cellular respiration, nerve impulse transmission	**Deficiency:** Confusion, disorientation, easily aroused anger, nervousness, irritability, rapid pulse, tremors, muscle control loss, neuromuscular dysfunction **Toxicity:** No known effects
Phosphorus *Main food sources: Eggs, fish, grains, meats, poultry, yellow cheese, milk, milk products*	
Bone and tooth formation, cell growth and repair, energy production, kidney function, metabolism, myocardial contraction, nerve and muscle activity, vitamin utilization, acid-base balance	**Deficiency:** Appetite loss, fatigue, irregular breathing, nervous disorders, muscle weakness **Toxicity:** No known effects
Potassium *Main food sources: Seafood, molasses, peaches, peanuts, raisins*	
Heartbeat, muscle contraction, nerve impulse transmission, rapid growth, fluid distribution and osmotic pressure balance, acid-base balance	**Deficiency:** Acne; constipation; dry skin; general weakness; insomnia; muscle damage; nervousness; persistent thirst; slow, irregular heartbeat; weak reflexes **Toxicity:** No known effects

(continued)

Guide to vitamins and minerals *(continued)*

Major functions	Deficiency and toxicity findings
Macronutrients *(continued)*	
Sodium	
Main food sources: Seafood, cheese, milk, salt	
Cellular fluid level maintenance, muscle contraction, acid-base balance, cell permeability, muscle function, nerve impulse transmission	**Deficiency:** Appetite loss, intestinal gas, muscle atrophy, vomiting, weight loss **Toxicity:** No known effects
Sulfur	
Main food sources: Milk, meats, legumes, eggs	
Collagen synthesis, vitamin B formation, enzyme and energy metabolism, detoxification reactions, blood clotting	**Deficiency:** No known effects **Toxicity:** No known effects
Micronutrients	
Chromium	
Main food sources: Clams, meats, cheese, corn oil, whole grains, brewer's yeast	
Carbohydrate and protein metabolism, serum glucose level maintenance	**Deficiency:** Glucose intolerance (in diabetic patients) **Toxicity:** No known effects
Cobalt	
Main food sources: Beef, eggs, fish, milk products, organ meats, pork	
Vitamin B_{12} formation	**Deficiency:** See Vitamin B_{12} deficiency **Toxicity:** No known effects
Copper	
Main food sources: Organ meats, raisins, seafood (especially oysters), nuts, molasses	
Bone formation, hair and skin color, healing processes, hemoglobin and RBC formation, mental processes, iron metabolism	**Deficiency:** Diarrhea (in infants), general weakness, impaired respiration, skin sores, bone disease **Toxicity:** Headache, dizziness, heartburn, weakness, nausea, vomiting, diarrhea

Guide to vitamins and minerals *(continued)*

Micronutrients *(continued)*	
Major functions	**Deficiency and toxicity findings**
Fluoride (fluorine) *Main food sources: Drinking water*	
Bone and tooth formation	**Deficiency:** Dental caries **Toxicity:** Tooth enamel mottling and discoloration, increased bone density and calcification
Iodine *Main food sources: Kelp, salt (iodized), seafood*	
Energy production, metabolism, physical and mental development	**Deficiency:** Cold hands and feet, dry hair, irritability, nervousness, obesity, simple goiter, cretinism (in infants and children) **Toxicity:** No known effects
Iron *Main food sources: Eggs, organ meats, poultry, wheat germ, liver, potatoes, enriched breads and cereals, green vegetables, molasses*	
Growth (in children), hemoglobin production, stress and disease resistance, cellular respiration, oxygen transport, energy production, regulation of biological and chemical reactions	**Deficiency:** Brittle nails, constipation, respiratory problems, tongue soreness or inflammation, anemia, pallor, weakness, cold sensitivity, fatigue **Toxicity:** Abdominal cramps and pains, nausea, vomiting, hemosiderosis, hemochromatosis (skin graying and pigmentation, liver and heart failure)
Manganese *Main food sources: Bananas, egg yolks, green leafy vegetables, liver, soybeans, nuts, whole grains, coffee, tea*	
Enzyme activation, fat and carbohydrate metabolism, reproduction and growth, sex hormone production, vitamin B_1 metabolism, vitamin E utilization	**Deficiency:** Ataxia, dizziness, hearing disturbances or loss **Toxicity:** Severe neuromuscular disturbances (similar to parkinsonian effects)

(continued)

Guide to vitamins and minerals *(continued)*

Micronutrients ***(continued)***

Major functions	Deficiency and toxicity findings
Molybdenum *Main food sources: Whole grains, legumes, organ meats*	
Body metabolism	**Deficiency:** No known effects **Toxicity:** See Copper deficiency
Selenium *Main food sources: Seafood, meats, liver, kidneys*	
Immune mechanisms, mitochondrial adenosine triphosphate synthesis, cellular protection, fat metabolism	**Deficiency:** No known effects **Toxicity:** No known effects
Zinc *Main food sources: Liver, mushrooms, seafood, soybeans, spinach, meat*	
Burn and wound healing, carbohydrate digestion, metabolism (carbohydrate, fat, protein), prostate gland function, reproductive organ growth and development, taste and smell	**Deficiency:** Delayed sexual maturity, fatigue, smell and taste loss, poor appetite, prolonged wound healing, retarded growth, skin disorders **Toxicity:** No known effects

compounds. The smaller units are then absorbed from the small intestine and transported to the liver through the portal venous system. (For more information on the role of the GI system in nutrition, see chapter 11, Gastrointestinal system.)

Carbohydrate digestion and absorption

Enzymes break down complex carbohydrates into hexoses by hydrolyzing the glycoside bonds; hydrolysis restores the water molecules that were released when the bonds were formed.

In the oral cavity, salivary amylase, or ptyalin, initiates starch hydrolysis into disaccharides. In the small intestine, pancreatic amylase continues this process.

Disaccharides in the intestinal mucosa hydrolyze disaccharides into monosaccharides. Lactase splits lactose into glucose and galactose, and sucrase hydrolyzes sucrose into glucose and fructose.

Monosaccharides, such as glucose, fructose, and galactose, are absorbed through the intestinal mucosa by diffusion and active transport and then are transported through the portal venous system to the liver. There, enzymes convert fructose and galactose to glucose.

Ribonucleases and deoxyribonucleases break down nucleotides from DNA and RNA into pentoses and nitrogen-containing compounds (nitrogen bases). These compounds are absorbed through the intestinal mucosa like glucose.

Protein digestion and absorption

Enzymes digest proteins by hydrolyzing the peptide bonds that link the amino acids of the protein chains. This process restores the water molecules released by formation of the peptide bonds.

Gastric pepsin breaks proteins into polypeptides; pancreatic trypsin, chymotrypsin, and carboxypeptidase convert polypeptides to peptides. Intestinal mucosal peptidases break down peptides into their constituent amino acids. After being absorbed through the intestinal mucosa by active transport mechanisms, these amino acids travel through the portal venous system to the liver, which converts the amino acids not needed for protein synthesis into glucose.

Lipid digestion and absorption

Insoluble in water, lipids must be emulsified into small droplets for digestion and eventual absorption in the small intestine. Pancreatic lipase breaks down fats and phospholipids into a mixture of glycerol, short- and long-chain fatty acids, and *monoglycerides* (fats composed of one molecule of a fatty acid and one molecule of glycerol). The portal venous system then carries these substances to the liver. Lipase hydrolyzes the bonds between glycerol and fatty acids—a process that restores the water molecules released when the bonds were formed.

Glycerol diffuses directly through the mucosa. Short-chain fatty acids diffuse into the intestinal epithelial cells and are carried to the liver through the portal venous system. Long-chain fatty acids and monoglycerides in the intestine dissolve in the bile salt micelles and then diffuse into the intestinal epithelial cells, where lipase breaks down absorbed monoglycerides into glycerol and fatty acids. In the smooth endoplasmic reticulum of the epithelial cells, fatty acids and glycerol recombine to form fats.

Along with a small amount of cholesterol and phospholipid, triglycerides are coated with a thin layer of protein to form lipoprotein particles called *chylomicrons.* Collecting in the intestinal lacteals (lymphatic vessels), chylomicrons are carried through lymphatic channels. After entering the circulation through the thoracic duct, they're distributed to body cells.

In the cells, fats are extracted from the chylomicrons and broken down by enzymes into fatty acids and glycerol. Then they're absorbed and recombined in fat cells, reforming triglycerides for storage and later use.

Carbohydrate metabolism

Carbohydrates are the preferred energy fuel of human cells. Most of the carbohydrate in absorbed food is quickly catabolized for the release of energy.

POINT TO REMEMBER

All ingested carbohydrates are converted to glucose, the body's main energy source. Glucose not needed for immediate energy is stored as glycogen or converted to lipids.

Energy from glucose catabolism is generated in three phases—glycolysis, Krebs cycle (also called the *citric acid cycle*) and the electron transport system. (See *Tracking the glucose pathway,* page 152.)

Glycolysis, which occurs in the cell cytoplasm, doesn't use oxygen. The other two phases, which occur in mitochondria, do use oxygen.

Glycolysis

Glycolysis refers to the process by which enzymes break down the six-carbon glucose molecule into two three-carbon molecules of pyruvic acid (pyruvate). Glycolysis yields energy in the form of adenosine triphosphate (ATP).

Next, pyruvic acid releases a carbon dioxide (CO_2) molecule and is converted in the mitochondria to a two-carbon acetyl fragment, which combines with

Tracking the glucose pathway

Glucose catabolism generates energy in three phases. This flowchart summarizes the first two phases.

Glycolysis, the first phase, breaks apart one molecule of glucose to form two molecules of pyruvate, which yields energy in the form of adenosine triphosphate and acetyl (acetyl CoA).

The second phase, Krebs cycle, continues carbohydrate metabolism. Fragments of acetyl CoA join to oxaloacetic acid to form citric acid. The CoA molecule breaks off from the acetyl group and may form more acetyl CoA molecules. Citric acid is first converted into intermediate compounds, and then back into oxaloacetic acid. Krebs cycle also liberates carbon dioxide (CO_2).

In the third phase of glucose catabolism, molecules on the inner mitochondrial membrane attract electrons from hydrogen atoms and carry them through oxidation-reduction reactions in the mitochondria. The hydrogen ions produced in Krebs cycle then combine with oxygen to form water (H_2O).

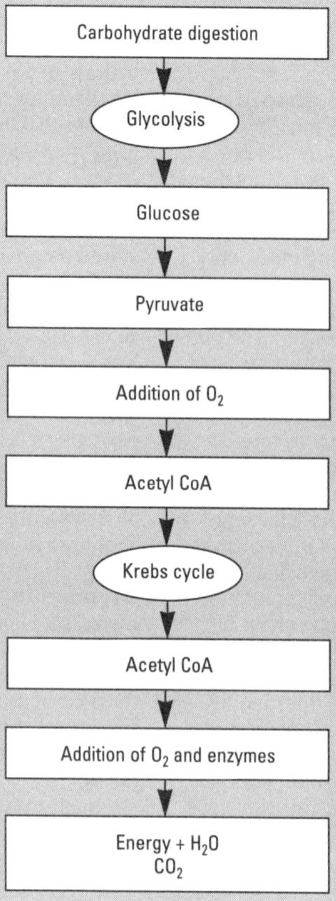

CoA (a complex organic compound) to form acetyl CoA.

Glycolysis is especially important when circulation and respiration can't supply the oxygen needed by muscle cells (such as during strenuous exercise). If tissues don't receive an adequate oxygen supply, cytoplasmic enzymes reduce pyruvic acid to lactic acid by the addition of two hydrogen atoms. When adequate oxygen becomes available, lactic acid is oxidized back to pyruvic acid.

Krebs cycle

The second phase in glucose catabolism, *Krebs cycle* is the pathway by which a molecule of acetyl coenzyme A (acetyl CoA) is oxidized by enzymes to yield energy.

The two-carbon acetyl fragments of acetyl CoA enter Krebs cycle by joining to the four-carbon compound oxaloacetic acid to form citric acid, a six-carbon compound. In this process, the CoA molecule detaches from the acetyl group, becoming available to form more acetyl CoA molecules. Enzymes convert citric acid into intermediate compounds and eventually convert it back into oxaloacetic acid. Then the cycle begins again.

Besides liberating CO_2 and generating energy, each turn of Krebs cycle releases hydrogen atoms, which are picked up by the coenzymes nicotinamide adenine dinucleotide (NAD) and flavin adenine dinucleotide (FAD).

Electron transport system

In the *electron transport system,* the last phase of carbohydrate catabolism, carrier molecules on the inner mitochondrial membrane pick up electrons from the hydrogen atoms carried by NAD and FAD. (Each hydrogen atom contains a hydrogen ion and an electron.) These carrier molecules transport the electrons through a series of enzyme-catalyzed oxidation-reduction reactions in the mitochondria.

Oxygen plays a crucial role by attracting electrons along the chain of carriers in the transport system. During *oxidation,* a chemical compound loses electrons; during *reduction,* it gains electrons. These reactions release the energy contained in the electrons and generate ATP.

After passing through the electron transport system, the hydrogen ions produced in Krebs cycle combine with oxygen to form water.

Role of the liver and muscle cells

The liver and muscle cells both help to regulate blood glucose levels.

Liver

When glucose levels exceed the body's immediate needs, hormones stimulate the liver to convert glucose into glycogen or lipids. Glycogen forms through *glycogenesis;* lipids form through *lipogenesis.*

When the blood glucose level drops excessively, the liver can form glucose by two processes:

- breakdown of glycogen to glucose through glycogenolysis
- synthesis of glucose from amino acids through gluconeogenesis.

Muscle cells

Muscle cells can convert glucose to glycogen for storage. However, they lack the enzymes to convert glycogen back to glucose when needed. During vigorous muscular activity, when oxygen requirements exceed the oxygen supply, muscle cells break down glycogen to yield lactic acid and energy. Lactic acid then builds up in the muscles, and muscle glycogen is depleted.

Some of the lactic acid diffuses from muscle cells, is transported to the liver, and is reconverted to glycogen. The liver converts the newly formed glycogen to glucose, which travels through the bloodstream to the muscles and reforms into glycogen.

When muscle exertion stops, some of the accumulated lactic acid converts back to pyruvic acid and then is oxidized completely to yield energy by means of Krebs cycle and the electron transport system.

Protein metabolism

Absorbed as amino acids, proteins are carried by the portal venous system to the liver and then throughout the body by blood. Absorbed amino acids mix with other amino acids in the body's amino acid pool. These other amino acids may be synthesized in the body from other substances such as keto-acids, or they may be produced by protein breakdown.

The body can't store amino acids. Instead, it converts them to protein or glucose or catabolizes them to provide energy. Before these changes can occur, however, amino acids must be transformed by deamination or transamination.

In *deamination*, an amino group ($-NH_2$) splits off from an amino acid molecule to form a molecule of ammonia and one of keto acid; most of the ammonia is converted to urea and excreted in the urine. In *transamination*, an amino group is exchanged for a keto group in a keto acid through the action of transaminase enzymes. During this process, the amino acid is converted to a keto acid and the original keto acid is converted to an amino acid.

Amino acid synthesis

Proteins are synthesized from 20 amino acids from the body's amino acid pool. The body can synthesize 11 amino acids from carbohydrates, fats, or other amino acids; these are called *nonessential* amino acids. (See *Essential and nonessential amino acids.*)

POINT TO REMEMBER
The other nine amino acids, called essential amino acids, can't be synthesized by the body and must be obtained from the diet.

Amino acid conversion

Amino acids not used for protein synthesis can be converted to keto acids and metabolized by Krebs cycle and the electron transport system to produce energy. Some keto acids can enter Krebs cycle directly by combining with an intermediate compound in the cycle. Other keto acids must undergo one of the following two conversions:

- conversion to pyruvic acid and then to acetyl CoA, which combines with oxaloacetic acid to form citric acid
- direct conversion to acetyl CoA, which combines with oxaloacetic acid to form citric acid.

Amino acids can also be converted to other nutrients such as fats. Those amino acids not used for protein synthesis may be converted to pyruvic acid and then to acetyl CoA. The acetyl CoA fragments condense to form long-chain fatty acids—a process that's the reverse of fatty acid breakdown. These fatty acids then combine with glycerol to form fats.

Amino acids can also be converted to glucose. They're first converted to pyruvic acid, which may then be converted to glucose.

Lipid metabolism

Until required for use as energy fuel, lipids are stored in adipose tissue within cells. When needed for energy, each fat molecule is hydrolyzed to glycerol and three molecules of fatty acids. Glycerol can be converted to pyruvic acid and then to acetyl CoA, which enters Krebs cycle.

Long-chain fatty acids are catabolized into two-carbon fragments, which combine with CoA to form acetyl CoA fragments. Acetyl CoA then enters Krebs cycle, yielding energy.

Ketone body formation

The liver normally forms ketone bodies from acetyl CoA fragments, which derive largely from fatty acid catabolism. Acetyl CoA molecules yield three types of ketone bodies: acetoacetic acid, betahydroxybutyric acid, and acetone.

Acetoacetic acid results from the combination of two acetyl CoA molecules and subsequent release of CoA from these molecules. Betahydroxybutyric acid forms when hydrogen is added to the oxygen atom in the acetoacetic acid molecule; the term *beta* indicates the location of the carbon

Essential and nonessential amino acids

Amino acids, the structural units of proteins, are classified as essential or nonessential based on whether the human body can synthesize them. The 9 amino acids that can't be synthesized must be obtained from the diet. The other 11 can be synthesized and are therefore nonessential in the diet; however, they're needed for protein synthesis.

Essential	Nonessential
Histidine	Alanine
Isoleucine	Arginine
Leucine	Asparagine
Lysine	Aspartic acid
Methionine	Cystine
Phenylalanine	Glutamic acid
Threonine	Glycine
Tryptophan	Hydroxyproline
Valine	Proline
	Serine
	Tyrosine

atom containing the OH group. Acetone forms when the COOH group of acetoacetic acid releases CO_2. Muscle tissue, brain tissue, and other tissues oxidize these ketone bodies for energy.

Excessive ketone formation

Under certain conditions, the body produces more ketone bodies than it can oxidize for energy. Such conditions include fasting, starvation, and uncontrolled diabetes (in which the body can't break down glucose). The body must then use fat instead of glucose as its primary energy source.

POINT TO REMEMBER

Use of fat instead of glucose for energy leads to an excess of ketone bodies. This condition disturbs normal acid-base balance and homeostatic mechanisms, leading to ketosis.

Lipid formation from proteins and carbohydrates

Excess amino acids can be converted to fat through keto acid–acetyl CoA conversion. Glucose may be converted to pyruvic acid and then to acetyl CoA, which is converted into fatty acids and then fat (in much the same way that amino acids are converted into fat).

Hormonal regulation of metabolism

Normal body functions necessitate that blood glucose levels stay within a certain range. Hormones regulate the blood glucose level by stimulating the metabolic processes that restore a normal level in response to blood glucose changes.

Focus on function
How insulin affects blood glucose level

Unlike most hormones, insulin tends to decrease the blood glucose level. It does this by helping glucose to enter cells, by promoting glycogenesis, and by stimulating glucose catabolism.

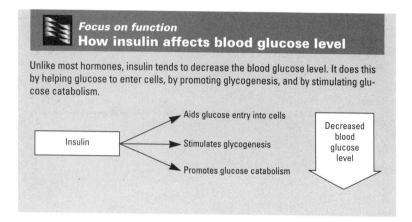

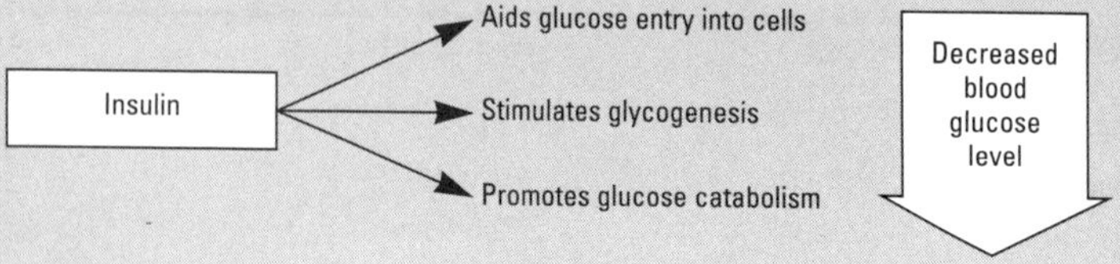

Hormones that raise the blood glucose level

Glucagon, a hormone produced in the pancreatic islets of Langerhans, promotes breakdown of glycogen to glucose (glycogenolysis), conversion of amino acids to glucose (gluconeogenesis), and breakdown of lipids (lipolysis). This breakdown results in liberation of free fatty acids and glycerol that can be converted to glucose. Epinephrine, a hormone secreted by the adrenal gland, promotes glycogenolysis, gluconeogenesis, and lipolysis.

Growth hormone, a peptide secreted by the anterior pituitary gland, has several effects on blood glucose:

- promotes protein synthesis by aiding amino acid entry into cells
- induces fat lipolysis from adipose tissue and promotes use of fat rather than carbohydrate as an energy source
- suppresses carbohydrate use for energy, leading to an increase in blood glucose through reduced glucose use
- promotes conversion of liver glycogen to glucose, which also tends to increase the blood glucose level.

Cortisol, a hormone secreted in the adrenal cortex, promotes protein hydrolysis to amino acids, which can be converted to glucose through gluconeogenesis.

Thyroxine, a thyroid gland hormone, typically raises the blood glucose level by aiding gluconeogenesis and lipolysis.

Hormones that decrease the blood glucose level

Insulin, produced by the pancreatic islet cells, is the only hormone that significantly reduces the blood glucose level. (See *How insulin affects blood glucose level.*) Besides promoting cell uptake and use of glucose as an energy source, insulin promotes glucose storage as glycogen (glycogenesis) and lipids (lipogenesis).

13 Urinary system

The urinary system consists of two kidneys, two ureters, the bladder, and the urethra. Working together, these structures remove wastes from the body, help govern acid-base balance by retaining or excreting hydrogen ions, and regulate fluid and electrolyte balance.

Kidneys

The *kidneys* are bean-shaped, highly vascular organs measuring approximately 4½″ (11.4 cm) long and 2½″ (6.4 cm) wide. Located retroperitoneally (at the small of the back), they lie on either side of the vertebral column, between the 12th thoracic and 3rd lumbar vertebrae. The right kidney, crowded by the liver, is positioned slightly lower than the left.

POINT TO REMEMBER
The kidneys are protected in front by the contents of the abdomen and behind by the muscles attached to the vertebral column. A layer of fat surrounding each kidney offers further protection.

Three layers of tissue surround each kidney:

- The *renal capsule* attaches directly to the kidney surface. This transparent capsule protects the kidney from infection.
- The middle layer, a fatty mass, is called the *adipose capsule.* The adipose capsule helps attach the kidney to the posterior wall of the body. It helps protect the kidney from trauma.
- The outermost layer is a dense fibrous connective tissue called the *renal fascia.* The renal fascia surrounds the kidney and the adrenal gland and anchors these organs to surrounding structures.

Atop each kidney lies an *adrenal gland.* These glands affect the renal system by influencing blood pressure and sodium and water retention by the kidneys.

Internal structures

The kidney has three regions: the renal cortex (outer region), renal medulla (middle region), and renal pelvis (inner region).

The *renal cortex,* which contains blood-filtering mechanisms, is protected by a fibrous capsule and by layers of fat *(perirenal fat).*

The *medulla* contains 8 to 12 *renal pyramids,* striated wedges composed mostly of tubular structures. The tapered portion of each pyramid *(apex)* empties into a cuplike *calyx.* The calyces channel formed urine from the pyramids into the *renal pelvis.* (See *Viewing the normal kidney,* page 158.)

Functions

Kidney functions include:

- elimination of wastes and excess ions (as urine)
- blood filtration (by regulating chemical composition and volume of blood)
- maintenance of fluid-electrolyte and acid-base balances
- production of *erythropoietin* (a hormone that stimulates red blood cell production) and enzymes (such as renin, which governs blood pressure and kidney function)
- conversion of vitamin D to a more active form.

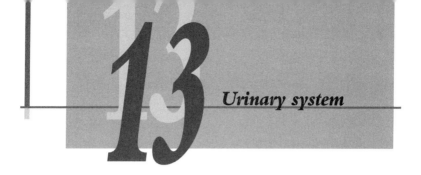

A structural view

Viewing the normal kidney

The kidneys are located retroperitoneally in the lumbar area, with the right kidney a bit lower than the left because of the liver mass above it. The kidneys assume different locations with changes in body position. Covering the kidneys are the true or fibrous capsule, perirenal fat, and renal fascia.

The kidneys receive waste-filled blood from the renal artery, which branches off the aorta. After passing through a complicated network of smaller blood vessels and nephrons, the filtered blood returns to the circulation by way of the renal vein, which empties into the inferior vena cava.

Urine excretion

Waste products that the nephrons remove from the blood are excreted by the kidneys, along with other fluids that constitute the formed urine. This urine passes through the ureters by peristalsis to the urinary bladder. When the bladder has filled, nerves in the bladder wall relax the sphincter. In conjunction with a voluntary stimulus, this relaxation causes urine to pass into the urethra for elimination from the body.

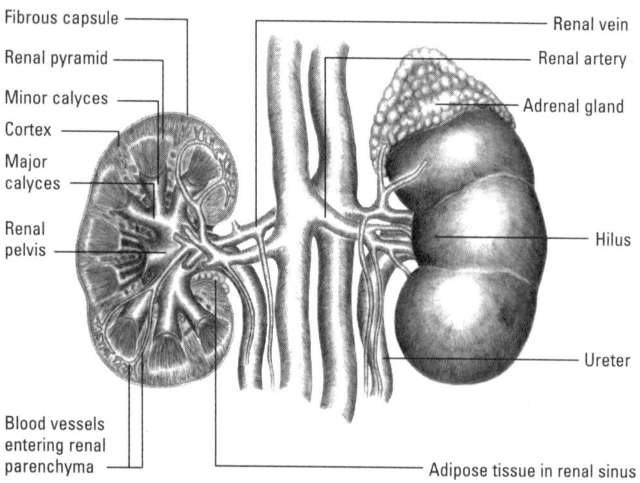

Nephron

The *nephron* is the kidney's basic structural and functional unit. Each nephron consists of a tubular apparatus called the *glomerulus*. Each glomerulus is located inside a glomerular capsule, or *Bowman's capsule*, and consists of a cluster of capillaries.

Parts of the nephron

The *nephron* is divided into three portions. The portion nearest the glomerular capsule is the *proximal convoluted tubule*. The second portion, the *loop of Henle,* has an ascending and a descending limb. The third portion, the one farthest from the glomerular capsule, is the *distal convoluted tubule.* Its distal end joins the distal ends of neighboring nephrons, forming a larger *collecting tubule.*

The glomeruli and proximal and distal tubules of the nephron are located in the renal cortex. The long loops of Henle, together with their accompanying blood vessels and collecting tubules, form the renal pyramids in the medulla.

Functions of the nephron

The nephrons perform two main functions:

- to mechanically filtrate fluids, wastes, electrolytes, acids, and bases into the tubular system
- to selectively reabsorb and secrete ions.

The proximal convoluted tubules have freely permeable cell membranes. This allows reabsorption of nearly all the filtrate's glucose, amino acids, metabolites, and electrolytes into nearby capillaries and the circulation. As these substances return to the circulation, they passively carry large amounts of water.

By the time the filtrate enters the descending limb of the loop of Henle, its water content has been reduced by 70%. At this point, the filtrate contains a high concentration of salts, chiefly sodium. As the filtrate moves deeper into the medulla and the loop of Henle, osmosis draws even more water into the extracellular spaces, further concentrating the filtrate.

Once the filtrate enters the ascending limb, its concentration is readjusted by the transport of ions into the tubule. This transport continues until the filtrate enters the distal convoluted tubule.

Vasculature

Blood enters the kidney from the *renal artery,* which subdivides into several branches. Some of these branches distribute blood within the kidney, while others nourish the kidney cells themselves. (See *Vasculature of the nephron,* page 160.)

Of the blood brought to the kidney for filtration, about 99% returns to general body circulation through the *renal vein.* The remaining 1% undergoes further processing, resulting in urine-containing waste products that flow to the calyx and renal pelvis.

Blood enters and leaves the glomerular capillaries by two small blood vessels, the *efferent* and *afferent arterioles.* The glomerular capillaries act as bulk filters and pass protein-free and red blood cell–free filtrate to the proximal convoluted tubules.

Ureters

The *ureters* are fibromuscular tubes that measure about 10" to 12" (25 to 30 cm) long in adults; their diameter ranges from 2 to 8 mm. Because the left kidney is higher than the right, the left ureter is usually slightly longer than the right ureter.

The ureters are narrowest where they join with the renal pelvis *(ureteropelvic junction)*. From their origins in this junction, the ureters travel in an oblique direction.

Internal structure

Ureters have three-layered walls. The *mucosa,* the innermost layer, contains transitional epithelium. The *muscularis,* the middle layer, contains smooth muscle layers. Extensions of the *fibrous coat,* the outer layer, hold the ureter in place.

Functions

The ureters act as ducts, allowing urine to pass from the kidneys to the bladder. Filling of the bladder constricts the ureters at their point of entry into the bladder. Peristaltic waves occurring about one to five times each minute channel urine along the ureters toward the bladder.

A structural view
Vasculature of the nephron

The kidneys are highly vascular, receiving about 20% of the blood pumped by the heart each minute. The renal artery, a large branch of the abdominal aorta, carries blood to each kidney. Then blood flows through the interlobular artery to the afferent arteriole, then through the glomerulus, efferent arteriole, peritubular capillaries, venules, and interlobular vein. The peritubular capillary network of vessels supplies blood to the tubules of the nephron—the kidney's basic functional unit and the site of urine formation.

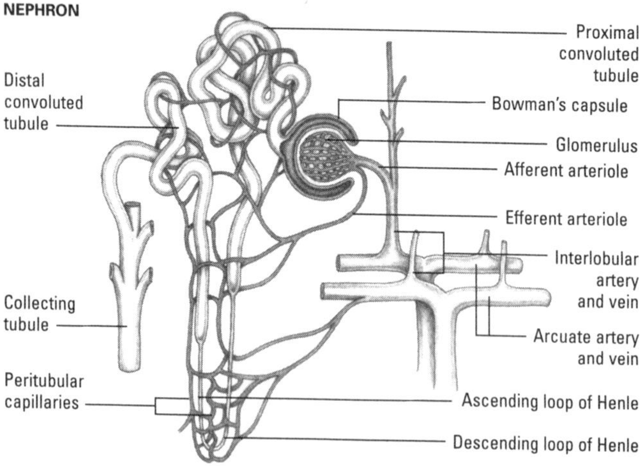

Bladder

A hollow, sphere-shaped, muscular organ in the pelvis, the *bladder* lies anterior and inferior to the pelvic cavity and posterior to the symphysis pubis. Its function is to store urine. If the amount of stored urine exceeds bladder capacity, the bladder distends above the symphysis pubis.

POINT TO REMEMBER
In a normal adult, bladder capacity ranges from 500 to 600 ml. It's less in children and elderly people.

Structure

The base of the bladder contains three openings that form a triangular area called the *trigone*. The two ureteral orifices act as the posterior boundary of the trigone; the urethral orifice forms its anterior boundary.

Bladder contraction and relaxation

Urination results from involuntary (reflex) and voluntary (learned or intentional) processes. When urine fills the bladder, parasympathetic nerve fibers in the bladder wall cause the bladder to contract and the internal sphincter (located at the internal urethral orifice) to relax. This is called the *micturition reflex.*

Then the cerebrum stimulates voluntary relaxation and contraction of the external sphincter (located about 3/4" [2 cm] beyond the internal sphincter).

Urethra

The *urethra* is a small tube that channels urine outside the body from the bladder.

Female urethra

In the female, the urethra is embedded in the anterior wall of the vagina behind the symphysis pubis. Ranging from 1" to 2" (2.5 to 5 cm) long, the urethra connects the bladder with an external opening, or urethral meatus, located anterior to the vaginal opening.

The female urethra is composed of an inner layer of mucous membrane, a middle layer of spongy tissue, and an outer layer of muscle.

Male urethra

In the male, the urethra passes vertically through the prostate gland and then extends through the urogenital diaphragm and the penis. Measuring approximately 8" (20 cm) long, it has three regions:

- *prostatic region,* which connects to the urinary bladder and passes through the prostate
- *membranous region,* which passes through the urogenital diaphragm
- *penile region,* which traverses the penis and ends at the external urethral orifice.

The male urethra serves as a passageway for semen as well as urine.

Urine formation

Three processes—glomerular filtration, tubular reabsorption, and tubular secretion—take place in the nephrons, ultimately leading to urine formation. (See *How the kidneys form urine,* page 162.)

Normal urine consists of sodium, chloride, potassium, calcium, magnesium, sulfates, phosphates, bicarbonates, uric acid, ammonium ions, creatinine, and urobilinogen. A few leukocytes and red blood cells and, in the male, some spermatozoa may enter the urine as it passes from the kidney to the urethral orifice. Urine may also contain drugs if the person is taking drugs that undergo urinary excretion.

The kidneys can vary the amount of substances reabsorbed and secreted in the nephrons, changing the composition of excreted urine.

POINT TO REMEMBER

Total daily urine output averages 720 to 2,400 ml, varying with fluid intake and climate. For example, after ingestion of a large volume of fluid, urine output increases as the body rapidly excretes excess water. If a person restricts water intake or has an excessive intake of such solutes as sodium, urine output decreases as the body retains water to restore normal fluid concentration.

Hormones and the urinary system

Hormones help regulate tubular reabsorption and secretion. For example, *antidiuretic hormone* (ADH) acts in the distal tubule and collecting ducts to increase water reabsorption and urine concentration. ADH deficiency decreases water reabsorption, causing dilute urine.

Another hormone, *aldosterone,* affects tubular reabsorption by regulating sodium retention and helping to control potassium secretion by epithelial cells in the tubules. When serum potassium levels rise, the adrenal cortex responds by increasing aldosterone secretion.

Renin-angiotensin system

By secreting the enzyme *renin,* the kidneys play a crucial role in blood pressure and fluid volume regulation. The *renin-angiotensin system* is an important homeostatic device for regulating the body's sodium and water levels and blood pressure. This system depends on feedback involving the *juxtaglomerular*

Focus on function
How the kidneys form urine

This diagram illustrates the three processes by which the kidneys secrete urine—glomerular filtration, tubular reabsorption, and tubular secretion.

From the proximal convoluted tubules, active transport leads to reabsorption of sodium (Na^+) and glucose into nearby circulation. Osmosis then causes water (H_2O) reabsorption.

From the distal convoluted tubules, active transport results in sodium reabsorption. The presence of antidiuretic hormone causes water reabsorption. Peritubular capillaries then secrete ammonia (NH_3) and hydrogen (H^+) into the distal tubules by active transport.

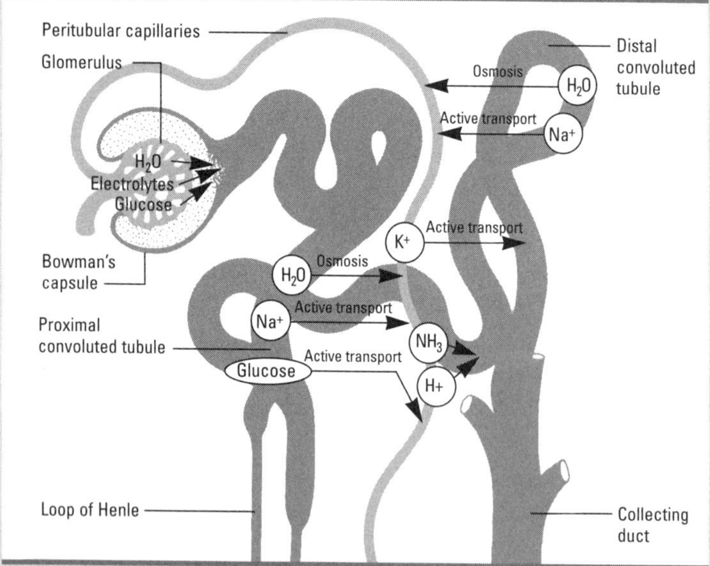

apparatus in the glomeruli and the liver, lungs, and adrenal cortex.

Juxtaglomerular cells near each glomerulus secrete renin into the blood. The rate of renin secretion depends on the rate of perfusion in the renal afferent arterioles and on the serum sodium level. A low sodium load and low perfusion pressure (as in hypovolemia) increase renin secretion; a high sodium load and high perfusion pressure decrease it.

Renin circulates throughout the body. In the liver, it converts *angiotensinogen,* a renin substrate, to the hormone *angiotensin I.* In the lungs, angiotensin I is converted by hydrolysis to *angiotensin II,* a potent vasoconstrictor. Angiotensin II acts on the adrenal cortex to stimulate production of the hormone aldosterone. Aldosterone, in turn, acts on the juxtaglomerular cells in the nephron to increase sodium and water retention and to stimulate or depress further renin secretion. This completes the feedback cycle that automatically readjusts homeostasis.

Other hormonal functions

The kidneys also secrete the hormone erythropoietin and regulate calcium and phosphorus balance. In response to low arterial oxygen tension, the kidneys produce erythropoietin, which travels to the bone marrow. There, it stimulates increased red blood cell production.

To help regulate calcium and phosphorus balance, the kidneys filter and reabsorb approximately half of unbound serum calcium and activate *vitamin* D_3, a compound that promotes intestinal calcium absorption and regulates phosphate excretion.

14 Fluid, electrolyte, and acid-base balance

The health and homeostasis of the human body depend on fluid, electrolyte, and acid-base balance. Factors that disrupt this balance, such as surgery, illness, and injury, may lead to potentially fatal changes in metabolic activity.

Fluid balance and electrolyte balance are highly interdependent: if one deviates from normal, so does the other. Acid-base balance is also vital to survival; even a slight imbalance can be life-threatening.

Body fluids

Water accounts for more than 50% of the average adult's body. Because fat contains no water, the proportion of body water varies inversely with the body's fat content. Consequently, an obese person has a lower percentage of body water than a lean person, and women have a lower percentage of body water than men (due to their higher percentage of body fat).

Body water contains *solutes,* or dissolved substances, that are necessary for physiologic functioning. Solutes include electrolytes, glucose, amino acids, and other nutrients.

Body fluid compartments

Fluid balance is a state in which the total amount of body water is normal. The term also indicates a relative constancy of the water distribution in the body's three fluid compartments. (See *Body fluid distribution.*)

Body fluid composition

Body fluid composition differs by compartment:

- The *intracellular fluid* (ICF) *compartment* consists of the fluid inside body cells.
- The *intravascular fluid compartment* includes the fluid in blood plasma and the lymphatic system.
- The *interstitial fluid compartment* consists of the fluid distributed through loose tissue in the spaces around the cells.

The intravascular and interstitial fluid compartments are commonly referred to collectively as the *extracellular fluid* (ECF) *compartment.* A capillary endothelium freely permeable to water, electrolytes, and other solutes separates the intravascular and interstitial fluids. For this reason, intravascular and interstitial fluids have a similar composition — a composition unlike that of the ICF.

For example, ICF has higher concentrations of protein, potassium, magnesium, phosphate, and sulfate and lower concentrations of sodium, calcium, chloride, and bicarbonate. Active transport mechanisms help maintain different concentrations of potassium and sodium in the ICF and ECF.

Body fluid osmolarity

When a semipermeable membrane separates two solutions of unequal solute concentration, water shifts by *osmosis* from the less concentrated solution to the more concentrated one. The more concentrated solution attracts water through a property called *osmotic activity.*

A solution's osmotic activity depends on the number of particles dissolved in it. Osmotic activity bears no relation to the particles' valence (combining capacity) or molecular weight. Thus, osmotic activity is the same in a

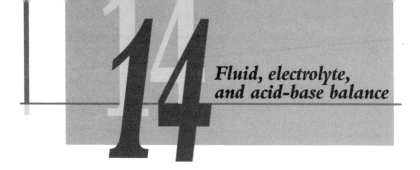

Body fluid distribution

Water in the body exists in two major compartments, separated by capillary walls and cell membranes. About two-thirds is found within cells as intracellular fluid (ICF). The other third remains outside cells as extracellular fluid (ECF).

The ECF includes both interstitial fluid (the fluid bathing the cells) and intravascular fluid (the fluid in blood plasma and the lymphatic system).

In an adult, interstitial fluid represents about 75% of ECF; intravascular fluid about 25%. ICF and ECF represent about 40% and 20% of an adult's total body weight, respectively.

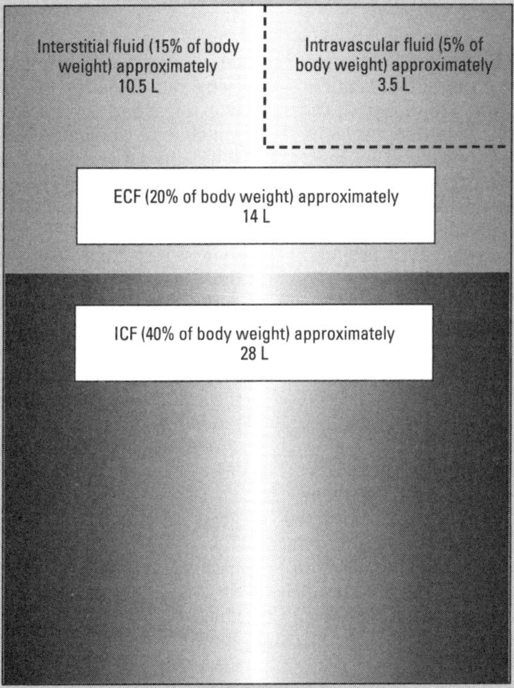

solution containing equal numbers of sodium ions (which are monovalent), calcium ions (which are divalent), or glucose molecules (which don't dissociate into ions).

Osmotic pressure

The *osmotic pressure* of a solution refers to the pressure that the solution exerts on a semipermeable membrane. This pressure is usually measured in terms of *osmolarity*. Examples include:

- A solution of 1 L (1 qt) of water containing 1 g molecular weight of a substance that doesn't dissociate in solution has an osmolarity of 1 Osm/L.
- A solution of 1 L of water containing 1 g molecular weight of an electrolyte

that dissociates into two ions has an osmolarity of 2 Osm/L.

- A solution of 1 L of water containing 1 g molecular weight of an electrolyte that dissociates into three ions has an osmolarity of 3 Osm/L.

Body fluid osmolarity is usually expressed in milliosmols per liter (mOsm/L) because of the low concentrations of dissolved particles.

Fluid balance

Fluid balance can exist only if fluid intake equals fluid output. Water enters the body through the GI tract and leaves through the skin, lungs, GI tract, and urinary tract. (See *How the body gains and loses fluids.*)

POINT TO REMEMBER
Fluid gains must equal fluid losses to stabilize the body's water content and to allow proper physiologic functioning.

Thirst (which regulates water intake) and the countercurrent mechanism (which governs urine concentration) help maintain the body's fluid balance.

Fluid intake

Water normally enters the body from the GI tract. The body obtains about 1,500 ml of water daily from consumed liquids and obtains about 800 ml from solid foods (which may contain up to 97% water). Oxidation of food in the body yields carbon dioxide and about 300 ml of water (water of oxidation).

Fluid output

Water leaves the body through the skin (in perspiration), lungs (in expired air), GI tract (in feces), and urinary tract (in urine). The main route of water loss is urine excretion; urine output typically varies from 1,000 to 1,500 ml daily. Water losses through the skin and lungs amount to 1,000 ml daily but may increase markedly with strenuous exertion, which predisposes a person to dehydration.

The body loses only about 100 ml of water in feces because the colon normally absorbs almost all the water contained in the contents of the GI tract.

Mechanisms of fluid balance

Interruption or dysfunction of one or both of the mechanisms that regulate fluid balance — thirst and the countercurrent mechanism — can lead to a fluid imbalance.

Thirst

Thirst — the conscious desire for water — primarily regulates fluid intake. Dehydration reduces ECF volume, which responds by increasing its sodium concentration and osmolarity. When the sodium concentration reaches about 2 mEq/L above normal, neurons of the thirst center in the hypothalamus are stimulated. The brain then directs motor neurons to satisfy thirst, causing the person to drink enough fluid to restore ECF to normal.

Countercurrent mechanism

Through the *countercurrent mechanism*, the kidneys regulate fluid output by modifying the urine concentration — that is, by excreting urine of greater or lesser concentration.

Electrolyte balance

Electrolytes are substances that break up, or dissociate, into electrically charged particles called *ions* when dissolved in water. Adequate amounts of each major electrolyte and a proper balance among the electrolytes must be present to maintain normal physiologic functioning.

The ICF and ECF normally have different concentrations of electrolytes. Various mechanisms govern electrolyte balance.

Electrolytes

Ions may be positively charged *cations* or negatively charged *anions*. Major cations include sodium, potassium, calcium, and magnesium. Major anions

How the body gains and loses fluids

Each day, the body takes in fluid from the GI tract (in foods, liquids, and water of oxidation) and loses fluids through the skin, lungs, intestine (feces), and urinary tract (urine). This illustration shows the primary sites involved in fluid gains and losses, along with the amount of normal daily fluid intake and output.

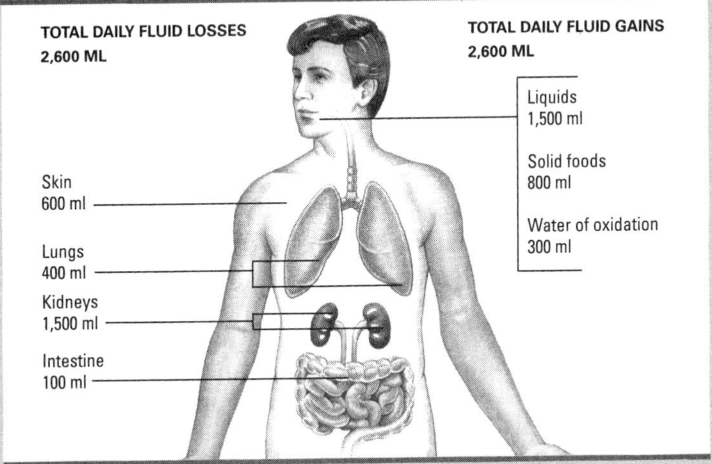

are chloride, bicarbonate, and phosphate. Normally, the electrical charges of cations balance the electrical charges of anions, keeping body fluids electrically neutral.

Blood plasma contains slightly more electrolytes than does interstitial fluid. Most notably, plasma contains a significant amount of protein anions, whereas interstitial fluid has hardly any because the capillary membrane is nearly impermeable to proteins. (See *Cations and anions in plasma,* page 168.)

Because of the proteins in plasma, certain other differences also distinguish plasma from interstitial fluid. For instance, plasma contains more sodium ions and fewer chloride ions than does interstitial fluid.

Ion concentration

Ion concentration is expressed in terms of the ion's *equivalent weight* (ability to combine with other ions). Equivalent weight equals the ion's gram molecular weight (amount of a substance whose weight in grams equals its molecular weight) divided by its chemical valence (numerical expression of chemical combining capacity). Ions with the same number of equivalents in a solution have equal combining powers; despite their different gram molecular weights, their concentrations are considered equal.

Because ions are present in such low concentrations in body fluids, they're usually expressed in milliequivalents per liter (mEq/L). ICF cells and ECF cells are permeable to different substances; therefore, these compartments normally have different electrolyte compositions. (See *Comparing electrolyte composition in ICF and ECF,* page 169.)

Cations and anions in plasma

Blood plasma contains varying amounts of cations (positively charged electrolytes) and anions (negatively charged electrolytes). However, cations and anions have the same total ionic charge (measured in milliequivalents [mEq]).

Cations	Anions
Sodium: 142 mEq	Chloride: 102 mEq
Calcium: 5 mEq	Bicarbonate: 26 mEq
Potassium: 4 mEq	Negatively charged proteins: 17 mEq
Magnesium: 2 mEq	Phosphate: 2 mEq
	Other: 6 mEq
Total: 153 mEq/L plasma	**Total: 153 mEq/L plasma**

Mechanisms of electrolyte balance

Electrolytes profoundly affect the body's water distribution, osmolarity, and acid-base balance. Various mechanisms help maintain electrolyte balance. Dysfunction or interruption of any of these mechanisms can produce an electrolyte imbalance.

For instance, the kidneys — through the action of aldosterone — are the chief regulators of sodium. Sodium and water balances are closely intertwined. (See *Osmotic regulation of sodium and water,* page 170.) The small intestine absorbs sodium readily from food and the skin and kidneys excrete sodium.

The kidneys also regulate potassium through aldosterone action. Most potassium is absorbed from food in the GI tract; normally, the amount excreted in urine equals dietary potassium intake. Because the body has no effective way to store potassium, it must be ingested daily to maintain adequate levels in the body.

Calcium in the blood normally is in equilibrium with calcium salts in bone. Parathyroid hormone (PTH) is the main regulator of calcium, controlling both calcium uptake from the GI tract and calcium excretion by the kidneys.

Magnesium is governed by aldosterone, which controls renal magnesium reabsorption. Absorbed from the GI tract, magnesium is excreted in urine, breast milk, and saliva.

Chloride also is regulated by the kidneys. Chloride ions move in conjunction with sodium ions.

The kidneys regulate bicarbonate, excreting, absorbing, or forming it. Bicarbonate, in turn, plays a vital part in acid-base balance.

Phosphate, too, is regulated by the kidneys. Absorbed well from food, phosphate is incorporated with calcium in bone. Along with calcium, phosphate levels are governed by PTH. Phosphate and calcium have an inverse relationship; when calcium levels become elevated, phosphate levels become decreased. When calcium levels become decreased, phosphate levels become increased.

Acid-base balance

Physiologic survival requires *acid-base balance* — a stable concentration of hydrogen ions in body fluids. An *acid* is a substance that yields hydrogen ions when dissociated in solution. A strong acid dissociates almost completely, releasing a large number of hydrogen ions. A weak acid, in contrast, dissociates less readily and releases fewer hydrogen ions.

A *base* dissociates in water, releasing ions that can combine with hydrogen ions such as hydroxyl ions. Like a strong acid, a strong base dissociates almost completely, releasing many ions. A weak base dissociates less readily and gives up fewer ions.

The hydrogen ion concentration of a fluid determines whether it's acidic or

Comparing electrolyte composition in ICF and ECF

This chart presents the electrolyte compositions of the intracellular fluid (ICF) compartment and extracellular fluid (ECF) compartment.

Electrolyte	ICF	ECF
Sodium	10 mEq/L	136 to 146 mEq/L
Potassium	140 mEq/L	3.6 to 5 mEq/L
Calcium	10 mEq/L	4.5 to 5.8 mEq/L
Magnesium	40 mEq/L	1.6 to 2.2 mEq/L
Chloride	4 mEq/L	96 to 106 mEq/L
Bicarbonate	10 mEq/L	24 to 28 mEq/L
Phosphate	100 mEq/L	1 to 1.5 mEq/L

basic (alkaline). A neutral solution such as pure water dissociates only slightly; it contains 0.0000001 (one ten-millionth) gram molecular weight (mol) of hydrogen ions per liter and the same amount of hydroxyl ions.

POINT TO REMEMBER
Hydrogen ion concentration is commonly expressed as pH. A neutral solution, for example, has a pH of 7.

An *acidic* solution contains more hydrogen ions; its pH is less than 7. An *alkaline* solution contains fewer hydrogen ions; its pH exceeds 7.

Because pH is an exponential expression, a change of one pH unit reflects a tenfold difference in actual hydrogen ion concentration. For instance, a solution with a pH of 7 has ten times more hydrogen ions than one with a pH of 8.

Hydrogen ion sources

The body produces acids through the following mechanisms:

- Protein catabolism yields nonvolatile acids, such as sulfuric, phosphoric, and uric acids.
- Fat oxidation produces acid ketone bodies.
- Anaerobic glucose catabolism produces lactic acid.
- Intracellular metabolism yields carbon dioxide as a by-product; carbon dioxide dissolves in body fluids to form carbonic acid.

Mechanisms of acid-base balance

Normally, the body's pH control mechanism is so effective that blood pH stays within a narrow range — 7.35 to 7.45. Acid-base balance is maintained by buffer systems and the lungs and kidneys, which neutralize and eliminate acids as rapidly as the acids are formed.

The lungs influence acid-base balance by excreting carbon dioxide and regulating the blood's carbonic acid content. The kidneys exert their effect by allowing tubular filtrate reabsorption of bicarbonate and by forming bicarbonate. Dysfunction or interruption of a buffer system or other governing mech-

Focus on function

Osmotic regulation of sodium and water

The flowchart here illustrates two compensatory mechanisms used to restore sodium and water balance.

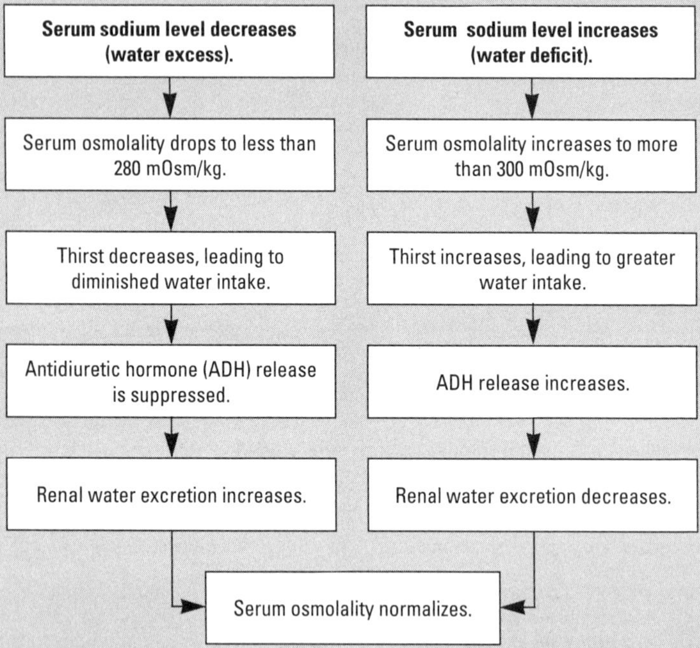
Serum sodium level decreases (water excess).
Serum osmolality drops to less than 280 mOsm/kg.
Thirst decreases, leading to diminished water intake.
Antidiuretic hormone (ADH) release is suppressed.
Renal water excretion increases.
Serum sodium level increases (water deficit).
Serum osmolality increases to more than 300 mOsm/kg.
Thirst increases, leading to greater water intake.
ADH release increases.
Renal water excretion decreases.
Serum osmolality normalizes.

anism can cause an acid-base imbalance. (See *Understanding respiratory and metabolic acidosis and alkalosis.*)

Buffer systems

Buffer systems — which consist of a weak acid and a salt of that acid, or a weak base and its salt — minimize pH changes brought about by an excess of acids or bases. These buffer systems reduce the effect of an abrupt change in hydrogen ion concentration by converting a strong acid or base (which normally would dissociate completely) into a weak acid or base (which releases a smaller number of free hydrogen or hydroxyl ions). The pH of a buffer system depends on the *ratio* of the two components in the buffer — not on their absolute amounts.

Sodium bicarbonate carbonic acid buffer system

The *sodium bicarbonate carbonic acid buffer system* is the major buffer in ECF. Sodium bicarbonate concentration is regulated by the kidneys and carbonic acid concentration, by the lungs. Both components of this buffer are replenished continually.

(Text continues on page 174.)

Understanding respiratory and metabolic acidosis and alkalosis

Metabolic buffer systems maintain the balance of acids and bases in the body. When the ratio is upset, either acidosis or alkalosis results. Depending on the cause of the condition, acidosis or alkalosis may be respiratory or metabolic.

Respiratory acidosis

When pulmonary ventilation decreases, retained carbon dioxide (CO_2) combines with water (H_2O) to form carbonic acid (H_2CO_3) in abnormally large amounts. Carbonic acid dissociates to release free hydrogen ions (H^+) and bicarbonate ions (HCO_3^-). Partial pressure of arterial carbon dioxide ($Paco_2$) rises above 45 mm Hg and blood pH falls below 7.35 creating an acidic environment.

The excessive carbonic acid causes a drop in pH. As the pH falls, 2,3-diphosphoglycerate (2,3-DPG) increases in the red blood cells, causing a change in hemoglobin (Hb) that makes Hb release oxygen (O_2). The altered Hb, now strongly alkaline, picks up hydrogen ions and carbon dioxide, thus eliminating some of the free hydrogen ions and excess carbon dioxide. Then oxygen saturation decreases.

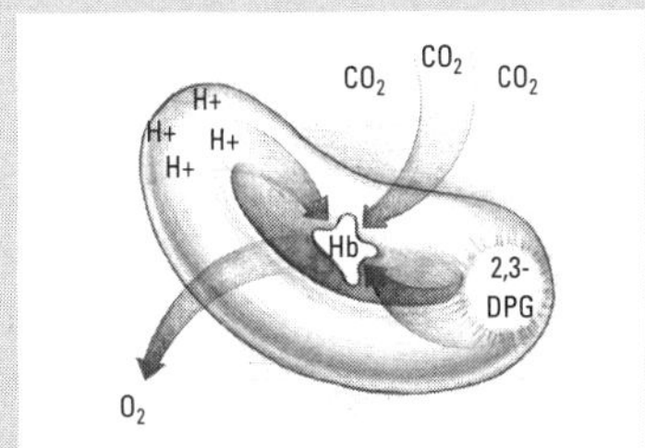

Whenever $Paco_2$ increases, carbon dioxide builds up in all tissues and fluids, including cerebrospinal fluid and the respiratory center in the medulla. carbon dioxide reacts with water to form carbonic acid, which then breaks into free hydrogen and bicarbonate ions. The increased amount of carbon dioxide and free hydrogen ions stimulate the respiratory center to speed the respiratory rate. This, in turn, leads to elimination of more carbon dioxide and helps to reduce the carbon dioxide level in the blood and other tissues. Respirations become rapid and shallow and $Paco_2$ decreases as the body attempts to compensate for the acidosis.

Eventually, carbon dioxide and hydrogen ions cause cerebral blood vessels to dilate, which increases blood flow to the brain. This heightened flow can cause cerebral edema and depress central nervous system (CNS) activity, leading to such signs and symptoms as headache, confusion, lethargy, nausea, and vomiting.

As respiratory mechanisms fail, the increasing $Paco_2$ stimulates the kidneys to retain bicarbonate and sodium ions and to excrete hydrogen ions, some of which are excreted in the form of ammonium (NH_4). The additional bicarbonate and sodium combine to form extra sodium bicarbonate ($NaHCO_3$), which can then buffer more free hydrogen ions. Urine acid content increases, blood pH

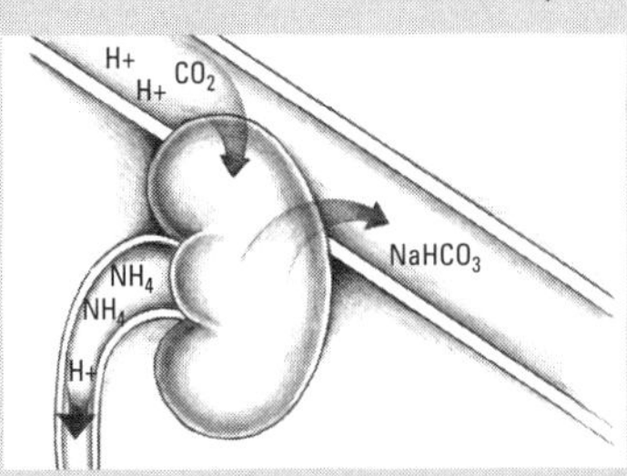

and bicarbonate levels rise, and respirations become shallow and depressed.

As the concentration of hydrogen ions overwhelms the body's compensatory mechanisms, these ions move into

(continued)

Understanding respiratory and metabolic acidosis and alkalosis *(continued)*

the cells and potassium ions (K^+) move out. Concurrent lack of oxygen boosts anaerobic production of lactic acid, further skewing the acid-base balance and critically depressing neurologic and cardiac functions. $Paco_2$ then increases and the patient experiences hyperkalemia, arrhythmias, reduced partial pressure of arterial oxygen and pH, and a decreased level of consciousness (LOC).

Respiratory alkalosis

When pulmonary ventilation increases above the amount needed to maintain normal carbon dioxide levels, excessive amounts of carbon dioxide are exhaled. This causes hypocapnia (a fall in $Paco_2$), which leads to a reduction in carbonic acid production, a loss of hydrogen and bicarbonate ions, and a subsequent rise in pH. Blood pH rises above 7.45, $Paco_2$ drops below 35 mm Hg, and bicarbonate falls below 24 mEq/L.

In defense against the rising pH, hydrogen ions leave the cells and enter the blood in exchange for potassium ions. Hydrogen ions entering the blood combine with bicarbonate ions to form carbonic acid, which lowers the pH level. Bicarbonate decreases further, blood pH falls, and the serum potassium level drops below normal (causing hypokalemia).

Hypocapnia stimulates the carotid and aortic bodies as well as the medulla, which speeds the heart rate without increasing blood pressure. The patient then experiences angina, electrocardiogram changes, restlessness, and anxiety. Simultaneously, hypocapnia produces cerebral vasoconstriction, which prompts a reduction in cerebral blood flow. Hypercapnia also overexcites the medulla, pons, and other parts of the autonomic nervous system. This causes such signs and symptoms as increasing

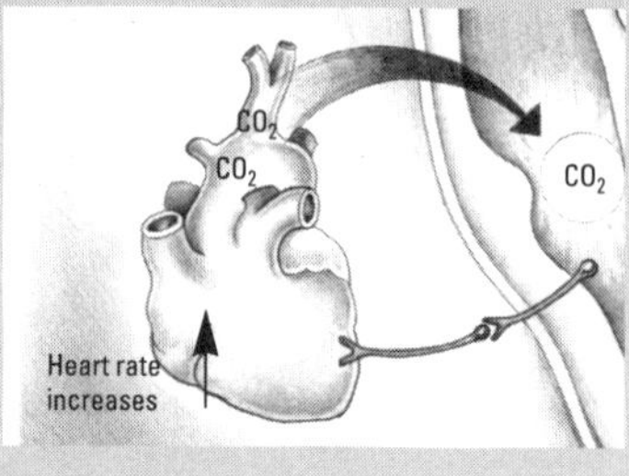

anxiety, diaphoresis, dyspnea, alternating periods of apnea and hyperventilation, dizziness, and tingling in the fingers or toes.

When hypocapnia lasts more than 6 hours, the kidneys increase secretion of bicarbonate and reduce hydrogen excretion. Periods of apnea may result if pH remains high and $Paco_2$ remains low. The respiratory rate slows and the patient experiences hypoventilation and Cheyne-Stokes respirations.

Continued low $Paco_2$ increases cerebral and peripheral hypoxia from vasoconstriction. Severe alkalosis inhibits calcium (Ca) ionization, in turn causing increased nerve excitability and muscle contractions. Eventually, alkalosis overwhelms the CNS and the heart. The patient's LOC decreases, and he exhibits hyperreflexia, carpopedal spasm, tetany, arrhythmias, seizures, and coma.

Metabolic acidosis

As hydrogen ions accumulate in the body, chemical buffers (plasma bicar-

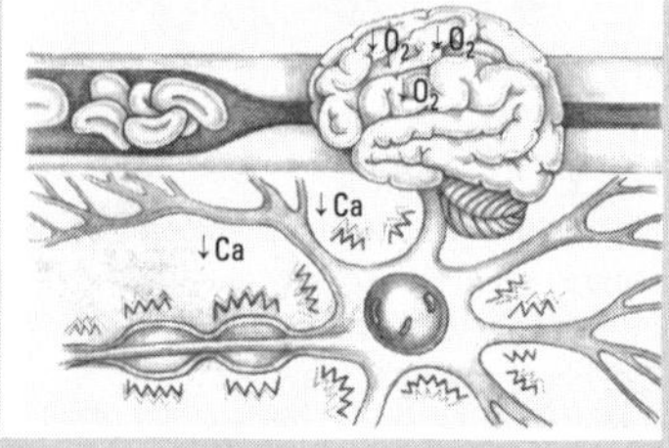

Understanding respiratory and metabolic acidosis and alkalosis *(continued)*

bonate and proteins) in the cells and extracellular fluid bind with them. No signs or symptoms are detectable at this stage.

Excess hydrogen ions that the buffers can't bind with decrease the pH level and stimulate chemoreceptors in the medulla to increase the respiratory rate. The increased respiratory rate lowers $Paco_2$, which allows more hydrogen ions to bind with bicarbonate ions. Respiratory compensation occurs within minutes but isn't sufficient to correct the imbalance. Blood pH drops below 7.35, bicarbonate level falls below 22 mEq/L, $Paco_2$ decreases, and rapid, deeper respirations occur.

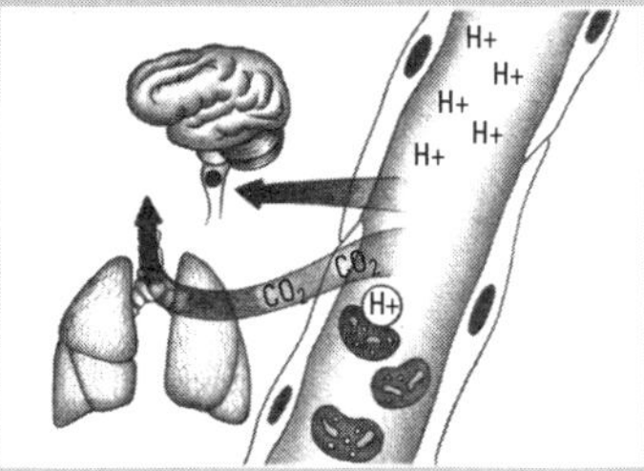

Healthy kidneys try to compensate for the acidosis by secreting excess hydrogen ions into the renal tubules. Those ions are buffered by phosphate or ammonia and then are excreted into the urine in the form of a weak acid. As a result, urine becomes acidic.

Each time a hydrogen ion is secreted into the renal tubules, a sodium ion and a bicarbonate ion are absorbed from the tubules and returned to the blood. The blood pH and bicarbonate levels slowly return to normal.

Excess hydrogen ions in the extracellular fluid diffuse into cells. To maintain the balance of the charge across the membrane, cells release potassium ions into the blood. The patient experiences signs and symptoms of hyperkalemia, including colic and diarrhea, weakness or flaccid paralysis, tingling and numbness in the extremities, bradycardia, a tall T wave, a prolonged PR interval, and a wide QRS complex.

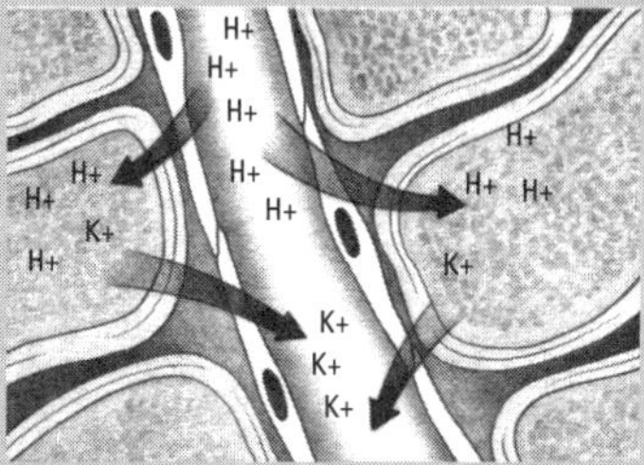

Excess hydrogen ions alter the normal balance of potassium, sodium, and calcium ions, reducing nerve cell excitability. Now the patient exhibits signs and symptoms of progressive CNS depression, including lethargy, dull headache, confusion, stupor, and coma.

Metabolic alkalosis

As bicarbonate ions start to accumulate in the body, chemical buffers (in extracellular fluid and cells) bind with the ions. No signs or symptoms are detectable at this stage.

Excess bicarbonate ions that don't bind with chemical buffers elevate serum pH, which in turn depresses chemoreceptors in the medulla. Depression of those chemoreceptors causes the respiratory rate to slow, which increases the $Paco_2$. The additional carbon dioxide combines with water to form carbonic acid. Lowered oxygen levels limit respiratory compensation. Blood pH rises above 7.45, bicarbonate level increases above 26 mEq/L, $Paco_2$ climbs, and respirations become slow and shallow.

When the bicarbonate level exceeds 28 mEq/L, the renal glomeruli can no longer reabsorb excess bicarbonate. The

(continued)

Understanding respiratory and metabolic acidosis and alkalosis *(continued)*

excess bicarbonate is excreted in the urine; hydrogen ions are retained. Urine becomes alkaline and pH and bicarbonate levels slowly return to normal.

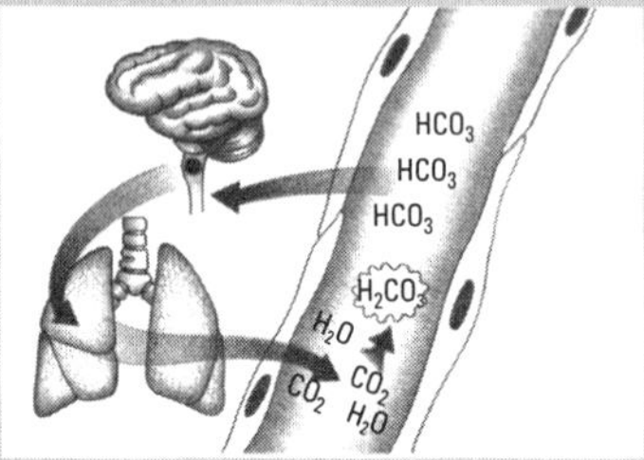

To maintain electrochemical balance, the kidneys excrete excess sodium ions, water, and bicarbonate. The patient initially experiences polyuria, then signs and symptoms of hypovolemia, including thirst and dry mucous membranes.

Lowered hydrogen ion levels in the extracellular fluid cause the ions to diffuse out of the cells. To maintain the balance of charges across the cell membrane, extracellular potassium ions move into the cells. Signs and symptoms of hypokalemia (such as anorexia, muscle weakness, and loss of reflexes) now arise.

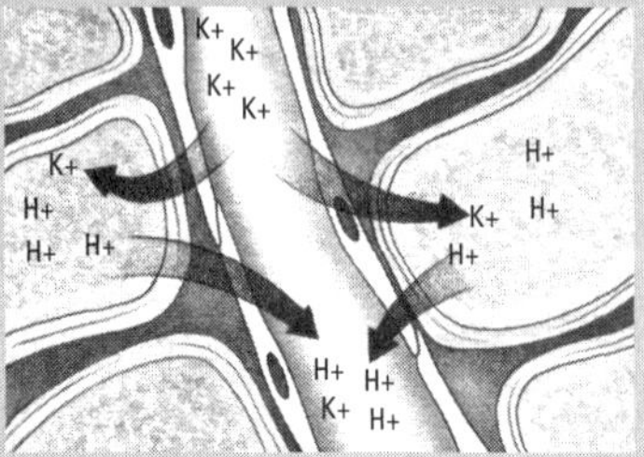

As hydrogen ion levels decline, calcium ionization decreases. Decreased ionization makes nerve cells more permeable to sodium ions. Sodium ions moving into nerve cells stimulate neural impulses and produce overexcitability of the CNS and peripheral nervous system. The patient experiences tetany, belligerence, irritability, disorientation, and seizures.

The normal ratio of the buffer components (20 parts sodium bicarbonate to 1 part carbonic acid) maintains a pH of 7.4. A change in this ratio would trigger a corresponding change in the pH of the buffer and the body fluids it governs.

Phosphate buffer system

The *phosphate buffer system* is especially important in the ECF. Its acidic component is sodium dihydrogen phosphate; its alkaline component is sodium monohydrogen phosphate. The phosphate buffer is crucial in neutralizing hydrogen ions secreted by the renal tubules.

Protein buffer system

In the *protein buffer system,* intracellular proteins absorb hydrogen ions generated by the body's metabolic processes.

Lungs

Respiration plays a crucial role in controlling pH. The lungs excrete carbon dioxide and regulate the carbonic acid content of the blood. Carbonic acid is derived from the carbon dioxide and water that are released as by-products of cellular metabolic activity.

Carbon dioxide (CO_2) is soluble in blood plasma. Some of the dissolved gas reacts with water (H_2O) to form carbonic acid (H_2CO_3), a weak acid that partially breaks apart to form hydrogen (H^+) and bicarbonate ions (HCO_3^-). These three substances are in equilibrium, as reflected in the following formula:

$$CO_2 + H_2O \leftrightarrow H_2CO_3 \leftrightarrow H^+ + HCO_3^-$$

Carbon dioxide dissolved in plasma is in equilibrium with carbon dioxide in the lung alveoli (expressed as a partial pressure [Pco_2]). Thus, an equilibrium exists between alveolar Pco_2 and the various forms of carbon dioxide present in the plasma, as expressed by the following formula:

$$Pco_2 \leftrightarrow CO_2 + H_2O \leftrightarrow H_2CO_3 \leftrightarrow H^+ + HCO_3^-$$

Role of respiratory rate and depth

A change in the rate or depth of respirations can alter the carbon dioxide content of alveolar air and the alveolar Pco_2. A change in alveolar Pco_2 produces a corresponding change in the amount of carbonic acid formed by dissolved carbon dioxide. In turn, these changes stimulate the respiratory center to modify respiratory rate and depth.

An increase in alveolar Pco_2 raises the blood concentration of carbon dioxide and carbonic acid. This, in turn, stimulates the respiratory center to increase respiratory rate and depth. As a result, alveolar Pco_2 decreases, which leads to a corresponding drop in the carbonic acid and carbon dioxide concentrations in blood. (See *How respiratory mechanisms affect blood pH,* page 176.)

A decrease in respiratory rate and depth has the reverse effect—it raises alveolar Pco_2, which in turn triggers an increase in the blood's carbon dioxide and carbonic acid concentrations.

Kidneys

Besides excreting various acid waste products, the kidneys regulate the blood's bicarbonate concentration by permitting bicarbonate reabsorption from tubular filtrate and by forming additional bicarbonate to replace that used in buffering acids.

Renal tubular ion secretion

Recovery and formation of bicarbonate in the kidneys hinge on hydrogen ion secretion by the renal tubules in exchange for sodium ions. The sodium ions are simultaneously reabsorbed into the circulation from the tubular filtrate.

Influenced by the enzyme carbonic anhydrase, tubular epithelial cells form carbonic acid from carbon dioxide and water. Carbonic acid quickly dissociates into hydrogen and bicarbonate ions. Hydrogen ions enter the tubular filtrate in exchange for sodium ions; bicarbonate ions enter the bloodstream along with the sodium ions that have been absorbed from the filtrate. Bicarbonate is then reabsorbed from the tubular filtrate.

Each hydrogen ion secreted into the tubular filtrate joins with a bicarbonate ion to form carbonic acid, which rapidly dissociates into carbon dioxide and water. The carbon dioxide diffuses into the tubular epithelial cell, where it can combine with more water and lead to the formation of more carbonic acid.

Bicarbonate reabsorption

The remaining water molecule in the tubular filtrate is eliminated in urine. As each hydrogen ion enters the tubular filtrate to combine with a bicarbonate ion, a bicarbonate ion in the tubular epithelial cell diffuses into the circulation. This process is termed *bicarbonate reabsorption.* (However, the bicarbonate ion that enters the circulation isn't the same one that's in the tubular filtrate.)

Formation of ammonia and phosphate salts

To form more bicarbonate, the kidneys must secrete additional hydrogen ions in exchange for sodium ions. For the renal tubules to continue secreting hydrogen ions, the excess ions must combine with other substances in the filtrate and be excreted. Excess hydrogen ions in the filtrate may combine with ammonia (produced by the renal tubules) or with phosphate salts (present in the tubular filtrate).

Ammonia forms in the tubular epithelial cells by removal of the amino groups from glutamine (an amino acid derivative) and from amino acids delivered to the tubular epithelial cells from

How respiratory mechanisms affect blood pH

A rise in the carbon dioxide (CO_2) content of arterial blood or a decrease in blood pH stimulates the respiratory center, causing hyperventilation. As a result, less carbon dioxide and therefore less carbonic acid and fewer hydrogen ions remain in the blood. Consequently, blood pH increases, possibly reaching a normal level.

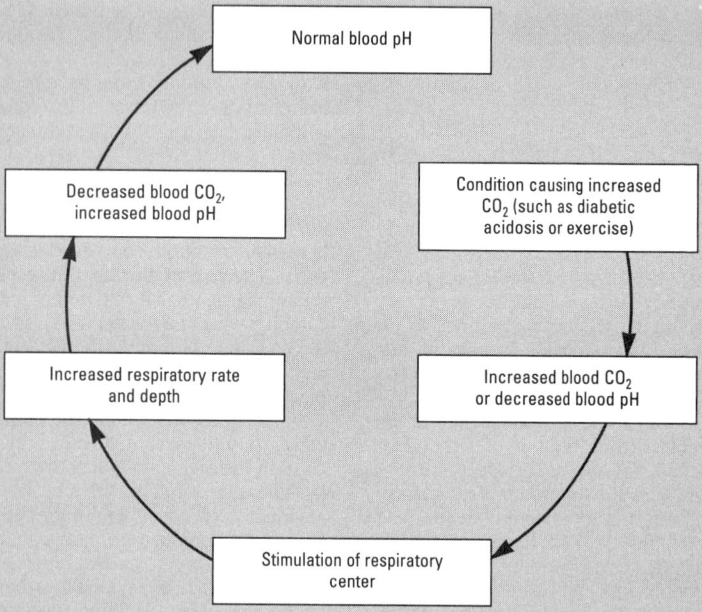

the circulation. After diffusing into the filtrate, ammonia joins with the secreted hydrogen ions, forming ammonium ions. These ions are excreted in the urine with chloride and other anions; each secreted ammonia molecule eliminates one hydrogen ion in the filtrate.

At the same time, sodium ions that have been absorbed from the filtrate and exchanged for hydrogen ions enter the circulation, as does the bicarbonate formed in the tubular epithelial cells. Some secreted hydrogen ions combine with sodium monohydrogen phosphate, a disodium phosphate salt in the tubular filtrate. Each of the secreted hydrogen ions that joins with the disodium salt changes it to the monosodium salt sodium dihydrogen phosphate. The sodium ion released in this reaction is absorbed into the circulation along with a newly formed bicarbonate ion.

Factors that affect the rate of bicarbonate formation

The rate of bicarbonate formation by renal tubular epithelial cells is affected by two factors:

- amount of dissolved carbon dioxide in the plasma
- potassium content of the tubular cells.

If the plasma carbon dioxide level rises, renal tubular cells form more bicarbonate. Increased plasma carbon dioxide encourages greater carbonic acid formation by renal tubular cells.

Partial dissociation of carbonic acid results in more hydrogen ions for excretion into the tubular filtrate and additional bicarbonate ions for entry into the circulation. This, in turn, increases the plasma bicarbonate level and reduces the plasma level of dissolved carbon dioxide toward normal. If the plasma carbon dioxide level decreases, renal tubular cells form less carbonic acid.

Because fewer hydrogen ions are formed and excreted, fewer bicarbonate ions enter the circulation. The plasma bicarbonate level then falls accordingly.

The potassium content of renal tubular cells also helps regulate plasma bicarbonate concentration by affecting the rate at which the renal tubules secrete hydrogen ions. Tubular cell potassium content and hydrogen ion secretion are interrelated; potassium and hydrogen ions are secreted at rates that vary inversely. Hydrogen ion secretion increases if tubular secretion of potassium ions falls; hydrogen ion secretion declines if tubular secretion of potassium ions increases.

For each hydrogen ion secreted into the tubular filtrate, an additional bicarbonate ion enters the blood plasma. Consequently, increased tubular secretion of hydrogen ions leads to a rise in the plasma bicarbonate content.

POINT TO REMEMBER

In a patient with potassium depletion from vomiting or diarrhea, potassium secretion by the tubular epithelial cells decreases and hydrogen ion secretion rises.

Depletion of body potassium causes more bicarbonate to enter the circulation; the plasma bicarbonate level then rises above normal. When the body contains excess potassium, the tubules excrete more potassium. As a result, fewer hydrogen ions are secreted, less bicarbonate forms, and the plasma bicarbonate concentration decreases.

15 Reproductive system

The reproductive system must function properly to ensure survival of the species. Anatomically, the main distinction between the male and female is the presence of conspicuous external genitalia in the male. In contrast, the major reproductive organs of the female lie within the pelvic cavity.

Male reproductive system

The male reproductive system consists of the organs that produce, transfer, and introduce mature sperm into the female reproductive tract, where fertilization occurs.

Besides supplying male sex cells (in a process called *spermatogenesis*), the male reproductive system plays a part in the secretion of male sex hormones. The penis also functions in urine elimination (as described in chapter 13, Urinary system).

The male reproductive organs include the penis, scrotum, testes, duct system, and accessory reproductive glands. (See *Structures of the male reproductive system.*)

Penis

The organ of copulation, the *penis* deposits sperm in the female reproductive tract and acts as the terminal duct for the urinary tract. It consists of an attached root, a free shaft, and an enlarged tip.

Internally, the cylinder-shaped penile shaft consists of three columns of erectile tissue bound together by heavy fibrous tissue. Two *corpora cavernosa* form the major part of the penis. On the underside, the *corpus spongiosum* encases the urethra. Its enlarged proximal end forms the bulb of the penis.

The *glans penis,* at the distal end of the shaft, is a cone-shaped structure formed from the corpus spongiosum. Its lateral margin forms a ridge of tissue known as the *corona*. The glans is highly sensitive to sexual stimulation.

Thin, loose skin covers the penile shaft. The *urethral meatus* opens through the glans to allow urination and ejaculation.

POINT TO REMEMBER

In an uncircumcised male, a skin flap — the foreskin, or prepuce — covers the corona and much of the glans.

Vasculature

The penis receives blood through the internal pudendal artery. Blood then flows into the corpora cavernosa through the penile artery. Venous blood returns through the internal iliac vein to the vena cava.

Scrotum

The penis meets the *scrotum,* or scrotal sac, at the penoscrotal junction. Located posterior to the penis and anterior to the anus, the scrotum is an extra-abdominal pouch consisting of a thin layer of skin overlying a tighter, musclelike layer. This musclelike layer, in turn, overlies the *tunica vaginalis,* a serous membrane covering the internal scrotal cavity. Externally, the *median raphe* separates the scrotal skin.

Internally, a septum divides the scrotum into two sacs, each containing a testis, an epididymis, and a *spermatic cord.* The spermatic cord is a connective

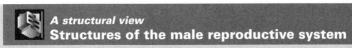

A structural view
Structures of the male reproductive system

The male reproductive system, pictured here, consists of the penis, the scrotum and its contents, the prostate gland, and the inguinal structures.

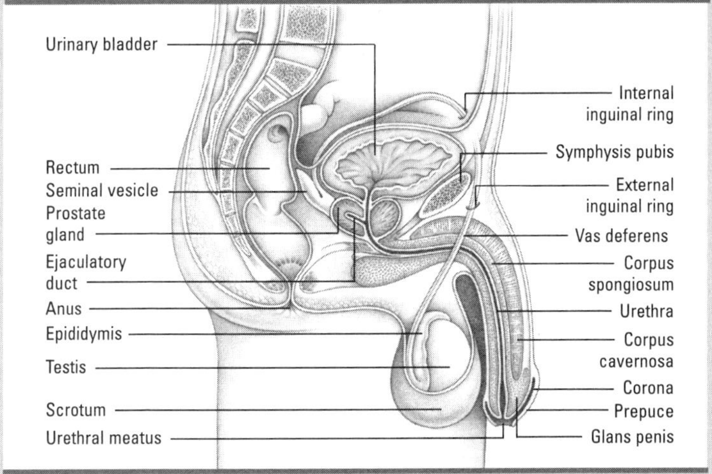

tissue sheath encasing autonomic nerve fibers, blood vessels, lymph vessels, and the *vas deferens* (also called *ductus deferens*). The spermatic cord travels from the testis through the *inguinal canal,* exiting the scrotum through the *external inguinal ring* and entering the abdominal cavity through the *internal inguinal ring*. The inguinal canal lies between the two rings.

Lymph nodes from the penis, scrotal surface, and anus drain into the inguinal lymph nodes. Lymph nodes from the testes drain into the lateral aortic and pre-aortic lymph nodes in the abdomen.

Testes

The *testes* (testicles) — paired oval structures in the scrotum — are the male gonads. Each testis measures about 2″ (5 cm) long by 1″ (2.5 cm) wide and weighs about ½ oz (14 g). The testes also function as part of the endocrine system. (See chapter 6, Endocrine system.)

The testes are enveloped in two connective tissue layers — the tunica vaginalis (outer layer) and the *tunica albuginea* (a deeper layer). Extensions of the tunica albuginea separate the testis into several hundred lobules. Each lobule contains one to four *seminiferous tubules,* small tubes where spermatogenesis takes place.

POINT TO REMEMBER

The apparent function of the scrotum is to keep the testes cool; spermatozoa development requires a temperature below that of the body. The dartos muscle, smooth muscle in the superficial fascia, causes scrotal skin to wrinkle, which helps regulate temperature. The cremaster

muscle, rising from the internal oblique muscle, helps to govern temperature by elevating the testes.

Spermatogenesis

Sperm formation, or *spermatogenesis,* begins when a male reaches puberty and normally continues throughout life. The process is stimulated by male sex hormones. Mature sperm cells form continuously within the seminiferous tubules.

Sperm formation occurs in several stages:

- In the first stage, the primary germinal epithelial cells, called *spermatogonia,* grow and develop into primary *spermatocytes*. Both spermatogonia and primary spermatocytes contain 46 chromosomes, consisting of 44 autosomes and the two sex chromosomes, X and Y.
- Next, primary spermatocytes divide to form secondary spermatocytes. No new chromosomes are formed in this stage; the pairs only divide. Each secondary spermatocyte contains half the number of autosomes, 22. One secondary spermatocyte contains an X chromosome; the other, a Y chromosome.
- In the third stage, each secondary spermatocyte divides again to form *spermatids* (also called spermatoblasts).
- Finally, the spermatids undergo a series of structural changes that transform them into mature *spermatozoa,* or sperm. Each spermatozoon has a head, neck, body, and tail. The head contains the nucleus; the tail, a large amount of *adenosine triphosphate,* which provides energy for sperm motility.

Newly mature sperm pass from the seminiferous tubules through the *vasa recta* into the *epididymis,* where they mature. Only a small number of sperm can be stored in the epididymis. Most of them move into the vas deferens, where they're stored until sexual stimulation triggers emission. Sperm cells retain their potency in storage for many weeks. After ejaculation, sperm survive for 24 to 72 hours at body temperature.

POINT TO REMEMBER

The number and motility of sperm affect fertility. A low sperm count (less than 20 million per milliliter of ejaculated semen) or poor sperm motility may cause infertility.

Duct system

The duct system — epididymis, vas deferens, and urethra — conveys sperm from the testes to the ejaculatory ducts near the bladder.

Epididymis

A coiled tube measuring about 20′ (6.1 m) long, the epididymis is located superior to and along the posterior border of the testis. At the lower border of the testis, the epididymis turns upward to join the vas deferens. During ejaculation, smooth muscle in the epididymis contracts, ejecting spermatozoa into the vas deferens.

Vas deferens

The vas deferens leads from the testes to the abdominal cavity. About 18″ (46 cm) long, it extends upward through the inguinal canal, arches over the urethra, and descends behind the bladder. Its enlarged portion, called the *ampulla,* merges with the duct of the seminal vesicle to form the *short ejaculatory duct*. After passing through the prostate gland, the vas deferens joins with the urethra.

Urethra

A small tube leading from the floor of the bladder to the exterior, the *urethra* consists of three parts:

- *prostatic urethra,* surrounded by the prostate gland, which drains the bladder
- *membranous urethra,* which passes through the urogenital diaphragm
- *spongy urethra,* which makes up about 75% of the entire urethra.

The function of the urethra is to convey urine and semen to the tip of the penis.

Accessory reproductive glands

The *accessory glands,* which produce most of the semen, include the seminal vesicles, bulbourethral glands (Cowper's glands), and prostate gland.

The *seminal vesicles* are paired sacs at the base of the bladder. The *bulbourethral glands,* also paired, are located inferior to the prostate.

Prostate gland

Lying under the bladder and surrounding the urethra, the walnut-sized *prostate gland* has a diameter of approximately 1½" (4 cm). It consists of three lobes — the left and right lateral lobes and the median lobe.

The prostate continuously secretes *prostatic fluid,* a thin, milky, alkaline fluid. During sexual activity, prostatic fluid adds volume to the semen. The fluid enhances sperm motility and may improve the chance for conception by neutralizing the acidity of the urethra and of the woman's vagina.

Semen

Consisting of spermatozoa and accessory gland secretions, *semen* is a viscous, white secretion with a slightly alkaline pH (7.8 to 8). The seminal vesicles produce roughly 60% of the fluid portion of the semen, while the prostate gland produces about 30%. A viscid fluid secreted by the bulbourethral glands also becomes part of the semen.

Hormonal control and sexual development

Male sex hormones *(androgens)* are produced in the testes and the adrenal glands. Located in the testes between the seminiferous tubules, *Leydig's cells* secrete *testosterone,* the most significant male sex hormone.

Effects of testosterone

Testosterone is responsible for the development and maintenance of male sex organs and secondary sex characteristics (such as facial hair and vocal cord thickness). Testosterone is also required for spermatogenesis.

Male sexuality is also affected by other hormones. Two of these — *luteinizing hormone* (LH), or interstitial cell-stimulating hormone, and *follicle-stimulating hormone* (FSH) — directly affect secretion of testosterone.

Testosterone secretion begins in utero, starting at approximately 2 months after conception, when the release of chorionic gonadotropins from the placenta stimulates Leydig's cells in the male fetus. The presence of testosterone directly affects sexual differentiation in the fetus. With testosterone, fetal genitalia develop into a penis, scrotum, and testes; without testosterone, genitalia develop into a clitoris, vagina, and other female organs.

During the last 2 months of gestation, testosterone normally causes the testes to descend into the scrotum. If the testes don't descend after birth, exogenous testosterone may correct the problem.

Puberty

During early childhood, a boy doesn't secrete gonadotropins and thus has little circulating testosterone. Secretion of gonadotropins from the pituitary gland, which usually occurs between ages 11 and 14, marks the onset of puberty. These pituitary gonadotropins stimulate testes functioning as well as testosterone secretion.

During puberty, the penis and testes enlarge and the male reaches full adult sexual and reproductive capability. Puberty also marks the development of male secondary sexual characteristics — distinct body hair distribution; skin changes (such as increased secretion by sweat and sebaceous glands), deepening of the voice (from laryngeal enlargement), increased musculoskeletal development, and other intracellular and extracellular changes.

Sexual maturity

After a male reaches full physical maturity — usually by age 20 — sexual and reproductive function remain fairly consistent throughout life. With aging, a man may experience subtle changes in

How exercise affects the reproductive system

Sexual maturation in the female, which is marked by the onset of menarche, typically occurs later in females who engage in such high-energy sports as swimming and running than in nonathletic females. *Amenorrhea* (the absence of menstruation) or *oligomenorrhea* (irregular or reduced menstruation), along with *anovulation* (absence of ovulation), are quite common in endurance athletes. These changes in the menstrual cycle may be related to low body fat levels, weight loss, and chronic high-energy expenditure.

sexual function, although he doesn't lose the ability to reproduce. For example, an elderly man may require more time to achieve an erection, experience less firm erections, and have reduced ejaculatory volume. After ejaculation, he may take longer to regain an erection.

Female reproductive system

Female reproductive structures include the external genitalia, internal genitalia, and mammary glands. Hormonal influences determine the development and function of these structures and affect fertility, childbearing, and the ability to experience sexual pleasure. (See *How exercise affects the reproductive system.*)

External genitalia

The *vulva* contains the external female genitalia visible on inspection. It includes the mons pubis, labia majora, labia minora, clitoris, and adjacent structures. (See *Structures of the female reproductive system.*)

Mons pubis

The *mons pubis* is a rounded cushion of fatty and connective tissue covered by skin and coarse, curly hair in a triangular pattern over the *symphysis pubis* (the joint formed by the union of the pubic bones anteriorly).

Labia majora

The *labia majora* are two raised folds of adipose and connective tissue that border the vulva on either side, extending from the mons pubis to the perineum. After *menarche* (onset of the first menstrual period), the outer surface of the labia is covered with pubic hair. The inner surface is pink and moist.

POINT TO REMEMBER

The labia are highly vascular and contain many nerve endings. This makes them sensitive to pain, pressure, touch, sexual stimulation, and temperature extremes.

Labia minora

The *labia minora* are two moist, dark pink to red folds of mucosal tissue that lie within and alongside the labia majora. Each labia minora has an upper and lower section; each upper section divides into an upper and lower *lamella.* The two upper lamellae join to form the *prepuce,* a hoodlike covering over the clitoris. The two lower lamellae form the *frenulum,* the posterior portion of the clitoris.

The lower labial sections taper down and back from the clitoris to the perineum, where they join to form the *fourchette,* a thin tissue fold along the anterior edge of the perineum.

The labia minora contain sebaceous glands, which secrete a lubricant that also acts as a bactericide. Like the labia majora, they're rich in blood vessels and nerve endings, making them highly responsive to stimulation. They swell in response to sexual stimulation — a reaction that triggers other changes that prepare the genitalia for coitus.

A structural view
Structures of the female reproductive system

These illustrations show the external and internal structures of the female reproductive system.

VIEW OF EXTERNAL GENITALIA IN LITHOTOMY POSITION

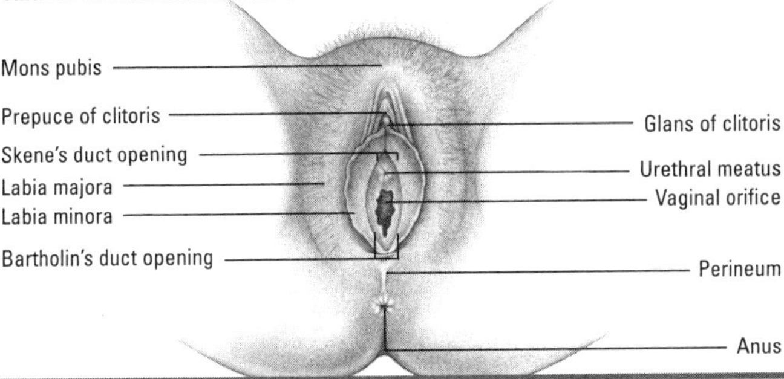

LATERAL VIEW OF INTERNAL GENITALIA

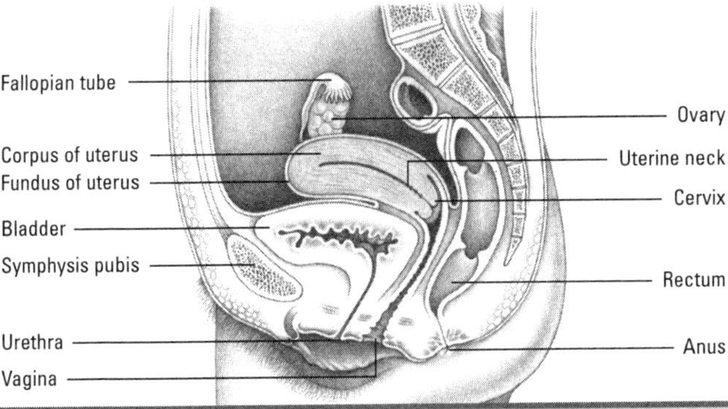

ANTERIOR CROSS-SECTIONAL VIEW OF INTERNAL GENITALIA

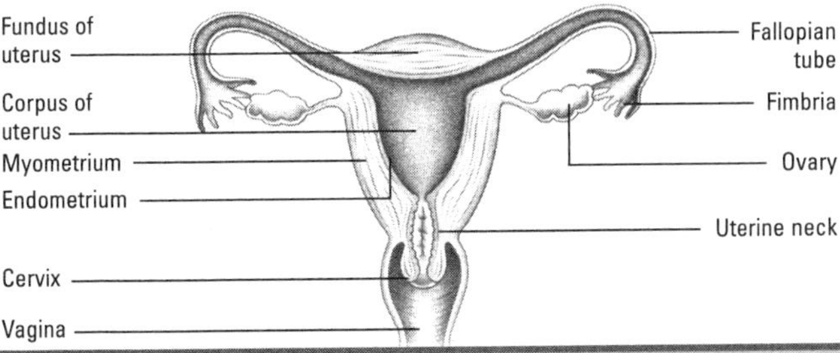

Clitoris

The *clitoris* is the small, protuberant organ just beneath the arch of the mons pubis. It contains erectile tissue, venous cavernous spaces, and specialized sensory corpuscles that are stimulated during sexual activity.

Vestibule

The *vestibule* is an oval area bounded anteriorly by the clitoris, laterally by the labia minora, and posteriorly by the fourchette. The mucus-producing *Skene's glands* are found on both sides of the urethral opening. Openings of the two mucus-producing *Bartholin's glands* are located laterally and posteriorly on either side of the inner vaginal orifice.

The *urethral meatus* is the slitlike opening below the clitoris through which urine leaves the body.

In the center of the vestibule is the *vaginal orifice.* It may be completely or partially covered by the *hymen,* a tissue membrane. Presence or absence of a hymen is no indication of whether a female has been sexually active. The hymen may rupture for any number of reasons — including tampon use, sexual activity, and other physical causes.

Perineum

Located between the lower vagina and the anal canal, the *perineum* is a complex structure of muscles, blood vessels, fascia, nerves, and lymphatics.

Internal genitalia

The female internal genitalia are specialized organs whose main function is reproduction. They include the vagina, uterus, fallopian tubes, ovaries, and related structures.

POINT TO REMEMBER

Hormones regulate the development and function of the internal genitalia.

Vagina

The *vagina,* a highly elastic muscular tube, is located between the urethra and the rectum. Approximately $2\frac{1}{2}$" to $2\frac{3}{4}$" (6 to 7 cm) long anteriorly and $3\frac{1}{2}$" (9 cm) long posteriorly, the vagina lies at a 45-degree angle to the long axis of the body. The vaginal wall has three tissue layers — epithelial tissue, loose connective tissue, and muscle tissue.

The uterine cervix connects the uterus to the vaginal vault. Four *fornices* — recesses in the vaginal wall — surround the cervix.

Functions

The vagina has three main functions:

- to accommodate the penis during coitus
- to channel blood discharged from the uterus during menstruation
- to serve as the birth canal during childbirth.

Vasculature

The upper, middle, and lower vaginal sections have separate blood supplies. Branches of the uterine arteries supply blood to the upper vagina; the inferior vesical arteries supply blood to the middle vagina; and the hemorrhoidal and internal pudendal arteries feed into the lower vagina.

Blood returns through a vast venous plexus to the hemorrhoidal, pudendal, and uterine veins and then to the hypogastric veins. This plexus merges with the vertebral venous plexus.

Uterus

The *uterus* is a small, firm, pear-shaped, muscular organ situated between the bladder and rectum. It usually lies at almost a 90-degree angle to the vagina (although other locations may be normal). The mucous membrane lining the uterus is called the *endometrium;* the muscular layer, the *myometrium.*

During pregnancy, the elastic, upper portion of the uterus, called the *fundus,* accommodates most of the growing fetus until term. The *uterine neck* joins the fundus to the *cervix,* the uterine part extending into the vagina. The fundus and neck make up the *corpus,* the main uterine body.

The cervix projects into the upper portion of the vagina. The lower cervical opening is the *external os;* the upper opening is the *internal os.*

POINT TO REMEMBER

Over a woman's lifetime, the size of the uterine corpus and the cervix changes, as does the percentage of space these parts occupy. For example, of the space filled by the whole uterus in a female before onset of the first menstrual period (menarche), one-third may be uterine corpus and two-thirds may be cervix. In the adult female who has borne children, the uterine corpus may occupy two-thirds of the space available, whereas the cervix may fill one-third.

Childbirth also permanently alters the cervix. In a female who hasn't delivered a child, the external os is a round opening about 3 mm in diameter; after the first childbirth, it becomes a small transverse slit with irregular edges.

Fallopian tubes

Two *fallopian tubes* attach to the uterus at the upper angles of the fundus. These narrow cylinders of muscle fibers, which measure $2\frac{3}{4}$" to $5\frac{1}{2}$" (7 to 14 cm) long, are the site of fertilization. The curved portion of the fallopian tube, called the *ampulla,* ends in the funnel-shaped *infundibulum.* Fingerlike projections in the infundibulum, called *fimbriae,* move in waves that sweep the mature ovum from the ovary into the fallopian tube.

Ovaries

The *ovaries* are almond-shaped organs located on either side of the uterus. They measure approximately $1\frac{1}{4}$" to $1\frac{1}{2}$" (3 to 4 cm) long, $\frac{3}{4}$" (2 cm) wide, and $\frac{1}{4}$" to $\frac{1}{2}$" (0.6 to 1.25 cm) thick.

The size, shape, and position of the ovaries vary with age. Round, smooth, and pink at birth, they grow larger, flatten, and turn grayish by puberty. During the childbearing years, they take on an almond shape and a rough, pitted surface; after menopause, they shrink and turn white.

Functions

The ovaries' main function is to produce mature ova. At birth, each ovary contains approximately 50,000 *graafian follicles.* During the childbearing years, one graafian follicle produces a mature ovum during the first half of each menstrual cycle. As the ovum matures, the follicle ruptures and the ovum is swept into the fallopian tube.

The ovaries also produce estrogen and progesterone as well as a small amount of androgens.

Mammary glands

Located in the breast, the *mammary glands* are specialized accessory glands that secrete milk. Although present in both sexes, they normally function only in the female.

Milk secretion

Each mammary gland contains 15 to 25 *lobes,* which are separated by fibrous connective tissue and fat. Within the lobes are clustered *acini*—tiny, saclike duct terminals that secrete milk during lactation.

The ducts draining the lobules converge to form *excretory (lactiferous) ducts* and *sinuses* (ampullae), which store milk during lactation. These ducts drain onto the nipple surface through 15 to 20 openings.

Large sebaceous glands in the central pigmented breast portion, or *areola,* produce *sebum* that lubricates the areola and nipple during breast-feeding. (See *The female breast,* page 186.)

Hormonal function and the menstrual cycle

The hypothalamus, ovaries, and pituitary gland secrete hormones that affect the buildup and shedding of the endometrium during the menstrual cycle. The average menstrual cycle usually occurs over 28 days, although the normal cycle may range from 22 to 34 days. The cycle is regulated by fluctuating hormone levels that, in turn, are regulated by negative and positive feedback mechanisms involving the hypothalamus, pituitary gland, and ovaries.

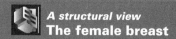

A structural view
The female breast

The breasts are located on either side of the anterior chest wall over the greater pectoral and the anterior serratus muscles. Within the areola—the pigmented area in the center of the breast—lies the nipple. Pigmented erectile tissue in the nipple responds to cold, friction, and sexual stimulation.

Breast tissue

Each breast is composed of glandular, fibrous, and adipose tissue. Glandular tissue contains 15 to 20 lobes made up of clustered acini, tiny saclike duct terminals that secrete milk. Fibrous *Cooper's ligaments* support the breasts; adipose tissue separates the two breasts.

Milk production and drainage

Acini draw the ingredients to make milk from the blood in surrounding capillaries. Lactiferous ducts and sinuses store milk during lactation, conveying milk to and through the nipples.

Sebaceous glands on the areolar surface, called *Montgomery's tubercles,* produce sebum, which lubricates the areola and nipple during breast-feeding.

LATERAL CROSS SECTION

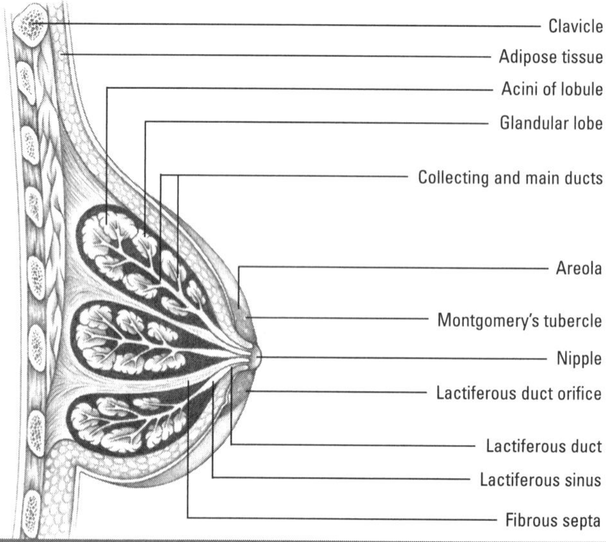

Menstrual (preovulatory) phase

The cycle starts with menstruation (cycle day 1), which usually lasts 5 days. As the cycle begins, low estrogen and progesterone levels in the bloodstream stimulate the hypothalamus to secrete

Focus on function

Events in the menstrual cycle

The female reproductive cycle, or menstrual cycle, typically lasts 28 days. Throughout the cycle, hormones influence the release of a mature ovum from a graafian follicle in the ovary. Hormones also stimulate changes in the endometrial layer of the uterus, preparing it for ovum implantation.

Hormones involved in this cycle are estrogen, progesterone, follicle-stimulating hormone (FSH), and luteinizing hormone (LH) The diagram here illustrates how hormones relate to various phases of the menstrual cycle.

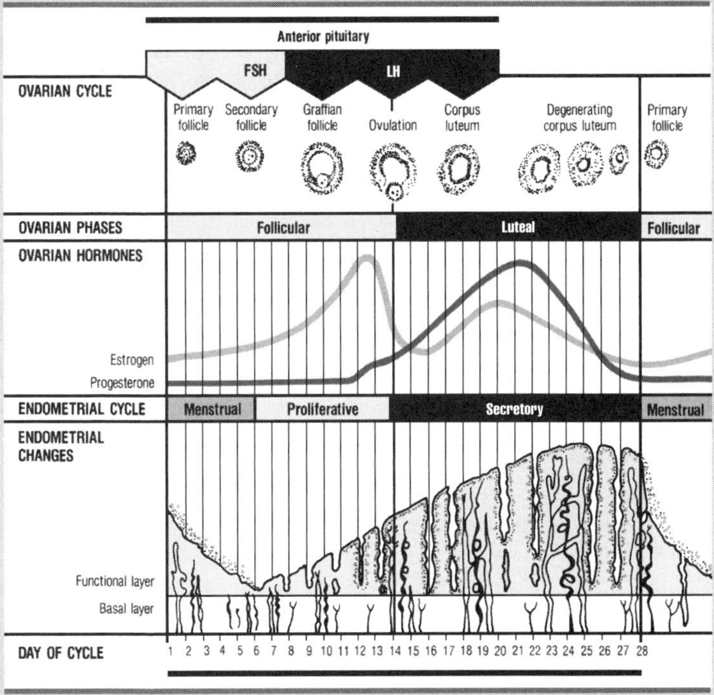

gonadotropin-releasing hormone (GnRH). In turn, GnRH stimulates the anterior pituitary to secrete FSH and LH. When the FSH level rises, LH output increases.

Proliferative (follicular) phase and ovulation

The *proliferative phase* lasts from cycle day 6 to day 14. During this phase, LH and FSH act on the *ovarian follicle* (mature ovarian cyst containing the ovum). This leads to estrogen secretion, which in turn stimulates buildup of the endometrium. Late in the proliferative phase, estrogen levels peak, FSH secretion declines, and LH secretion increases, surging at midcycle (around day 14). Then estrogen production decreases, the follicle matures, and ovulation occurs. Normally, one follicle matures during the ovulatory process and is released from the ovary during each cycle.

Luteal (secretory) phase

During the *luteal phase,* which lasts about 14 days, FSH and LH levels drop. Estrogen levels decline initially, then increase along with progesterone levels as the *corpus luteum* (a progesterone-producing structure that develops after the follicle ruptures) begins functioning. During this phase, the endometrium responds to progesterone stimulation by becoming thick and secretory to prepare for implantation of a fertilized ovum.

About 10 to 12 days after ovulation, the corpus luteum begins to diminish if ovum fertilization hasn't occurred. At the same time, estrogen and progesterone levels decrease until their levels are too low to keep the endometrium in a fully developed secretory state. Then the endometrial lining is shed as menstrual fluid during menstruation, or *menses.*

Decreasing estrogen and progesterone levels stimulate the hypothalamus to produce GnRH, and the cycle begins again. (See *Events in the menstrual cycle,* page 187.)

Menopause

Cessation of menses usually occurs between ages 40 and 55 because the body has exhausted the supply of ovarian follicles that respond to FSH and LH released by the pituitary gland. The term *menopause* applies if menses are absent for 1 year. *Climacteric* refers to the transitional years from reproductive fertility to infertility during which several physiologic changes, including menopause, occur.

16 Fertilization, pregnancy, labor, and lactation

Production of a new human being begins when a spermatozoon and an ovum unite to form a single cell. Fertilization of an ovum triggers dramatic changes inside a woman's body. The cells of the fertilized ovum begin dividing as the ovum travels to the uterine cavity, where it implants in the uterine lining.

Fertilization

Fertilization — the union of a *spermatozoon* and an *ovum* — can take place only when the following conditions are present:

- Spermatozoa are adequate in function and number.
- A mature ovum is available and ready to be fertilized.
- Spermatozoa are transported effectively through the female reproductive tract.

Transport of spermatozoa

Spermatozoa move through the female reproductive tract by two mechanisms. First, using flagellar movements, they propel themselves several millimeters per hour. Second, rhythmic contractions of uterine muscles transport spermatozoa into the uterus and fallopian tubes.

Although a single ejaculation deposits several hundred million spermatozoa, many are destroyed by acidic vaginal secretions. The only spermatozoa that survive are those that enter the cervical canal, where cervical mucus protects them.

Role of the menstrual cycle

The menstrual cycle plays a role in the ability of spermatozoa to penetrate the cervical mucus.

Early in the cycle, estrogen and progesterone levels are lowest and menstruation occurs. During midcycle, however, when the mucus is relatively thin, spermatozoa can pass readily through the cervix. Later in the cycle, the cervical mucus thickens in response to increased progesterone levels, hindering spermatozoa passage.

Role of uterine contractions

Once spermatozoa pass through the cervical mucus, they enter the uterus, where uterine contractions help them to penetrate the fallopian tubes. Spermatozoa can probably fertilize the ovum for up to 2 days after ejaculation, although they may survive for 3 to 4 days in the reproductive tract.

Zygote creation

Fertilization is possible, based on the viability of the germ cells, when sexual intercourse takes place near the time of ovulation. The ovum remains viable for 24 to 36 hours; spermatozoa, for 48 hours or longer.

Before a spermatozoon can penetrate the ovum, it must disperse the granulosa cells and penetrate the *zona pellucida*, the thick, transparent layer surrounding the incompletely developed ovum. Enzymes in the *acrosome* (head cap) of the spermatozoon permit this penetration. After penetration, the ovum completes its second meiotic division and the zona pellucida prevents penetration by other spermatozoa.

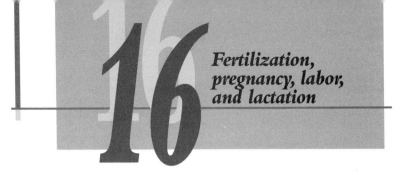

The spermatozoon head then fuses with the ovum nucleus, creating a cell nucleus with 46 chromosomes. The fertilized ovum is called a *zygote.* (See *How fertilization occurs.*)

Pregnancy

Pregnancy starts with fertilization and ends with childbirth; typically, its duration is 38 to 40 weeks. During this time (also called *gestation*), the zygote divides as it passes through the fallopian tube and attaches to the uterine lining by *implantation.* A complex sequence of preembryonic, embryonic, and fetal development transforms the zygote into a full-term fetus.

Because the uterus grows throughout pregnancy, uterine size serves as a rough estimate of the duration of pregnancy. The actual fertilization date is rarely known, so the woman's expected delivery date is typically calculated from the beginning of her last menstrual period (LMP).

POINT TO REMEMBER

The length of gestation calculated from the LMP is 40 weeks — not 38 — because the 1st day of the calculation is about 2 weeks before ovulation.

Preembryonic development

The first stage of prenatal development, preembryonic development starts with ovum fertilization and lasts 3 weeks. As the zygote passes through the fallopian tube, it undergoes a series of mitotic divisions, or cleavage.

About 30 hours after fertilization, the first cell division is completed. During subsequent divisions occurring in rapid succession, the zygote is transformed into a ball of cells called a *morula,* which reaches the uterus about 3 days after fertilization. Fluid that builds up in the center of the morula forms a central cavity; the structure now is called a *blastocyst.*

Blastocyst cells differentiate in two ways:

- The *trophoblast,* a peripheral rim of cells, gives rise to the fetal membranes and contributes to placenta formation.
- The *inner cell mass,* a discrete cluster of cells in the trophoblast, eventually forms the embryo.

The blastocyst, enclosed in the zona pellucida, remains unattached to the uterus for several days. During the week after fertilization, the zona pellucida degenerates, permitting the blastocyst to attach to the endometrium and become implanted. (See *Events leading to ovum implantation,* page 192.)

The inner cell mass becomes the *germ disc* — a flat structure that differentiates into three germ layers. A cleft separating the ectoderm of the germ disc and the surrounding trophoblast forms the *amniotic cavity* (amniotic sac). The *yolk sac,* a second cavity, forms on the opposite side of the germ disc.

A connective tissue layer lines the enlarging blastocyst cavity and covers the amniotic and yolk sacs. The blastocyte cavity, which now contains the germ disc, amniotic sac, and yolk sac, is called the *chorionic cavity* (chorionic sac); its wall is called a *chorion.* The entire chorionic sac and developing embryo is termed the *chorionic vesicle.* Anchoring the chorionic vesicle to the endometrium, fingerlike columns of cells called *chorionic villi* extend from the chorion.

Embryonic development

During the embryonic period (from the 4th through the 7th week of gestation), the developing zygote starts to take on a human shape and is now called an *embryo.* Each germ layer, the *ectoderm, mesoderm,* and *endoderm,* eventually forms specific tissues in the embryo. (See *How germ layers develop,* page 193.) The ectoderm primarily forms the external embryonic covering and the structures that will come in contact with the environment.

The mesoderm forms the circulatory system, muscles, supporting tissues, and most of the urinary and reproductive systems. The endoderm gives rise to the internal linings of the embryo,

How fertilization occurs

1. When a spermatozoon meets an ovum after several hours in the female reproductive tract, the spermatozoon undergoes activation.

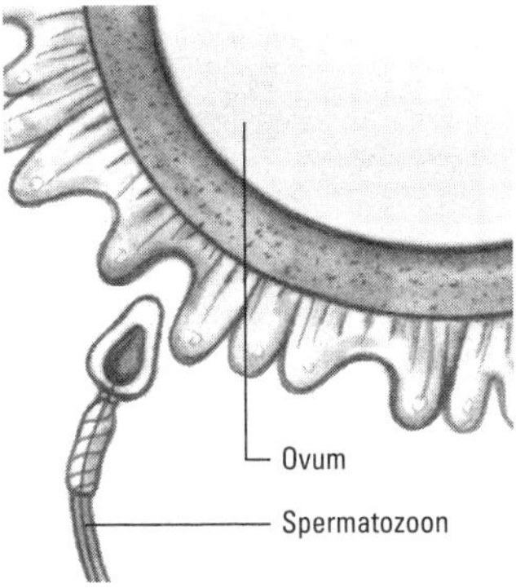

2. The covering of its acrosome develops small perforations. Enzymes released through these perforations disperse the ovum's granulosa cells.

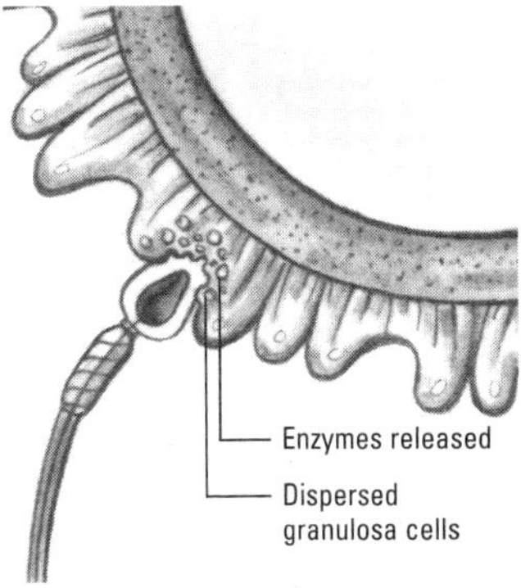

3. The spermatozoon then penetrates the zona pellucida. This triggers the ovum's second meiotic division, making the zona pellucida impenetrable to other spermatozoa.

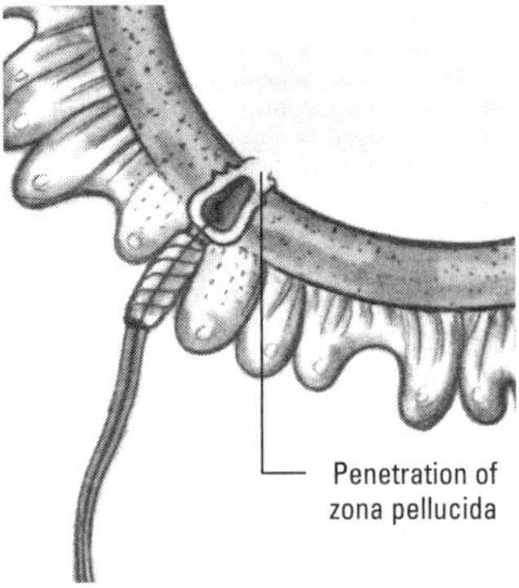

4. After the spermatozoon penetrates the ovum, its nucleus is released into the ovum, its tail degenerates, and its head enlarges and fuses with the nucleus of the ovum. This fusion provides the fertilized ovum, called a zygote, with 46 chromosomes.

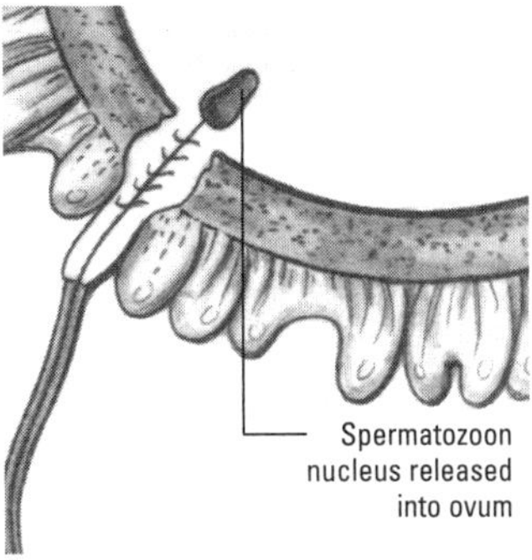

such as the epithelial lining of the pharynx and respiratory and GI tracts.

POINT TO REMEMBER

During embryonic development, when all organ systems

Focus on function

Events leading to ovum implantation

As the fertilized ovum advances through the fallopian tube toward the uterus, it undergoes mitotic division, forming daughter cells (initially called *blastomeres*). The first cell division ends about 30 hours after fertilization; subsequent divisions occur rapidly. The zygote develops into a small mass of cells, called a *morula,* which reaches the uterus about the third day after fertilization. Fluid that amasses in the center of the morula forms a central cavity.

At this point, the structure is called a *blastocyst.* Its cells differentiate either into a trophoblast, which gives rise to fetal membranes and contributes to placenta formation (early blastocyte), or the inner cell mass, a discrete cell cluster enclosed within the trophoblast, that will form the embryo (late blastocyst).

For several days, the blastocyst stays within the zona pellucida, unattached to the uterus. Then the zona pellucida degenerates and, by the end of the first week after fertilization, the blastocyst attaches to the endometrium. The part of the blastocyst adjacent to the inner cell mass is the first part to become attached. The trophoblast, in contact with the endometrial lining, proliferates and invades the underlying endometrium by separating and dissolving endometrial cells.

During the next week, the invading blastocyst sinks below the surface of the endometrium. The site of penetration becomes sealed over, restoring the continuity of the endometrial surface.

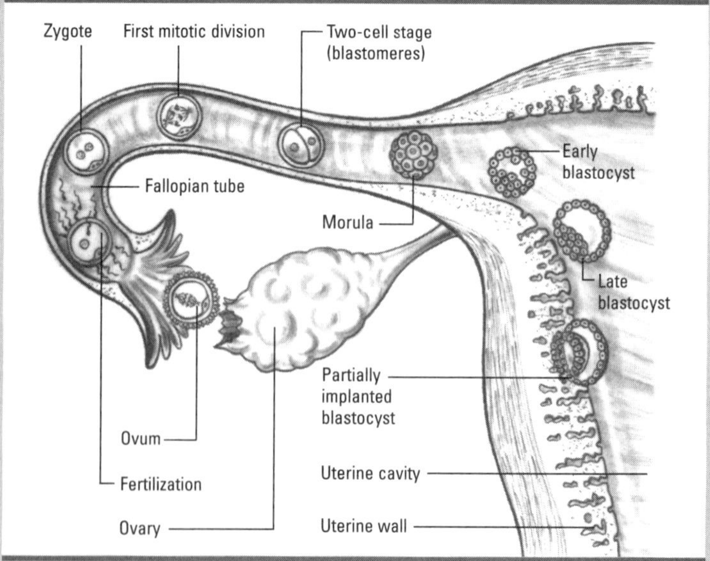

How germ layers develop

Each of the three germ layers—ectoderm, mesoderm, and endoderm—forms specific tissues and organs in the developing embryo.

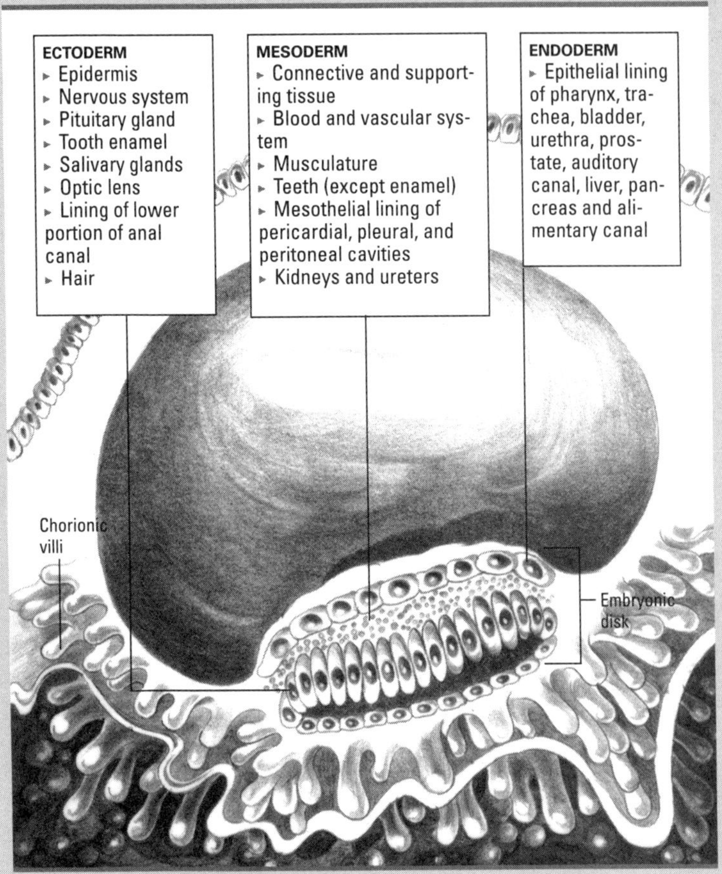

form, the embryo is vulnerable to injury by maternal drug use, certain maternal infections, and other factors.

Fetal development

During the fetal period, which extends from the 8th week until birth, the maturing fetus enlarges and grows heavier—yet experiences no major changes in its basic structure comparable to those that occur during the embryonic period. (See *Embryonic and fetal growth and development,* page 194.)

Two unusual fetal features appear during this stage:

▸ disproportionately large head—a condition that changes after birth as the infant grows

▸ lack of subcutaneous fat (fat starts to accumulate shortly before birth).

Embryonic and fetal growth and development

At the end of 1 month, the embryo has a definite form. The head, the trunk, and the tiny buds that will become the arms and legs are discernible. The cardiovascular system has begun to function, and the umbilical cord is visible in its most primitive form.

1 MONTH

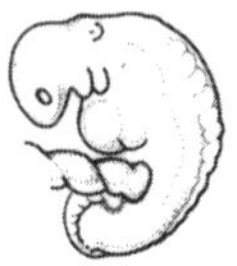

During the next month, the embryo, called a fetus from the 8th week, grows to 1" (2.5 cm) in length and weighs 1/30 oz. The head and facial features develop as the eyes, ears, nose, lips, tongue, and tooth buds form. The arms and legs also take shape. Although the gender of the fetus isn't yet discernible, all external genitalia are present. Cardiovascular function is complete and the umbilical cord has a definite form. At the end of 2 months, the fetus resembles a full-term neonate except for size.

2 MONTHS

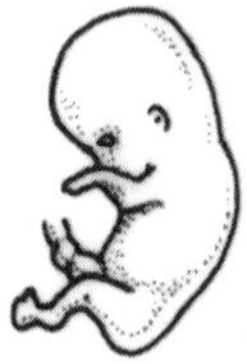

During the 3rd month, the fetus grows to 3" (7.5 cm) in length and weighs 1 oz (28.4 g). Teeth and bones begin to appear, and the kidneys start to function. The fetus opens its mouth to swallow, grasps with its fully developed hands, and prepares for breathing by inhaling and exhaling (although its lungs aren't functioning). At the end of the 1st trimester, its gender is distinguishable.

3 MONTHS

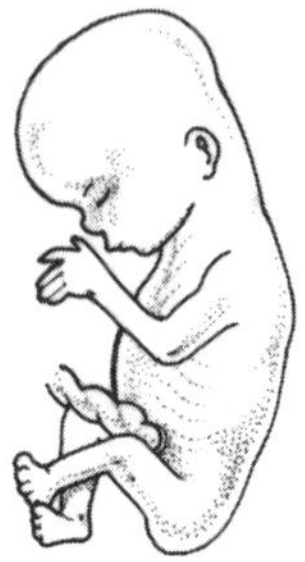

Over the remaining 6 months, fetal growth continues as internal and external structures develop at a rapid rate. In the 3rd trimester, the fetus stores the fats and minerals it will need to live outside the womb. At birth, the average full-term fetus measures 20" (51 cm) and weighs 7 to 7 ½ lbs (3.2 to 3.4 kg).

9 MONTHS

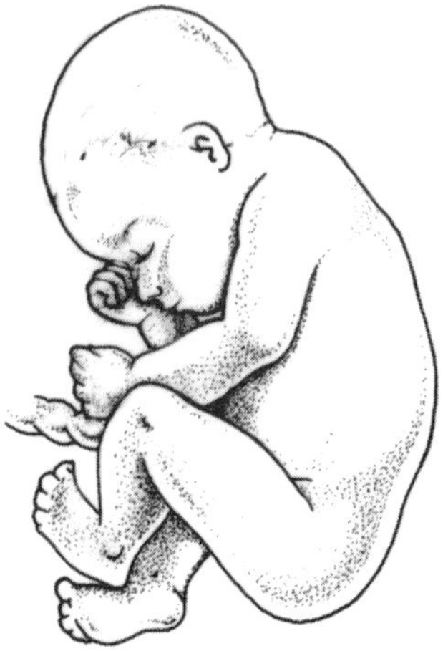

Structural development during pregnancy

Pregnancy changes the usual development of the *corpus luteum* and results in development of such structures as the *decidua, amniotic sac and fluid, yolk sac,* and *placenta*.

Corpus luteum

Normal functioning of the corpus luteum requires continual stimulation by luteinizing hormone (LH). Progesterone produced by the corpus luteum suppresses LH release by the pituitary gland.

With age, the corpus luteum grows less responsive to LH. For this reason, the mature corpus luteum degenerates unless stimulated by progressively increasing amounts of LH.

Pregnancy stimulates the placental tissue to secrete large amounts of human chorionic gonadotropin (HCG), which resembles LH and follicle-stimulating hormone (FSH), also produced by the pituitary gland. HCG prevents corpus luteum degeneration, stimulating the corpus luteum to produce large amounts of estrogen and progesterone.

For the first 3 months of pregnancy, the corpus luteum is the main source of estrogen and progesterone — hormones required during pregnancy. Later, the placenta produces most of the hormones; the corpus luteum persists but is no longer needed to maintain the pregnancy.

Decidua

The *decidua* is the endometrial lining that has undergone the hormone-induced changes of pregnancy. Enveloping the embryo and fetus during gestation, the decidua has several portions:

- The *decidua basalis* lies beneath the chorionic vesicle and eventually merges with the placenta.
- The *decidua capsularis* lies above the chorionic vesicle.
- The *decidua parietalis* (also called the *decidua vera*) lines the remainder of the endometrial cavity. (See *Development of the decidua and fetal membranes*, page 196.)

Decidual secretions

Decidual cells secrete three substances:

- The hormone *prolactin* promotes lactation.
- *Relaxin*, a peptide hormone, induces relaxation of the connective tissue of the symphysis pubis and pelvic ligaments; it also promotes cervical dilation.
- *Prostaglandin* is a potent hormone-like fatty acid that mediates several physiologic functions.

Amniotic sac and fluid

Enclosed within the chorion, the amniotic sac gradually increases in size and surrounds the embryo. As it enlarges, the amniotic sac expands into the chorionic cavity, eventually filling the cavity and fusing with the chorion by the 8th week of gestation. The decidua capsularis stretches and thins, eventually fusing with the decidua parietalis on the opposite wall of the uterus.

The amniotic sac and amniotic fluid serve two crucial functions:

- During gestation, they guard the fetus by producing a buoyant, temperature-controlled environment.
- During delivery, they form a fluid wedge that helps open the cervix.

Amniotic fluid source and volume

The source and volume of amniotic fluid vary with the gestational stage. Amniotic fluid derives from both maternal and fetal sources. Early in pregnancy, it comes chiefly from three sources:

- fluid filtering into the amniotic sac from maternal blood as it passes through the uterus
- fluid filtering into the sac from fetal blood passing through the placenta
- fluid diffusing into the amniotic sac from the fetal skin and respiratory tract.

Later in pregnancy, when the fetal kidneys begin to function, the fetus urinates into the amniotic fluid. Fetal urine then becomes the major source of amniotic fluid.

Development of the decidua and fetal membranes

Specialized tissues support, protect, and nurture the embryo and fetus throughout its development. Among these, the decidua and fetal membranes begin to develop shortly after conception. These illustrations highlight their development at approximately 4 and 16 weeks.

Decidua

During pregnancy, the endometrial lining is called the *decidua.* It provides a nesting place for the developing conceptus and has some endocrine functions. Based primarily on its position relative to the embryo, the decidua may be known as the *decidua basalis* (which lies beneath the chorionic vesicle), *decidua capsularis* (which stretches over the vesicle), or *decidua parietalis* (which lines the rest of the endometrial cavity).

Chorion and chorionic villi

The chorionic villi arise from the periphery of the chorion. However, as the chorionic vesicle enlarges, villi arising from the superficial portion of the chorion atrophy. This part of the chorion, which becomes smooth, is called the *chorion laeve.* Villi arising from the deeper part of the chorion proliferate; this part of the chorion is called the *chorion frondosum.* Its villi project into the large blood vessels within the decidua basalis through which the maternal blood flows.

Blood vessels form within the villi as they grow, and become connected with blood vessels that form in the chorion, body stalk, and within the body of the embryo. Blood begins to flow through this developing network of vessels as soon as the embryo's heart starts to beat.

APPROXIMATELY 4 WEEKS

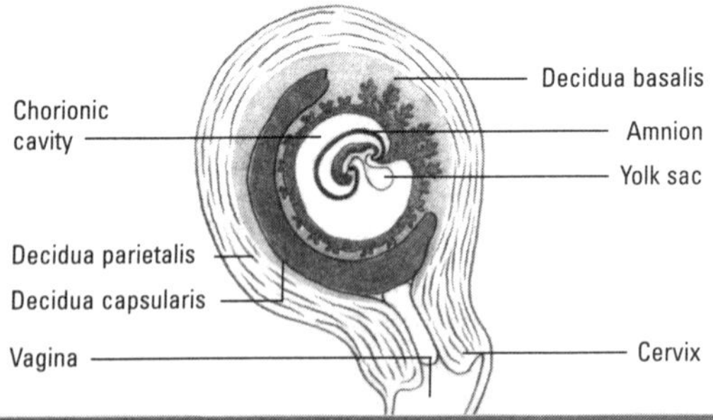

APPROXIMATELY 16 WEEKS

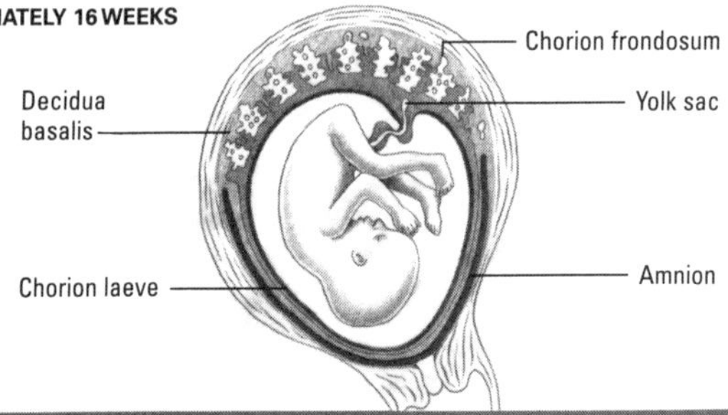

Blood filtered from maternal and fetal sources and fetal urine excretion continually add to amniotic fluid volume. From about $1\frac{5}{8}$ oz (48 ml) at 12 weeks' gestation, this volume gradually increases to 27 to 34 oz (798 to 1,005 ml) at term.

Production of amniotic fluid from maternal and fetal sources balances out amniotic fluid loss through the fetal GI tract. Normally, the fetus swallows up to several hundred milliliters of amniotic fluid each day. The fluid is absorbed into the fetal circulation from the fetal GI tract; some is transferred from the fetal circulation to the maternal circulation and excreted in maternal urine.

Yolk sac

The yolk sac forms next to the endoderm of the germ disc; a portion of it is incorporated in the developing embryo and forms the GI tract. Another portion of the sac gives rise to primitive germ cells, which travel to the developing gonads and eventually form oocytes or spermatocytes. During early embryonic development, the yolk sac also forms blood cells. Eventually, it undergoes atrophy and disintegrates.

Placenta

The flattened, disk-shaped *placenta* forms from the chorion and its chorionic villi as well as from the adjacent decidua basalis. A highly vascular organ, the placenta provides nutrients to and removes wastes from the fetus from the 3rd month of pregnancy until childbirth. At delivery, it weighs about $17\frac{5}{8}$ oz (500 g).

Linking the fetus and placenta, the *umbilical cord* contains two arteries and one vein. The umbilical arteries, which transport blood from the fetus to the placenta, take a spiral course on the cord, divide on the placental surface, and branch off to the chorionic villi. (See *Picturing the placenta and umbilical cord,* page 198.)

Large veins on the placental surface gather blood returning from the villi and then join to form the single umbilical vein. This vein enters the cord, returning blood to the fetus.

Placental circulation

The placenta has a specialized circulation consisting of two separate circulatory systems. The *uteroplacental circulation* carries oxygenated arterial blood from the maternal circulation to the intervillous spaces — large spaces separating chorionic villi in the placenta. Blood *enters* the intervillous spaces from uterine arteries that penetrate the basal part of the placenta; it *leaves* the intervillous spaces and flows back into the maternal circulation through veins in the basal part of the placenta near arteries.

The *fetoplacental circulation* transports oxygen-depleted blood from the fetus to the chorionic villi by the umbilical arteries and returns oxygenated blood to the fetus through the umbilical vein.

POINT TO REMEMBER

Even though the maternal and fetal circulations exchange oxygen, nutrients, and wastes, fetal and maternal blood don't mix.

Placental hormones

The placenta produces several hormones — among them the peptide hormones HCG and human placental lactogen (HPL). Until the placenta assumes hormone production, HCG stimulates the corpus luteum to produce the estrogen and progesterone needed to maintain the pregnancy. HCG can be detected as early as 9 days after fertilization. Its level gradually increases, peaks at about 10 weeks' gestation and then gradually declines. Highly sensitive pregnancy tests can detect HCG in the blood and urine even before the first missed menstrual period.

HPL, which resembles growth hormone, stimulates maternal protein and fat metabolism to ensure a sufficient supply of amino acids and fatty acids for the mother and fetus. HPL antagonizes the action of insulin, reducing maternal glucose metabolism and freeing up more glucose for the fetus. HPL

Picturing the placenta and umbilical cord

Normally, the placenta has many lobes with smooth, rounded edges. Its color is consistent throughout, indicating adequate tissue perfusion. At term, the placenta is flat, cakelike, round or oval, measuring 6" to 7 ¾" (15 to 20 cm) in diameter and ¾" to 1 ¼" (2 to 3 cm) in breadth at its thickest parts. The maternal side is lobulated; the fetal side is shiny.

NORMAL PLACENTA

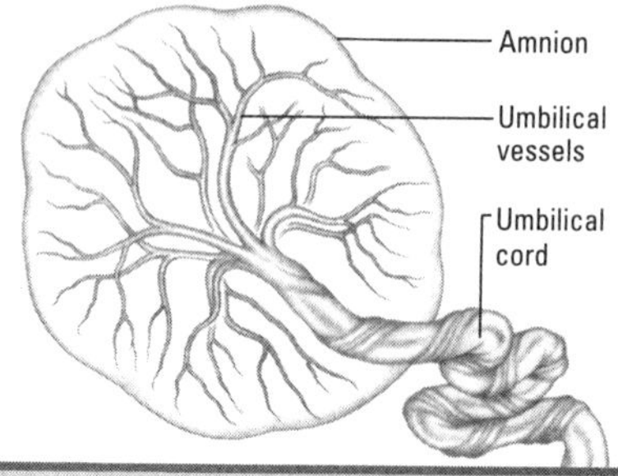

Umbilical cord

The normal umbilical cord contains three vessels—two arteries and one vein.

NORMAL UMBILICAL VESSELS

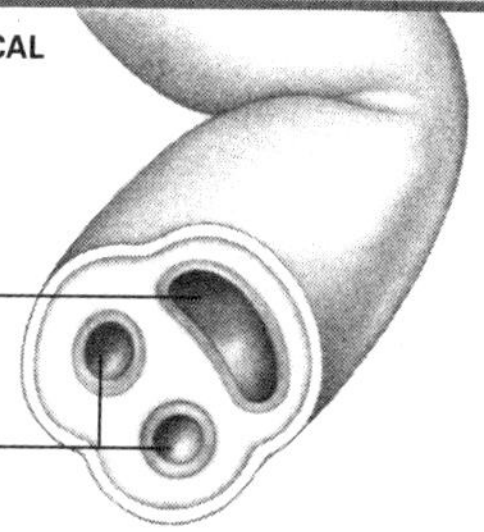

also stimulates breast growth in preparation for lactation. Throughout pregnancy, HPL levels rise progressively.

Estrogen and progesterone are steroid hormones produced by the placenta. As with HPL, their levels increase progressively throughout pregnancy.

Estrogen

Estrogen heightens uterine muscle irritability and contractility. The placenta produces three estrogens, which differ in the number of hydroxyl groups attached to the steroid nucleus:

- Estrone (E_1) has one hydroxyl group.
- Estradiol (E_2) has two hydroxyl groups.
- Estriol (E_3) has three hydroxyl groups.

Lacking some of the enzymes needed to complete estrogen synthesis, the placenta requires some precursor compounds produced by the fetal adrenal glands. Neither the fetus nor the placenta can synthesize estrogens independently; thus, estrogen production reflects the functional activity of the fetus and placenta.

Progesterone

Synthesized by the placenta from maternal cholesterol, progesterone reduces uterine muscle irritability. The fetus plays no role in progesterone production.

Labor and the postpartum period

Childbirth *(parturition)*, or delivery of the fetus, is achieved through *labor*—the process in which uterine contractions force the fetus to be expelled from the uterus.

Weak uterine contractions take place irregularly throughout pregnancy. When labor begins, these contractions become strong and regular. Eventually, voluntary bearing-down efforts supplement the contractions, resulting in expulsion of the fetus and placenta.

The head of the fetus usually occupies the lowest part of the uterus; in this *cephalic presentation,* the fetus is delivered head-first. Occasionally, the head occupies the upper part of the uterus; in this *breech presentation,* the fetus may be delivered buttocks-, knees-, or feet-first.

Rarer types of presentation include shoulder presentation (shoulder-first delivery) and compound presentation, in which two presenting parts are delivered first. (See *Comparing fetal presentations,* page 200.)

Onset of labor

The onset of labor results from several factors:

- The number of oxytocin receptors on uterine muscle fibers, which progressively increases during pregnancy, peaks just before labor onset. This makes the uterus more sensitive to the effects of oxytocin.
- Stretching of the uterus over the course of the pregnancy initiates nerve impulses that stimulate oxytocin secretion from the posterior pituitary lobe.

Fetal role

The fetus also may play a part in labor initiation. Near term, the fetal pituitary gland secretes more adrenocorticotropic hormone. This increased secretion, in turn, causes the fetal adrenal glands to secrete more cortisol, which diffuses into the maternal circulation through the placenta. Cortisol heightens oxytocin and estrogen secretion and reduces progesterone secretion. These changes intensify uterine muscle irritability and make the uterus more sensitive to oxytocin stimulation.

Role of prostaglandins

Prostaglandins also contribute to labor initiation. The effect of declining progesterone levels is to convert esterified arachidonic acid into a nonesterified form. The nonesterified arachidonic acid undergoes biosynthesis to form prostaglandins which, in turn, induce uterine contractions.

Maintenance of labor

Several factors maintain labor once it begins. As the cervix dilates, nerve impulses are transmitted to the central nervous system, causing an increase in oxytocin secretion from the pituitary gland. Acting as a positive feedback mechanism, increased oxytocin secretion stimulates more uterine contractions, which further dilate the cervix and lead the pituitary to secrete more oxytocin.

Oxytocin secretions may also stimulate prostaglandin formation by the decidua. Prostaglandins diffuse into the uterine myometrium, enhancing contractions.

Stages of labor

Childbirth can be divided into three stages. The duration of each stage varies with the size of the uterus, the woman's age, and the number of previous pregnancies.

POINT TO REMEMBER

The first and second stages are commonly shorter in women who have previously given birth (multiparous women) than in those who have not (primiparous women).

First stage

The first stage of labor, in which the fetus begins its descent, is marked by *cervical effacement* (thinning) and *dilation* (widening). Before labor begins, the cervix isn't dilated; by the end of the first stage, it's dilated fully. (See *Cervical effacement and dilation,* page 202.)

As uterine muscles contract actively, the cervix and the lower part of the uterus dilate and thin. The amniotic sac and fluid help to dilate the cervix by

Comparing fetal presentations

Fetal presentation may be broadly classified as cephalic, breech, shoulder, or compound. Cephalic presentations comprise almost all deliveries. Of the remaining three presentations, breech deliveries are the most common.

Cephalic presentation

In this head-down presentation, the position of the fetus may be further classified by the presenting skull landmark, such as the vertex (the area between the anterior and posterior fontanel), brow, sinciput, or face.

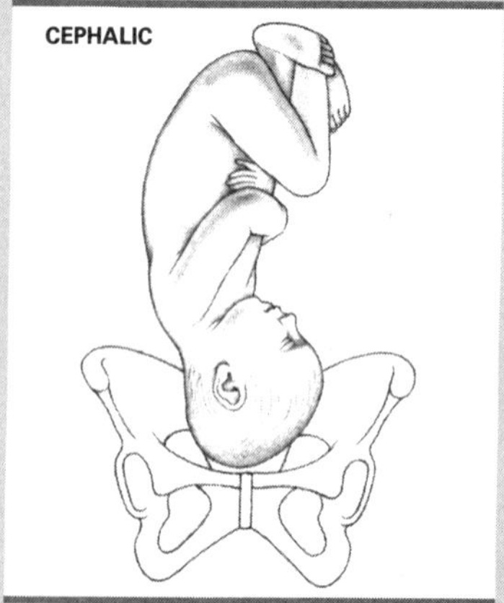

Breech presentation

In the head-up presentation, the position of the fetus may be further classified as frank (hips flexed, knees straight), complete (knees and hips flexed), and footling (knees and hips of one or both legs extended).

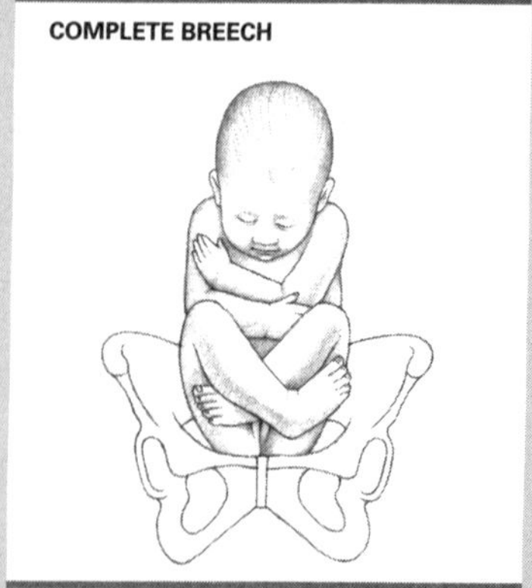

Shoulder presentation

Although a fetus may adopt one of several shoulder presentations, examination can't differentiate among them. Thus, all transverse lies are called shoulder presentations.

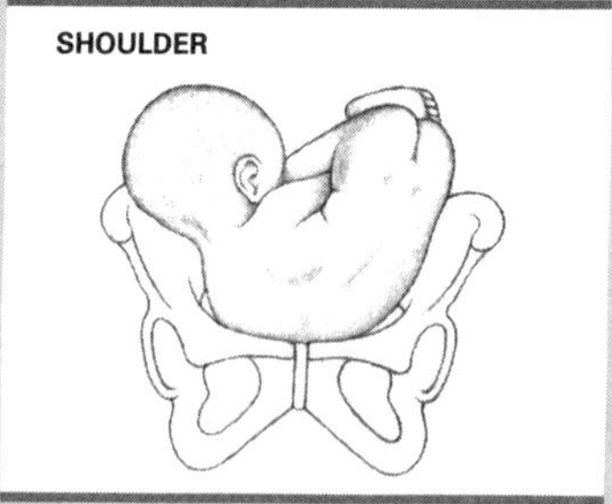

Compound presentation

In the compound presentation, an extremity prolapses alongside the major presenting part so that two presenting parts appear in the pelvis at the same time.

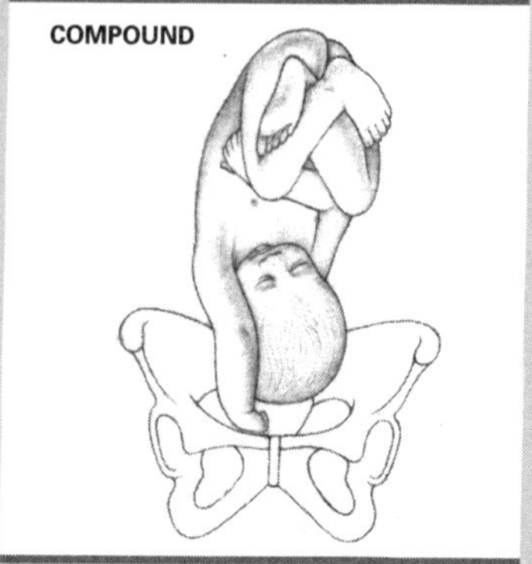

serving as a hydrostatic wedge. The first stage lasts from 6 to 24 hours in primiparous women but is much shorter in multiparous women.

Second stage

The second stage of labor begins with full cervical dilation and ends with expulsion of the fetus. During this stage, uterine contractions grow more frequent and more intense, and the amniotic sac ruptures. As the flexed head of the fetus enters the pelvis, the mother's pelvic muscles force the head to rotate anteriorly and cause the back of the head to move under the symphysis pubis.

As the uterus contracts, the flexed head of the fetus is forced deeper into the pelvis; resistance of the pelvic floor gradually forces the head to extend. As the head presses against the pelvic floor, vulvar tissues stretch and the anus dilates. At this point, the vulvovaginal orifice may be enlarged surgically by an *episiotomy,* a small incision.

With delivery of the head, the face of the fetus passes over the perineum, and maternal tissues retract under the chin. The head of the fetus now rotates back to its former position after passing through the vulvovaginal orifice. Usually, head rotation is lateral (external) as the anterior shoulder rotates forward to pass under the pubic arch. Delivery of the shoulders and the rest of the fetus follows.

The second stage of labor averages about 45 minutes in primiparous women; it may be much shorter in multiparous women.

Third stage

The third stage of labor starts immediately after childbirth and ends with placenta expulsion. After the neonate is delivered, the uterus continues to contract intermittently and grows smaller.

The area of placental attachment also decreases. The placenta, which can't decrease in size, separates from the uterus, and blood seeps into the area of placental separation.

With the uterus still contracting, retroplacental blood is compressed and acts as a fluid wedge, cleaving the placenta from the uterus. Commonly, the middle portion of the placenta, covered by the fetal membrane, is expelled first, while the edges of the placenta are the last to separate from the uterine wall. Less commonly, the lower edge of the placenta separates and is expelled first.

The third stage of labor averages about 10 minutes in both primiparous and multiparous women.

Fourth stage

The fourth stage of labor begins after delivery of the placenta and ends within 2 hours. During this time, physiologic hemostasis is reestablished.

Postpartum period

After childbirth, the reproductive tract takes about 6 weeks to revert to its former condition — a process called *involution.*

Immediately following delivery of the placenta, the uterus is firm, midline, and midway between the umbilicus and the symphysis pubis. It's approximately the size of a grapefruit and weighs approximately 1,000 grams. Within 12 hours after delivery, the fundus lies approximately 1 cm above the umbilicus. The fundus descends about 1 cm per day and is no longer palpable 10 days after delivery. The stretched tissues of the vulva, pelvis, and rectum return to their former state, though more slowly.

Postpartum vaginal discharge *(lochia)* persists for several weeks after childbirth. During the postpartum period, lochia changes in appearance and consistency:

- *Lochia rubra,* a bloody discharge, appears 1 to 4 days postpartum.
- *Lochia serosa,* a pinkish brown, serous discharge, occurs from 5 to 7 days postpartum.
- *Lochia alba,* a grayish white or colorless discharge, appears from 1 to 3 weeks postpartum.

Focus on function
Cervical effacement and dilation

Cervical effacement refers to progressive shortening of the vaginal portion of the cervix and thinning of its walls during labor as it's stretched by the fetus. Effacement is described as a percentage, ranging from 0% (noneffaced and thick) to 100% (fully effaced and paper-thin).

Cervical dilation refers to progressive enlargement of the cervical os to allow the fetus to pass from the uterus into the vagina. Dilation ranges from less than 1 cm to about 10 cm (full dilation).

NO EFFACEMENT OR DILATION

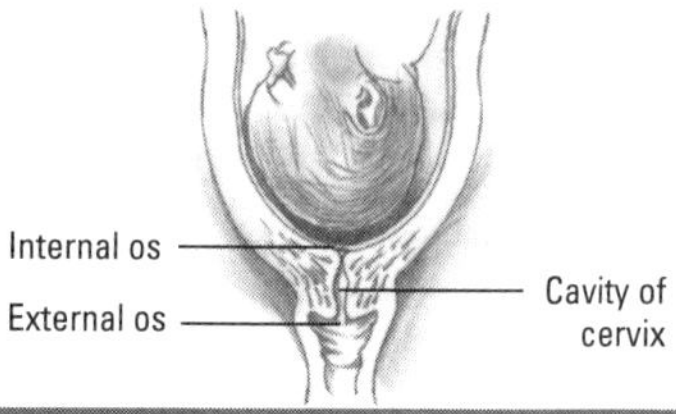

EARLY EFFACEMENT AND DILATION

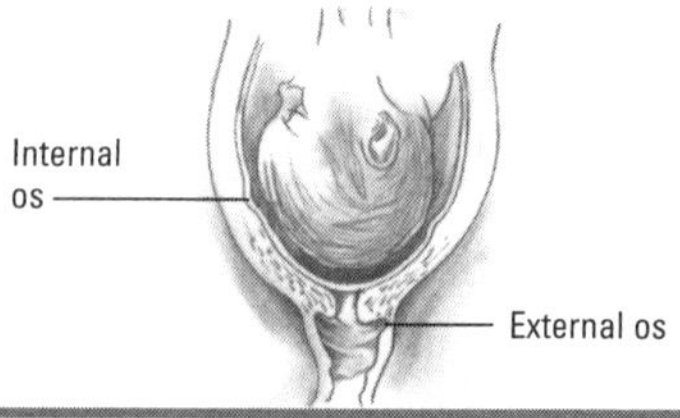

COMPLETE EFFACEMENT AND DILATION

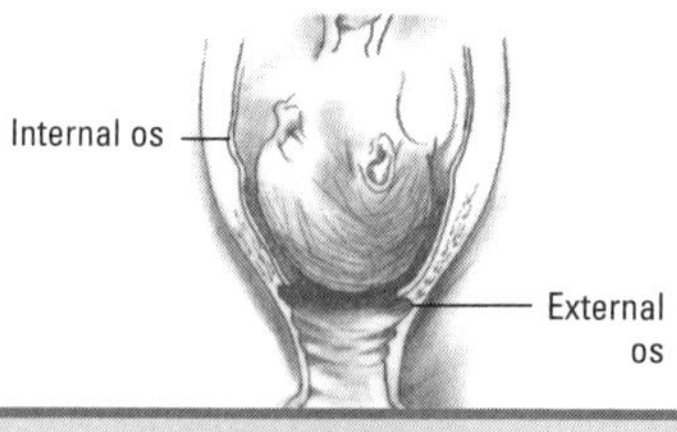

Events leading to cervical dilation

Because uterine muscle fibers remain shortened even after a contraction stops, the uterus elongates and the uterine cavity becomes smaller. These actions force the fetus downward toward the cervix.

This pressure, along with the upward pulling of longitudinal muscle fibers over the fetus, results in cervical dilation.

Lactation

Lactation — milk synthesis and secretion by the breasts — is governed by interactions involving four hormones:

- estrogen and progesterone, produced by the ovaries and placenta during pregnancy
- prolactin and oxytocin, produced by the pituitary under hypothalamic control (some prolactin is also produced by decidual cells during pregnancy).

As pregnancy progresses, placental production of estrogen and progesterone increases, causing glandular and ductal tissue in the breasts to proliferate. After breast stimulation by estrogen and progesterone, prolactin causes milk secretion.

Prolactin secretion also increases throughout pregnancy in response to high estrogen levels. However, the high estrogen and progesterone levels present during pregnancy suppress milk

Breast milk composition

The composition of breast milk undergoes various changes—both over the course of a feeding and during the first few days after delivery. Initial feedings provide a thin, serous fluid called *colostrum*. Unlike mature breast milk, which has a bluish tinge, colostrum is yellow.

Colostrum contains high concentrations of protein, fat-soluble vitamins, minerals, and immunoglobulins, which function as antibodies. Its laxative effect promotes early passage of meconium—the greenish black material that collects in the fetal intestines and forms the neonate's first stool. Because colostrum is produced in low volumes, it doesn't tax the neonate's limited stomach capacity or cause fluid overload.

The breasts may contain colostrum for up to 96 hours after delivery. The maturation rate from colostrum to breast milk varies. Colostrum matures to milk more rapidly with increased breast-feeding frequency and duration over the first 48 hours.

From foremilk to hindmilk

Breast milk composition also changes over the course of a feeding. The foremilk—the thin, watery milk secreted when a feeding begins—is low in calories but abounds in water-soluble vitamins. It accounts for about 60% of the total volume of a feeding. Next, whole milk is released. The hindmilk, available 10 to 15 minutes after a breast-feeding session begins, has the highest concentration of calories; this helps to satisfy the neonate's hunger between feedings.

secretion by the prolactin-stimulated breast.

Oxytocin from the posterior pituitary lobe causes contraction of specialized cells in the breast, producing a squeezing effect that forces milk down the ducts. Breast-feeding, in turn, stimulates prolactin secretion, resulting in a high prolactin level that induces changes in the menstrual cycle.

Hormonal initiation of lactation

After the placenta is expelled, progesterone and estrogen levels fall dramatically. With estrogen and progesterone no longer inhibiting prolactin's effects on milk production, the mammary glands start to secrete milk.

Nipple stimulation during breast-feeding results in transmission of sensory impulses from the nipples to the hypothalamus. This, in turn, stimulates prolactin release from the anterior pituitary lobe. If the nipples aren't stimulated by breast-feeding, prolactin secretion declines after delivery.

Milk secretion continues as long as breast-feeding regularly stimulates the nipples. If breast-feeding stops, the stimulus for prolactin release is eliminated and milk production ceases.

Breast-feeding also stimulates oxytocin. Sensory impulses from the nipples to the hypothalamus result in oxytocin release from the posterior pituitary lobe. Oxytocin, in turn, causes contraction of the myoepithelial cells surrounding the breast lobules, resulting in *milk ejection*. The breast-feeding infant readily obtains the breast milk expelled from the secretory lobules into larger ducts. (See *Breast milk composition*.)

Effects of breast-feeding on the menstrual cycle

During the postpartum period, the woman's high prolactin level inhibits FSH and LH release. If she doesn't breast-feed, her prolactin output soon drops, ending inhibition of FSH and LH production by the pituitary. Subsequently, cyclic release of FSH and LH occurs, initiating the menstrual cycle.

POINT TO REMEMBER
Normal menstrual cycles typically resume about 6 weeks after delivery in a woman who doesn't breast-feed.

In a breast-feeding woman, the menstrual cycle doesn't resume because prolactin inhibits the cyclic release of FSH and LH necessary for ovulation. This explains why a breast-feeding woman usually doesn't become pregnant.

Prolactin release in response to breast-feeding gradually declines, as does the inhibitory effect of prolactin on FSH and LH release. Consequently, ovulation and the menstrual cycle may resume. Pregnancy may occur after this, even if the woman continues to breast-feed.

17 Normal aging process

Aging is a normal part of human development. The patterns of aging—what happens, how, and when—vary greatly. Although specific changes are part of the normal aging process, each person ages in his own way. As the years accumulate, people become more diverse rather than more alike, each influenced by physical, social, and environmental factors.

How a person ages depends on life experiences, available support systems, and previous coping skills. In addition, not all body systems age from the same functional level or at the same rate.

Definitions of aging

Aging and *old age* are highly subjective terms. *Aging* is defined as the time from birth to the present for a living individual, as measured in specific units. *Old* is defined as having lived for a long time. The meanings of old and aging depend to a great extent on the age of the speaker and on that person's experiences. For adults, aging is negatively associated with being old.

Descriptions of aging

Aging is a complex process that can be described chronologically, physiologically, and functionally.

Chronological age

Chronological age refers to the number of years a person has lived. Easy to identify and measure, it's the most commonly used objective method. In addition, chronological age serves as a criterion in society for certain activities, such as driving, employment, and the collection of retirement benefits.

With the passage of the Social Security Act and the establishment of Medicare, age 65 became the minimum age of eligibility for retirement benefits. In the United States, therefore, 65 is a commonly accepted age for becoming a senior citizen. However, because of a change in law in 1983, the full retirement age will gradually increase to age 67 for people born in 1960 and later.

Physiologic age

Physiologic age refers to the determination of age by body function. Although age-related changes affect everyone, it's impossible to pinpoint exactly when these changes occur. Therefore, physiologic age isn't useful in determining a person's age.

Functional age

Functional age refers to a person's ability to contribute to society and benefit others and himself. The concept is based on the fact that not all individuals of the same chronological age function at the same level. A person may be chronologically older but remain a physically fit, mentally active, and productive member of society. Another individual may be chronologically young but physically or functionally old.

Chronological categories of aging

In an attempt to further define the aging population, old age has been divided into chronological categories. One such classification uses three categories:

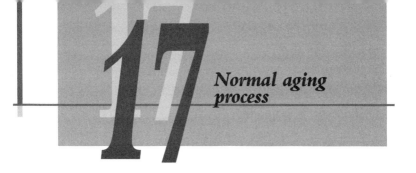

> **Profile of the frail elderly**
>
> Characteristics common to the frail elderly include:
> - poor mental and physical health
> - low socioeconomic status
> - predominantly female
> - possibly isolated living conditions
> - more and longer hospital stays with more money spent on health care and drugs
> - more frequent visits to the doctor
> - increased use of nursing home beds, rather than hospital beds.

- young-old (ages 65 to 74)
- middle-old (ages 75 to 84)
- old-old (age 85 and older).

Frail elderly

The fastest growing segment of the older population is over age 75. Those in this group who require help are called the *frail elderly.* Of those noninstitutionalized adults ages 75 to 84, about 25% need help with daily activities. Of those age 85 and older, nearly one-half need help with daily activities. (See *Profile of the frail elderly*.)

Demographics of aging

The older adult population is growing rapidly. In 2000, 34.9 million older adults accounted for approximately 12.5% of the U.S. population. By the year 2030, older adults are projected to make up about 22% of the U.S. population.

Since 1900, the percentage of older adults in the population has tripled. The greatest increase occurred in the 65-to-74 age-group, which is eight times larger now than in 1900. The current 75-to-84 age-group is 13 times larger, and the age-85-and-older group is 24 times larger.

According to projections, the growth of the elderly population will peak in 2030. The most rapid increase will occur from 2005 to 2030, as the baby boom generation reaches age 65.

Theories of aging

Various theories have been proposed to explain the process of normal aging and to help dispel some of the myths. A set of biological, psychosocial, and developmental theories of aging provides guidelines to determine how well a person is adjusting to aging. No single theory of aging is universally accepted.

Biological theories attempt to explain physical aging as an involuntary process, which eventually leads to cumulative changes in cells, tissues, and fluids. Intrinsic biological theory maintains that aging changes arise from internal, predetermined causes. Extrinsic biological theory maintains that environmental factors lead to structural alterations which, in turn, cause degenerative changes.

Psychological theories of aging attempt to explain age-related changes in cognitive function, such as intelligence, memory, learning, and problem solving.

Sociologic theories attempt to explain changes that affect socialization and life satisfaction. Sociologic theories maintain that as social expectations change, people assume new roles, which leads to changes in identity.

Finally, *developmental theories* describe specific life stages and tasks associated with each stage. (See *Comparing selected theories of aging*.)

Normal physiologic changes of aging

The loss of some body cells and reduced metabolism in other cells characterize aging. These processes cause a decline in body function and changes in body composition.

Although an older person's body tends to work less efficiently than a younger person's, illness doesn't inevitably accompany old age; however, a person's heart, lungs, kidneys, and other organs are less efficient at age 60 than at age 20.

Despite normal physiologic changes, aging shouldn't be equated

Comparing selected theories of aging

This chart discusses some of the common biological and psychosocial theories of aging. For each theory, proposed aging sources and age-retarding factors are listed.

Theory	Description
Biological theories	
Cross-link theory	Strong chemical bonding between organic molecules in the body causes increased stiffness, chemical instability, and insolubility of connective tissue and deoxyribonucleic acid. Thus, restricting calories and lathyrogens (antilink agents) may retard aging.
Free-radical theory	Unstable free radicals (such as from environmental pollutants) increase and produce effects harmful to biological systems, such as chromosomal changes, pigment accumulation, and collagen alteration. Improving environmental monitoring, decreasing intake of free-radical–stimulating foods and increasing intake of vitamins A and C (mercaptans) and vitamin E may retard aging.
Immunologic theory	An aging immune system is less able to distinguish body cells from foreign cells; as a result, it begins to attack and destroy body cells as if they were foreign. This may explain the adult onset of certain conditions, such as diabetes mellitus, rheumatic heart disease, and arthritis. Theorists have speculated on several erratic cellular mechanisms capable of precipitating attacks on various tissues through autoaggression or immunodeficiencies. Immunoengineering—selective alteration and replenishment or rejuvenation of the immune system—may slow aging.
Wear-and-tear theory	Body cells, structures, and functions wear out or are overused through exposure to internal and external stressors. Effects from the residual damage accumulate, the body can no longer resist stress, and death occurs. Reevaluating and possibly adjusting lifestyle may help slow aging.
Psychosocial theories	
Activity theory	Successful aging and life satisfaction depend on maintaining a high level of activity. Increasing activities in other areas when activities in one area decrease may retard aging.

(continued)

Comparing selected theories of aging *(continued)*

Theory	Description
Psychosocial theories *(continued)*	
Continuity theory	Individual remains essentially the same, despite life changes; the focus is more on personality and individual behavior over time. Taking into account the impact of major societal changes, which can alter individual expectations and behaviors, may slow aging.
Disengagement theory	Progressive social disengagement occurs with age because of age-related changes in health, energy, income, and social roles. Taking into account diversity of individual outlook and lifestyle and social structure variables, such as economy and social organizations, may retard aging.
Social exchange theory	Social behavior involves doing what's valued and rewarded by society. With age comes diminished resources and increased dependency, leading to unequal contribution to society, reduced power and value, and a decreased number of roles available in society. Assuming new roles and friendships with other older adults can help socialize the older person and help him adjust to age-related norms; this may help to slow aging.

with the unavoidable breakdown of body systems. Even laboratory test values change to reflect the aging process. Values considered abnormal in younger adults may be perfectly normal in older adults. (See *How laboratory values change with age.*)

Nutrition

A person's protein, vitamin, and mineral requirements usually remain the same as he ages, whereas caloric needs decrease.

POINT TO REMEMBER
Diminished activity may lower energy requirements by about 200 calories per day for men and women ages 51 to 75, 400 calories per day for women over age 75, and 500 calories per day for men over age 75.

Other physiologic changes that can affect nutrition in an older patient include:

- decreased renal function, causing greater susceptibility to dehydration and formation of renal calculi
- loss of calcium and nitrogen (in persons who aren't ambulatory)
- diminished enzyme activity and gastric secretions
- reduced pepsin and hydrochloric acid secretion, which tends to diminish the absorption of calcium and vitamins B_1 and B_2
- decreased salivary flow and diminished sense of taste, which may reduce the appetite and increase a person's consumption of sweet and spicy foods
- diminished intestinal motility and peristalsis of the large intestine
- thinning of tooth enamel, causing teeth to become more brittle
- decreased biting force

(Text continues on page 212.)

How laboratory values change with age

Standard normal laboratory values reflect the physiology of 20 to 40 year olds. However, normal values for older patients commonly differ because of age-related physiologic changes.

Certain test results, though, remain unaffected by age. These include partial thromboplastin time (PTT), prothrombin time (PT), serum acid phosphatase, serum carbon dioxide, serum chloride, aspartate aminotransferase, and total serum protein. This chart lists other test values that change with age.

Test values at ages 20 to 40	Changes in older adults	Considerations
Blood tests		
Albumin 3.5 to 5.0 g/dl	Under age 65: Higher in men Over age 65: Levels equalize, then decrease at same rate	Increased dietary protein intake needed in older patients if liver function is normal; edema a sign of low albumin level
Alkaline phosphatase 13 to 39 IU/L	Increases 8 to 10 IU/L	May reflect liver function decline or vitamin D malabsorption and bone demineralization
Beta globulin 2.3 to 3.5 g/dl	Increases slightly	Increases in response to decrease in albumin if liver function is normal; increased dietary protein intake needed
Blood urea nitrogen Men: 10 to 25 mg/dl Women: 8 to 20 mg/dl	Increases, possibly to 69 mg/dl	Slight increase acceptable in absence of stressors, such as infection or surgery
Cholesterol 120 to 220 mg/dl	Men: Increases to age 50, then decreases Women: Lower than men until age 50, increases to age 70, then decreases	Rise in cholesterol level (and increased cardiovascular risk) in women as a result of postmenopausal estrogen decline; dietary changes, weight loss, and exercise needed
Creatine kinase 17 to 148 U/L	Increases slightly	May reflect decreasing muscle mass and liver function
Creatinine 0.6 to 1.5 mg/dl	Increases, possibly to 1.9 mg/dl in men	Important factor in preventing toxicity when giving drugs that are excreted in urine

(continued)

How laboratory values change with age *(continued)*

Test values at ages 20 to 40	Changes in older adults	Considerations
Blood tests ***(continued)***		
Creatinine clearance 104 to 125 ml/min	Men: Decreases; formula: (140 − age × kg body weight)/72 × serum creatinine Women: 85% of men's rate	Reflects reduced glomerular filtration rate; important factor in preventing toxicity when giving drugs that are excreted in urine
Glucose tolerance (fasting plasma glucose) 1 hour: 160 to 170 mg/dl 2 hour: 115 to 125 mg/dl 3 hour: 70 to 110 mg/dl	Rises faster in first 2 hours, then drops to baseline more slowly	Reflects declining pancreatic insulin supply and release and diminishing body mass for glucose uptake (rapid rise can quickly trigger hyperosmolar hyperglycemic nonketotic syndrome; rapid decline can result from certain drugs, such as alcohol, beta-adrenergic blockers, and MAO inhibitors)
Hematocrit Men: 45% to 52% Women: 37% to 48%	May decrease slightly (unproven)	Reflects decreased bone marrow and hematopoiesis, increased risk of infection (fewer and weaker lymphocytes, and immune system changes that diminish antigen-antibody response)
Hemoglobin Men: 13 to 18 g/100 ml Women: 12 to 16 g/100 ml	Men: Decreases by 1 to 2 g/dl Women: Unknown	Reflects decreased bone marrow, hematopoiesis, and (for men) androgen levels
High-density lipoproteins 80 to 310 mg/dl	Levels higher in women than in men; levels equalize with age	Compliance with dietary restrictions required for accurate interpretation of test results
Lactate dehydrogenase 45 to 90 U/L	Increases slightly	May reflect declining muscle mass and liver function
Leukocyte count 4,300 to 10,800/mm^3	Drops to 3,100 to 9,000/mm^3	Decrease proportionate to lymphocytes

How laboratory values change with age *(continued)*

Test values at ages 20 to 40	Changes in older adults	Considerations
Blood tests *(continued)*		
Lymphocyte count T: 500 to 2,400/mm^3 B: 50 to 200/mm^3	Decreases	Decrease proportionate to leukocytes
Platelet count 150,000 to 350,000/mm^3	Change in characteristics: decreased granular constituents, increased platelet-release factors	May reflect diminished bone marrow, increased fibrinogen levels
Potassium 3.5 to 5.5 mEq/L	Increases slightly	Requires avoidance of salt substitutes composed of potassium, food-label vigilance, and knowledge of hyperkalemia signs and symptoms
Thyroid-stimulating hormone 0.3 to 5.0 microIU/ml	Increases slightly	Suggests primary hypothyroidism or endemic goiter at much higher levels
Thyroxine 4.5 to 13.5 mcg/dl	Decreases 25%	Reflects declining thyroid function
Triglycerides 40 to 150 mg/dl	Range widens: 20 to 200 mg/dl	Suggests abnormality at any other levels, requiring additional tests such as serum cholesterol
Triiodothyronine 90 to 220 ng/dl	Decreases 25%	Reflects declining thyroid function
Urine tests		
Glucose 0 to 15 mg/dl	Decreases slightly	May reflect renal disease or urinary tract infection (UTI); unreliable check for older diabetic patients because glycosuria may not occur until plasma glucose level exceeds 300 mg/dl

(continued)

How laboratory values change with age *(continued)*

Test values at ages 20 to 40	Changes in older adults	Considerations
Urine tests ***(continued)***		
Protein 0 to 5 mg/dl	Increases slightly	May reflect renal disease or UTI
Specific gravity 1.032	Decreases to 1.024 by age 80	Reflects 30% to 50% decrease in number of nephrons available to concentrate urine

- diminished gag reflex.

Some common conditions found in older people can affect nutritional status by limiting mobility and, therefore, the ability to obtain or prepare food or feed oneself.

Diminished intestinal motility typically accompanies aging and may cause GI disorders such as constipation. Fecal incontinence may also occur. Physical inactivity, emotional stress, certain medications, or nutritionally inadequate diets of soft, refined foods low in dietary fiber can also cause constipation. Laxative abuse results in the rapid transport of food through the GI tract, decreasing digestion and absorption.

Socioeconomic and psychological factors that affect nutritional status include loneliness, decline of the older person's importance in the family, susceptibility to nutritional quackery, and lack of money or transportation to buy nutritious foods.

Skin, hair, and nails

Skin changes, such as facial lines around the eyes (crow's feet), mouth, and nose, noticeably show aging. These lines result from subcutaneous fat loss, dermal thinning, decreasing collagen and elastin, and a 50% decline in cell replacement.

Women's skin shows signs of aging about 10 years earlier than men's because it's thinner and drier.

POINT TO REMEMBER
With the decreased rate of skin cell replacement, an older person's wounds may heal more slowly and he may be more susceptible to infection.

In very old people, the skin loses its elasticity until it may seem almost transparent. The supraclavicular and axillary regions, knuckles, and hand tendons and vessels are more prominent, as are fat pads over bony prominences.

Mucous membranes become dry, and sweat gland output decreases as the number of active sweat glands declines. Body temperature becomes more difficult to regulate because of the decrease in size, number, and function of sweat glands and loss of subcutaneous fat. Although melanocyte production decreases as a person ages, localized melanocyte proliferations are common and cause brown spots (senile lentigo) to appear, especially in areas regularly exposed to the sun.

Hair pigment decreases with age, and hair may turn gray or white. Hair also thins as the number of melanocytes declines; by age 70, it's baby fine again. Hormonal changes cause pubic hair loss. Facial hair commonly increases in postmenopausal women and decreases in aging men.

Aging also may alter nails. They may grow at different rates, and longitudinal ridges, flaking, brittleness, and malformations may increase. Toenails may discolor.

Other common hyperplastic skin conditions in older people include senile keratosis (dry, harsh skin) and senile angioma (a benign tumor of dilated blood vessels caused by weakened capillary walls).

Eyes and vision

Eye structure and visual acuity change with age. The eyes sit deeper in their sockets and the eyelids lose their elasticity, becoming baggy and wrinkled. The conjunctivae become thinner and yellow, and pingueculae — fat pads that form under the conjunctivae — may develop. As the lacrimal apparatus gradually loses fatty tissue, the quantity of tears decreases and evaporation occurs more quickly.

With age, the cornea loses its luster and flattens, while the iris fades or develops irregular pigmentation. Increased connective tissue may cause sclerosis of the sphincter muscles. The pupil becomes smaller, reducing the amount of light that reaches the retina. Aging diminishes night vision and depth perception.

POINT TO REMEMBER
Older adults need about three times as much light as younger people to see objects clearly.

The sclera becomes thick and rigid, and fat deposits cause yellowing. The vitreous can degenerate over time, revealing opacities and floating vitreous debris, and can also detach from the retina. Through the ophthalmoscope, the vitreous, detached from the area of the optic disk, looks like a dark ring in front of the disk. With age, the lens enlarges and loses transparency. Accommodation decreases because of impaired lens elasticity (presbyopia).

Many older adults experience impaired color vision, especially in the blue and green ranges, because cones in the retina deteriorate. They also experience decreased reabsorption of intraocular fluid, which predisposes them to glaucoma.

Ears and hearing

Many older people lose some degree of hearing. Sometimes, gradual buildup of cerumen in the ear is the cause. Usually, however, hearing loss results from the slowly progressing deafness of aging, called *presbycusis* or senile deafness.

Presbycusis

An irreversible, bilateral, sensorineural hearing loss, presbycusis usually starts during middle age, slowly worsens, and affects more men than women.

Presbycusis appears in four forms. The most common form, sensory presbycusis, is caused by atrophy of the organ of Corti and the auditory nerve. The accompanying hearing loss occurs mostly in the high-pitch ranges. By age 60, most adults have difficulty hearing above 4,000 Hz. (The normal range for speech recognition is 500 to 2,000 Hz.) Older adults can't easily distinguish the high-pitched consonants s, z, t, f, and g.

Aging causes degenerative structural changes in the entire auditory system. The incidence of hearing loss in older people is probably higher than statistics indicate. In many cases, the older person isn't immediately aware of a hearing defect's onset or progression. Later the person may recognize the problem but, accepting it as a natural aspect of aging, may not seek medical help.

Respiratory system

Age-related anatomic changes in the upper airways include nose enlargement from continued cartilage growth, general atrophy of the tonsils, and tracheal deviations from changes in the aging spine. Possible thoracic changes include increased anteroposterior chest diameter (resulting from altered calcium metabolism) and calcification of costal cartilages, which reduces mobility of the chest wall. Kyphosis advances with age because of such factors as osteoporosis and vertebral collapse.

Pulmonary function changes

Pulmonary function decreases in older people as a result of respiratory muscle degeneration or atrophy. Ventilatory capacity diminishes for several reasons:

- The lungs' diffusing capacity declines; decreased inspiratory and expiratory muscle strength diminishes vital capacity.
- Lung tissue degeneration causes a decrease in the lungs' elastic recoil capability, which results in an elevated residual volume. Thus, aging alone can cause emphysema.
- Closing of some airways produces poor ventilation of the basal areas, resulting in both a decreased surface area for gas exchange and reduced partial pressure of oxygen. The normal partial pressure of oxygen in arterial blood decreases to 70 to 85 mm Hg. Oxygen saturation decreases by 5%.

The lungs become more rigid, and the number and size of alveoli decline with age. In addition, a 30% reduction in respiratory fluids heightens the risk of pulmonary infection and mucus plugs.

POINT TO REMEMBER
Because maximum breathing capacity, forced vital capacity, vital capacity, and inspiratory reserve volume diminish with age, the older person has a lower tolerance for oxygen debt.

Cardiovascular system

As a person ages, his heart usually becomes slightly smaller and loses its contractile strength and efficiency (although exceptions occur in people with hypertension or heart disease). By age 70, cardiac output at rest has diminished by about 30% to 35% in many people.

Fibrotic and sclerotic changes thicken the heart valves and reduce their flexibility, leading to rigidity and incomplete closure of the heart valves, which may result in systolic murmurs. In addition, the thickness of the left ventricular wall increases by 25% between ages 30 and 80. Older people may also develop obstructive coronary disease and fibrosis of the cardiac skeleton.

As the myocardium of the aging heart becomes more irritable, extra systoles may occur, along with sinus arrhythmias and sinus bradycardias. In addition, increased fibrous tissue infiltrates the sinoatrial node and internodal atrial tracts, which may cause atrial fibrillation and flutter.

The veins also dilate and stretch with age, and coronary artery blood flow decreases 35% between ages 20 and 60. The aorta becomes more rigid, causing systolic blood pressure to rise disproportionately higher than the diastolic, resulting in a widened pulse pressure. Electrocardiogram changes include a shift of the QRS axis to the left, decreased amplitude of the QRS complex, and increased PR, QRS, and QT intervals.

Decreased response to stress

The heart's ability to respond to physical and emotional stress also may decrease markedly with age. The heart rate takes longer to return to normal after exercise.

Usually, aging also contributes to arterial and venous insufficiency as the strength and elasticity of blood vessels decrease. All these factors contribute to increased incidence of cardiovascular disease, particularly coronary disease, in elderly people.

GI system

The physiologic changes that accompany aging usually prove less debilitating in the GI system than in most other body systems. Normal changes include diminished mucosal elasticity and reduced GI secretions which, in turn, modify some processes — for example, digestion and absorption. GI tract motility, bowel wall and anal sphincter tone, and abdominal muscle strength also may decrease with age. Any of these changes may cause complaints in an older patient, ranging from loss of appetite to constipation.

Changes also occur in the oral cavity. Tooth enamel wears away, leaving the teeth prone to cavities. Periodontal disease increases and the number of taste buds declines. The sense of smell diminishes and salivary gland secretion decreases, leading to appetite loss.

Liver changes

Normal physiologic changes in the liver include decreased liver weight, reduced regenerative capacity, and decreased blood flow to the liver. Because hepatic enzymes involved in oxidation and reduction markedly decline with age, the liver metabolizes drugs and detoxifies substances less efficiently.

Renal system

After age 40, a person's renal function may diminish; if he lives to age 90, it may decrease by as much as 50%. This change is reflected in a decline in the glomerular filtration rate caused by age-related changes in renal vasculature that disturb glomerular hemodynamics. Renal blood flow decreases 53% from reduced cardiac output and age-related atherosclerotic changes. In addition, tubular reabsorption and renal concentrating ability decline because the size and number of functioning nephrons decrease.

As a person ages, his bladder muscles weaken. This may lead to incomplete bladder emptying and chronic urine retention—predisposing the bladder to infection.

Other age-related changes that affect renal function include diminished kidney size, impaired renal clearance of drugs, reduced bladder size and capacity, and decreased renal ability to respond to variations in sodium intake. By age 70, blood urea nitrogen levels rise by 21%. Residual urine, frequency, and nocturia also increase with age.

Male reproductive system

Physiologic changes in older men include reduced testosterone production which, in turn, may cause a decrease in libido. A reduced testosterone level also causes the testes to atrophy and soften and decreases sperm production by 48% to 69% between ages 60 and 80.

Normally, the prostate gland enlarges with age and its secretions diminish. Seminal fluid also decreases in volume and becomes less viscous.

Sexual changes

During intercourse, older men experience slower and weaker physiologic reactions. However, these changes don't necessarily weaken a man's sex drive or lessen his sexual satisfaction. (See *Understanding the male climacteric,* page 216.)

Female reproductive system

Declining estrogen and progesterone levels cause numerous physical changes in an aging woman. Significant emotional changes also take place during the transition from childbearing years to infertility.

Because a woman's breasts and internal and external reproductive structures are estrogen-dependent, aging takes a more conspicuous toll on the female than the male. As estrogen levels decrease and menopause approaches, usually at about age 50, changes affect most parts of the female reproductive system.

Ovaries

Ovulation usually stops 1 to 2 years before menopause. As the ovaries reach the end of their productive cycle, they become unresponsive to gonadotropic stimulation. With aging, the ovaries atrophy and become thicker and smaller.

Vulva

The vulva atrophies with age. Changes include pubic hair loss and flattening of the labia majora. Vulval tissue shrinks, exposing the sensitive area around the urethra and vagina to abrasions and irritation — for example, from undergarments. The introitus also constricts, tissues lose their elasticity, and the epidermis thins from 20 layers to about 5.

Vagina

Atrophy causes the vagina to shorten and the mucous lining to become thin, dry, less elastic, and pale from de-

Understanding the male climacteric

This list reviews the physiologic changes that characterize the male climacteric:

- Testosterone production declines.
- Pleasure sensations become less genitally localized and more generalized.
- Erections require more time and stimulation to achieve.
- Erections aren't as full or as hard.
- The prostate gland enlarges and its secretions diminish.
- Seminal fluid decreases.
- Ejaculatory force diminishes.
- Contractions in the prostate gland and penile urethra during orgasm vary in length and quality.
- The refractory period following ejaculation may lengthen from minutes to days.

creased vascularity. In this state, the vaginal mucosa is highly susceptible to abrasion. In addition, the pH of vaginal secretions increases, making the vaginal environment more alkaline. The type of flora also changes, increasing the older woman's risk for vaginal infections.

Uterus

After menopause, the uterus shrinks rapidly to half its premenstrual weight then continues to shrink until the organ reaches approximately one-fourth its premenstrual size. The cervix atrophies and no longer produces mucus for lubrication, and the endometrium and myometrium become thinner.

Breasts

Glandular, supporting, and fatty tissues atrophy. As Cooper's ligaments lose their elasticity, the breasts become pendulous. The nipples decrease in size and become flat. Fibrocystic disease that may have been present at menopause usually diminishes and disappears with increasing age. The inframammary ridges become more pronounced.

Pelvic support structures

Relaxation of these structures occurs commonly among postreproductive women. Initial relaxation usually occurs during labor and delivery, but clinical effects commonly go unnoticed until the process accelerates with menopausal estrogen depletion and loss of connective tissue elasticity and tone. Signs and symptoms include pressure and pulling in the area above the inguinal ligaments, lower backache, a feeling of pelvic heaviness, and difficulty in rising from a chair. Urinary stress incontinence may also become a problem if urethrovesical ligaments weaken.

Neurologic system

Aging affects the nervous system in many ways. Neurons of the central and peripheral nervous systems undergo degenerative changes. After about age 50, the number of brain cells decreases at a rate of about 1% per year. Yet clinical effects usually aren't noticeable until aging is more advanced.

POINT TO REMEMBER

Because nerve transmission typically slows down, the older person may react sluggishly to external stimuli.

As a person ages, the hypothalamus becomes less effective at regulating body temperature. The cerebral cortex undergoes a 20% neuron loss. The corneal reflex becomes slower, and the pain threshold increases. An older person experiences a decrease in stages III and IV sleep, causing frequent awakenings; rapid-eye-movement sleep also decreases.

Illness and injury: Why older adults are at increased risk

The normal aging process places older adults at risk for certain diseases and injuries. Here are some examples:

- Decreased cerebral blood flow increases the risk of stroke.
- An older person's spinal cord is tightly encased in vertebrae that may be studded with bony spurs or shrunken around the cord. For this reason, even a minor fall can cause severe cord damage.
- In older women, osteoporosis can cause compression fractures even without a history of trauma.
- Brittle bones make an older person especially prone to fractures. Falling on an outstretched arm or hand or experiencing a direct blow to the arm or shoulder is likely to fracture the shoulder or humerus.
- Diminished cardiac rate and stroke volume place an older person at risk for developing heart failure, hypertensive crisis, arterial occlusion, and myocardial infarction.
- Weakened chest musculature reduces an older person's ability to clear lung secretions and increases his risk of developing pneumonia, tuberculosis, and other respiratory diseases.
- In older men, prostatic hypertrophy is a common cause of urinary tract obstruction and acute urine retention.
- A weakened immune system increases an older, debilitated person's risk of acquiring almost any infection he's exposed to.

Musculoskeletal system

Adipose tissue stores usually increase with age; lean body mass and bone mineral contents usually diminish. The most apparent change is decreasing height. This results from exaggerated spinal curvatures and narrowing intervertebral spaces, which shorten the trunk and make the arms appear relatively long.

Other changes include decreased bone mass, muscle mass (which may result in muscle weakness), and collagen formation, which causes loss of resilience and elasticity in joints and supporting structures. Synovial fluid becomes more viscous, and the synovial membranes become more fibrotic.

In addition, aging may cause difficulty in tandem walking. Usually the person walks with shorter steps and a wider leg stance to achieve better balance and stable weight distribution.

Immune system

Immune function starts declining at sexual maturity and continues declining with age. During this decline, the immune system begins losing its ability to differentiate between self and nonself, and the incidence of autoimmune disease increases. The immune system also begins losing its ability to recognize and destroy mutant cells, which presumably accounts for the increase in cancer among older people.

Decreased antibody response in older people makes them more susceptible to infection. (See *Illness and injury: Why older adults are at increased risk.*) Tonsillar atrophy and lymphadenopathy commonly occur.

Total and differential leukocyte counts don't change significantly with age. However, some people over age 65 may exhibit a slight decrease in the leukocyte count. When this happens, the number of B cells and total lymphocytes decreases, and T cells decrease in number and become less effective. Also, the size of the lymph nodes and spleen reduces slightly.

Fatty bone marrow replaces some active blood-forming marrow first in the long bones and later in the flat bones. The altered bone marrow can't increase erythrocyte production as readily as before in response to such stimuli as hormones, anoxia, hemorrhage, and hemolysis. With age, vitamin B_{12} absorption may also diminish, resulting in reduced erythrocyte mass and decreased hemoglobin levels and hematocrit.

Endocrine system

Normal variations in endocrine function include reduced progesterone production, a 50% decline in serum aldosterone levels, and a 25% decrease in cortisol secretion rate.

A common and important endocrine change in older people is decreased ability to tolerate stress. The most obvious and serious indication of this diminished stress response occurs in glucose metabolism.

Changes in glucose metabolism

Normally, fasting blood glucose levels aren't significantly different in young and old adults. However, when stress stimulates an older person's pancreas, the blood glucose concentration increases more and remains elevated longer than in a younger adult. This diminished glucose tolerance occurs as a normal part of aging.

Changes related to sex hormones

In women, ovarian senescence at menopause causes permanent cessation of menstrual activity. Changes in endocrine function during menopause vary from woman to woman, but normally estrogen levels diminish and follicle-stimulating hormone production increases.

This estrogen deficiency may result in either or both of two key metabolic effects: coronary thrombosis and osteoporosis. Some symptoms characteristic of menopause (such as depression, insomnia, headaches, fatigue, palpitations, and irritability) may also be associated with endocrine disorders.

In men, the climacteric stage lowers testosterone levels and seminal fluid production.

Appendices, suggested readings, index

Appendix A: Table of equivalents

Metric system equivalents

Metric weight		*Household*	*Metric*
1 kilogram (kg or Kg)	= 1,000 grams (g or gm)	1 teaspoon (tsp)	= 5 ml
1 gram	= 1,000 milligrams (mg)	1 tablespoon (T or tbs)	= 15 ml
1 milligram	= 1,000 micrograms (µg or mcg)	2 tablespoons	= 30 ml
0.6 g	= 600 mg	8 ounces	= 236 ml
0.3 g	= 300 mg	1 pint (pt)	= 473 ml
0.1 g	= 100 mg	1 quart (qt)	= 946 ml
0.06 g	= 60 mg	1 gallon (gal)	= 3,785 ml
0.03 g	= 30 mg		
0.015 g	= 15 mg		
0.001 g	= 1 mg		

Metric volume	
1 liter (l or L)	= 1,000 milliliters (ml)*
1 milliliter	= 1,000 microliters (µl)

Temperature conversions

Fahrenheit	*Celsius*	*Fahrenheit*	*Celsius*	*Fahrenheit*	*Celsius*
106.0	41.1	103.0	39.4	100.0	37.8
105.8	41.0	102.8	39.3	99.8	37.7
105.6	40.9	102.6	39.2	99.6	37.6
105.4	40.8	102.4	39.1	99.4	37.4
105.2	40.7	102.2	39.0	99.2	37.3
105.0	40.6	102.0	38.9	99.0	37.2
104.8	40.4	101.8	38.8	98.8	37.1
104.6	40.3	101.6	38.7	98.6	37.0
104.4	40.2	101.4	38.6	98.4	36.9
104.2	40.1	101.2	38.4	98.2	36.8
104.0	40.0	101.0	38.3	98.0	36.7
103.8	39.9	100.8	38.2	97.8	36.6
103.6	39.8	100.6	38.1	97.6	36.4
103.4	39.7	100.4	38.0	97.4	36.3
103.2	39.6	100.2	37.9	97.2	36.2

Temperature conversions ***(continued)***

Fahrenheit	*Celsius*	*Fahrenheit*	*Celsius*	*Fahrenheit*	*Celsius*
97.0	36.1	94.6	34.8	92.2	33.4
96.8	36.0	94.4	34.7	92.0	33.3
96.6	35.9	94.2	34.6	91.8	33.2
96.4	35.8	94.0	34.4	91.6	33.1
96.2	35.7	93.8	34.3	91.4	33.0
96.0	35.6	93.6	34.2	91.2	32.9
95.8	35.4	93.4	34.1	91.0	32.8
95.6	35.3	93.2	34.0	90.8	32.7
95.4	35.2	93.0	33.9	90.6	32.6
95.2	35.1	92.8	33.8	90.4	32.4
95.0	35.0	92.6	33.7	90.2	32.3
94.8	34.9	92.4	33.6	90.0	32.2

Weight conversions

1 oz = 30 g	1 lb = 453.6 g	2.2 lb = 1 kg

* 1 ml = 1 cubic centimeter (cc); however, ml is the preferred measurement term used today.

Appendix B: Findings in acid-base disorders

Disorder and arterial blood gas findings	Possible causes	Signs and symptoms
Respiratory acidosis (excess CO_2 retention) pH < 7.35 HCO_3^- > 26 mEq/L (if compensating) $Paco_2$ > 45 mm Hg	▸ Central nervous system depression from drugs, injury, or disease ▸ Asphyxia ▸ Hypoventilation due to pulmonary, cardiac, musculoskeletal, or neuromuscular disease	▸ Diaphoresis, headache, tachycardia, confusion, restlessness, apprehension
Respiratory alkalosis (excess CO_2 excretion) pH > 7.42 HCO_3^- < 22 mEq/L (if compensating) $Paco_2$ < 35 mm/Hg	▸ Hyperventilation due to anxiety, pain, or improper ventilator settings ▸ Respiratory stimulation by drugs, disease, hypoxia, fever, or high room temperature ▸ Gram-negative bacteremia	▸ Rapid, deep respirations; paresthesia; light-headedness; twitching; anxiety; fear
Metabolic acidosis (HCO_3^- loss, acid retention) pH < 7.35 HCO_3^- < 22 mEq/L $Paco_2$ < 35 mm Hg (if compensating)	▸ HCO_3^- depletion due to renal disease, diarrhea, or small-bowel fistulas ▸ Excessive production of organic acids due to hepatic disease, endocrine disorders (including diabetes mellitus), hypoxia, shock, or drug intoxication ▸ Inadequate excretion of acids due to renal disease	▸ Rapid, deep breathing; fruity breath odor; fatigue; headache; lethargy; drowsiness; nausea and vomiting; coma (if severe)
Metabolic alkalosis (HCO_3^- retention, acid loss) pH > 7.42 HCO_3^- > 26 mEq/L $Paco_2$ > 45 mm Hg (if compensating)	▸ Loss of hydrochloric acid from prolonged vomiting, gastric suctioning ▸ Loss of potassium from increased renal excretion, steroid overdose ▸ Excessive alkali ingestion	▸ Slow, shallow breathing; restlessness; twitching; confusion; irritability; apathy, tetany; seizures; coma (if severe)

Glossary

Abdomen: area of the body between the diaphragm and pelvis
Abduct: to move away from the midline of the body; the opposite of adduct
Acetabulum: hip joint socket into which the head of the femur fits
Acromion: bony projection of the scapula
Adduct: to move toward the midline of the body; the opposite of abduct
Adenoids: paired lymphoid structures located in the nasopharynx
Adrenal gland: one of two secretory organs that lie atop the kidneys; consists of a medulla and a cortex
Afferent neuron: nerve cell that conveys impulses from the periphery to the central nervous system; the opposite of efferent neuron
Alveolus: in the lung, a small saclike dilation of the terminal bronchioles
Ampulla: saclike dilation of a tube or duct
Anterior: front or ventral; the opposite of posterior or dorsal
Antibody: immunoglobulin produced by the body in response to exposure to a specific foreign substance (antigen)
Antigen: foreign substance that causes antibody formation when introduced into the body
Anus: distal end or outlet of the rectum
Aorta: main trunk of the systemic arterial circulation, originating from the left ventricle and eventually branching into the two common iliac arteries
Arachnoid: delicate middle membrane of the meninges
Areola: pigmented ring around the nipple
Arteriole: small branch of an artery
Artery: vessel that carries blood away from the heart
Arthrosis: joint or articulation
Atrium: chamber or cavity
Auricle: part of the ear that's attached to the head
Axon: extension of a nerve cell that conveys impulses away from the cell body
Bladder: membranous sac that holds secretions
Bone: dense, hard connective tissue that composes the skeleton
Bone marrow: soft tissue in the cancellous bone of the epiphyses; crucial for blood cell formation and maturation
Bronchiole: small branch of the bronchus
Bronchus: larger air passage of the lung
Buccal: pertaining to the cheek
Bursa: fluid-filled sac lined with synovial membrane
Capillary: microscopic blood vessel that links arterioles with venules
Carpal: pertaining to the wrist
Cartilage: connective supporting tissue occurring mainly in the joints, thorax, larynx, trachea, nose, and ear
Cecum: pouch located at the proximal end of the large intestine
Celiac: pertaining to the abdomen
Central nervous system: one of the two main divisions of the nervous system; consists of the brain and spinal cord
Cerebellum: portion of the brain situated in the posterior cranial fossa, behind the brain stem; coordinates voluntary muscular activity

Cerebrum: largest and uppermost section of the brain, divided into hemispheres
Cilia: small, hairlike projections on the outer surfaces of some cells
Cochlea: spiral tube that makes up a portion of the inner ear
Colon: part of the large intestine that extends from the cecum to the rectum
Condyle: rounded projection at the end of a bone
Contralateral: on the opposite side; the opposite of ipsilateral
Cornea: convex, transparent anterior portion of the eye
Coronary: pertaining to the heart or its arteries
Cortex: outer part of an internal organ; the opposite of medulla
Costal: pertaining to the ribs
Cricoid: ring-shaped cartilage found in the larynx
Cutaneous: pertaining to the skin
Deltoid: shaped like a triangle (as in the deltoid muscle)
Dendrite: branching process extending from the neuronal cell body that directs impulses toward the cell body
Dermis: skin layer beneath the epidermis
Diaphragm: membrane that separates one part from another; the muscular partition separating the thorax and abdomen
Diaphysis: shaft of a long bone
Diarthrosis: freely movable joint
Diencephalon: part of the brain located between the cerebral hemisphere and the midbrain
Distal: far from the point of origin or attachment; the opposite of proximal
Diverticulum: outpouching from a tubular organ such as the intestine
Dorsal: pertaining to the back or posterior; the opposite of ventral or anterior
Duct: passage or canal
Duodenum: shortest and widest portion of the small intestine, extending from the pylorus to the jejunum
Dura mater: outermost layer of the meninges
Ear: organ of hearing
Efferent neuron: nerve cell that conveys impulses from the central nervous system to the periphery; the opposite of afferent neuron
Endocardium: interior lining of the heart
Endocrine: pertaining to secretion into the blood or lymph rather than into a duct; the opposite of exocrine
Epidermis: outermost layer of the skin; lacking vessels
Epiglottis: cartilaginous structure overhanging the larynx that guards against entry of food into the lung
Epiphyses: ends of a long bone
Erythrocyte: red blood cell
Esophagus: muscular canal that transports nutrients from the pharynx to the stomach
Exocrine: Pertaining to secretion into a duct; the opposite of endocrine
Eye: one of two organs of vision
Fallopian tube: one of two ducts extending from the uterus to the ovary
Fontanel: incompletely ossified area of a neonate's skull
Foramen: small opening
Fossa: hollow or cavity
Fundus: base of a hollow organ; the part farthest from the organ's outlet
Gallbladder: excretory sac lodged in the visceral surface of the liver's right lobe
Ganglion: cluster of nerve cell bodies found outside the central nervous system
Genitalia: reproductive organs; may be external or internal
Gland: organ or structure body that secretes or excretes substances
Glomerulus: compact cluster; the capillaries of the kidney
Gonad: sex gland in which reproductive cells form
Heart: muscular, cone-shaped organ that pumps blood throughout the body
Hemoglobin: protein found in red blood cells that contains iron
Hormone: substance secreted by an endocrine gland that triggers or regulates the activity of an organ or cell group
Hyoid: shaped like the letter U; the U-shaped bone at the base of the tongue
Hypothalamus: structure in the diencephalon that secretes vasopressin and oxytocin

Ileum: distal part of the small intestine extending from the jejunum to the cecum
Incus: one of three bones in the middle ear
Inferior: lower; the opposite of superior
Intestine: portion of the GI tract that extends from the stomach to the anus
Intima: innermost structure
Ipsilateral: on the same side; the opposite of contralateral
Jejunum: one of three portions of the small intestine; connects proximally with the duodenum and distally with the ileum
Joint: fibrous, cartilaginous, or synovial connection between bones
Kidney: one of two urinary organs on the dorsal part of the abdomen
Labia: lips
Lacrimal: pertaining to tears
Larynx: voice organ; joins the pharynx and trachea
Lateral: pertaining to the side; the opposite of medial
Leukocyte: white blood cell
Ligament: band of white fibrous tissue that connects bones
Liver: large gland in the right upper abdomen; divided into four lobes
Lobe: defined portion of any organ, such as the liver or brain
Lobule: small lobe
Lumbar: pertaining to the area of the back between the thorax and the pelvis
Lungs: organs of respiration found in the chest's lateral cavities
Lymph: watery fluid in lymphatic vessels
Lymph node: small oval structure that filters lymph, fights infection, and aids hematopoiesis
Lymphocyte: white blood cell; the body's immunologically competent cells
Malleolus: projections at the distal ends of the tibia and fibula
Malleus: tiny hammer-shaped bone in the middle ear
Mammary: pertaining to the breast
Manubrium: upper part of the sternum
Meatus: opening or passageway
Medial: pertaining to the middle; the opposite of lateral
Mediastinum: middle portion of the thorax between the pleural sacs that contain the lungs
Medulla: inner portion of an organ; the opposite of cortex
Membrane: thin layer or sheet
Metacarpals: bones of the hand located between the wrist and the fingers
Metatarsals: bones of the foot located between the tarsal bones and the toes
Muscle: fibrous structure whose contraction initiates movement
Myocardium: thick, contractile layer of muscle cells that forms the heart wall
Nares: nostrils
Nephron: structural and functional unit of the kidney
Nerve: cordlike structure consisting of fibers that convey impulses from the central nervous system to the body
Neuron: nerve cell
Neutrophil: white blood cell that removes and destroys bacteria, cellular debris, and solid particles
Occiput: back of the head
Olfactory: pertaining to the sense of smell
Ophthalmic: pertaining to the eye
Ossicle: small bone, especially of the ear
Ovary: one of two female reproductive organs found on each side of the lower abdomen, next to the uterus
Palate: roof of the mouth
Pancreas: secretory gland in the epigastric and hypogastric regions
Parotid: located near the ear (as in the parotid gland)
Patella: floating bone that forms the kneecap
Pectoral: pertaining to the chest or breast
Pelvis: funnel-shaped structure; lower part of the trunk
Pericardium: fibroserous sac that surrounds the heart and the origin of the great vessels
Phalynx: one of the tapering bones that makes up the fingers and toes
Pharynx: tubular passageway that extends from the base of the skull to the esophagus
Phrenic: pertaining to the diaphragm

Pia mater: innermost covering of the brain and spinal cord
Pituitary gland: gland attached to the hypothalamus that stores and secretes hormones
Plantar: pertaining to the sole of the foot
Plasma: colorless, watery fluid portion of lymph and blood
Platelet: small, disk-shaped blood cell necessary for coagulation
Pleura: thin serous membrane that encloses the lung
Plexus: network of nerves, lymphatic vessels, or veins
Pons: portion of the brain that lies between the medulla and the mesencephalon
Popliteal: pertaining to the back of the knee
Posterior: back or dorsal; the opposite of anterior or ventral
Pronate: to turn the palm downward; the opposite of supinate
Prostate: male gland that surrounds the bladder neck and urethra
Proximal: situated nearest the center of the body; the opposite of distal
Pupil: circular opening in the iris of the eye through which light passes
Reflex: involuntary action
Renal: pertaining to the kidney
Scrotum: skin pouch that houses the testes and parts of the spermatic cords
Semen: male reproductive fluid
Sphenoid: wedged-shaped bone at the base of the skull
Spleen: highly vascular organ between the stomach and diaphragm
Stapes: tiny stirrup-shaped bone in the middle ear
Sternum: long, flat bone that forms the middle portion of the thorax
Stomach: major digestive organ, located in the right upper abdomen
Striated: marked with parallel lines such as striated (skeletal) muscle
Superior: higher; the opposite of inferior
Supinate: to turn the palm of the hand upward; the opposite of pronate
Symphysis: growing together; a type of cartilaginous joint in which fibrocartilage firmly connects opposing surfaces
Synapse: point of contact between adjacent neurons
Systole: contraction of the heart muscle
Talus: anklebone
Tarsus: instep
Tendon: band of fibrous connective tissue that attaches a muscle to a bone
Testis: one of two male gonads that produce semen
Thyroid: secretory gland located at the front of the neck
Tibia: shinbone
Tongue: chief organ of taste, found in the floor of the mouth
Trachea: nearly cylindrical tube in the neck, extending from the larynx to the bronchi, that serves as a passageway for air
Turbinate: shaped like a cone or spiral; a bone located in the posterior nasopharynx
Ureter: one of two thick-walled tubes that transport urine to the bladder
Urethra: small tubular structure that drains urine from the bladder
Uterus: hollow, internal female reproductive organ in which the fertilized ovum is implanted and the fetus develops
Uvula: tissue projection that hangs from the soft palate
Vagina: sheath; the canal in the female extending from the vulva to the cervix
Valve: structure that permits fluid to flow in only one direction
Vein: vessel that carries blood to the heart
Vena cava: one of two large veins that returns blood from the peripheral circulation to the right atrium
Ventral: pertaining to the front or anterior; the opposite of dorsal or posterior
Ventricle: small cavity, such as one of several in the brain or one of the two lower chambers of the heart
Venule: small vessel that connects a vein and capillary plexuses
Vertebra: any of the 33 bones that make up the spinal column
Viscera: internal organs
Xiphoid: sword-shaped; the lower portion of the sternum

Suggested readings

Anatomy & Physiology Made Incredibly Easy, 2nd ed. Springhouse, Pa.: Lippincott Williams & Wilkins, 2002.

Baggaley, A. *Human Body: An Illustrated Guide to Every Part of the Human Body and How It Works.* New York: Dorling Kindersley Publishing, Inc., 2001.

Berne, R.M., and Levy, M.N. *Cardiovascular Physiology,* 8th ed. St. Louis: Mosby–Year Book, Inc., 2001.

Guyton, A.C., and Hall, J.E. *Textbook of Medical Physiology,* 10th ed. Philadelphia: W.B. Saunders Co., 2000.

Herlihy, B., and Maebius, N. *The Human Body in Health and Illness.* Philadelphia: W.B. Saunders Co., 2000.

Johnson, L.R., and Gerwin, T., eds. *Gastrointestinal Physiology,* 6th ed. St. Louis: Mosby–Year Book, Inc., 2001.

Levitzky, M. *Pulmonary Physiology,* 5th ed. New York: McGraw-Hill Professional, 1999.

Mackie, J., and Greig, J. *Anatomy & Physiology Applied to Health Professions,* 7th ed. Philadelphia: W.B. Saunders Co., 2002.

Marieb, E. *Human Anatomy & Physiology,* 5th ed. San Francisco: Benjamin Cummings, 2001.

Porterfield, S. *Endocrine Physiology,* 2nd ed. St. Louis: Mosby–Year Book, Inc., 2001.

Thibodeau, G.A., and Patton, K.T. *The Human Body in Health & Disease,* 3rd ed. St. Louis: Mosby–Year Book, Inc., 2002.

Thibodeau, G.A., and Patton, K.T. *Structure and Function of the Body,* 11th ed. St. Louis: Mosby–Year Book, Inc., 2000.

Index

i refers to an illustration; t refers to a table; **boldface** refers to full-color insert.

F

i refers to an illustration; t refers to a table; **boldface** refers to full-color insert.

i refers to an illustration; t refers to a table; **boldface** refers to full-color insert.

M

N

i refers to an illustration; t refers to a table; **boldface** refers to full-color insert.

Q

R

i refers to an illustration; t refers to a table; **boldface** refers to full-color insert.

T

i refers to an illustration; t refers to a table; **boldface** refers to full-color insert.

U

V

W

X

Y

Z